HOW TO BE
A SUCCESSFUL
FERTILITY PATIENT

Also by Peggy Robin

Outwitting Toddlers (with Bill Adler, Jr.)
Saving the Neighborhood

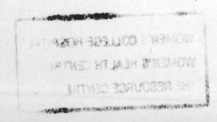

HOW TO BE A SUCCESSFUL FERTILITY PATIENT

YOUR GUIDE TO
GETTING THE BEST POSSIBLE
MEDICAL HELP TO HAVE A BABY

Peggy Robin

WILLIAM MORROW AND COMPANY, INC.
NEW YORK

Copyright © 1993 by Adler & Robin Books, Inc.

All rights reserved. No part of this book may be reproduced or utilized in any form or by any means, electronic or mechanical, including photocopying, recording, or by any information storage or retrieval system, without permission in writing from the Publisher. Inquiries should be addressed to Permissions Dept., William Morrow and Company, Inc., 1350 Avenue of the Americas, New York, N.Y. 10019.

It is the policy of William Morrow and Company, Inc., and its imprints and affiliates, recognizing the importance of preserving what has been written, to print the books we publish on acid-free paper, and we exert our best efforts to that end.

Library of Congress Cataloging-in-Publication Data

Robin, Peggy.
    How to be a successful fertility patient : your guide to getting
the best possible medical help to have a baby / Peggy Robin. — 1st
ed.
        p.   cm.
    Includes bibliographical references and index.
    ISBN 0–688–11732–5
    1. Infertility—Popular works.   I. Title.
RC889.R75   1993
616.6'92—dc20   92–41043
                                        CIP

Printed in the United States of America

11 12 13 14 15 16 17 18 19 20

BOOK DESIGN BY MICHAEL MENDELSOHN, MM DESIGN 2000, INC.

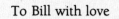

To Bill with love

CONTENTS

❧

CHAPTER EIGHT
"It Doesn't Work!"
301

About Doctor-switching and Clinic-hopping • About Breaks in Treatment

CHAPTER NINE
Coping with Stress
326

Prepare as for War • Sex and the Infertile Couple • To Tell or Not to Tell • Knowing When It's Time to Quit—and What You'll Do Next • Three Nonmedical Approaches • When the Couple Cannot Agree

CHAPTER TEN
Fertility and the Nontraditional Patient
367

The Single Woman • The Single Man • The Unmarried Heterosexual Couple • The Gay Male Couple • The Lesbian Couple • The Postmenopausal Woman • Disabled or Seriously Ill • The Couple Who Already Have One Child (Secondary Infertility) • Member of a Religion That Restricts or Forbids Fertility Treatment

.CHAPTER ELEVEN
Pregnancy After Infertility
401

Are You or Aren't You? • Finding the Right OB • The Critical First Three Months • Coping with the Fear of Miscarriage • How Many Are There? • Parenthood After Infertility

Conclusion
416

Glossary
419

ACKNOWLEDGMENTS

When struggling to overcome infertility, you come to depend upon many other people for help. When writing a book about the struggle to overcome infertility, you depend on even more people for help. Much gratitude is in order.

First, thanks are due to more than a hundred women and men who shared their stories with me—painful, touching, sad, funny, happy, bittersweet, and sometimes a mixture of all of these—though it was difficult for many to talk about such an intimate subject with a stranger. I am moved by their courage.

My thanks as well to the national office of RESOLVE, that infinitely helpful organization, for allowing me to use the organization's newsletter as a means of seeking contact with infertile couples from all over the country. RESOLVE of Metropolitan Washington, D.C., also was the source of much valuable information, especially about dealing with health insurance companies and other financial matters.

My very special gratitude goes to Bill Adler, who is not only the most wonderful husband I could possibly imagine, but also an excellent and supportive book agent. His expert handling of computer data bases netted much useful information for this book; his skill at debugging computer programs kept me more than once from losing all my text (not to mention my sanity).

Elizabeth Prungel made it so much easier for me to get my day's quota of writing done by leaving me with the knowledge that my baby was in the best possible hands. I must also credit my daughter Karen for understanding, at the young age of eighteen months, that Mommy couldn't come and play when she was in her "offa, wooking."

Much of my desire to write this book sprang out of my own experience when trying to have Karen. I was extremely fortunate to have found, on my first try, expert medical professionals to help me—though I'm sure I was never the easiest patient to work with. Dr. Paul R. Gindoff nevertheless managed to find time to answer my endless questions and prescribe the right medications at the right time. I thank him especially for his compassion at the time of my miscarriage. I am also grateful to Drs. Robert Stillman, Vanessa Barnabei, and Susanne Bathgate, all of

11

the George Washington University Hospital Center Department of Obstetrics/Gynecology and Reproductive Endocrinology. The nursing and other support staff also have my deep appreciation, especially Mark Ivey in the blood lab, whose good humor and gentleness with a needle got me through more difficult mornings than I care to remember. I must also thank Lois, Shelby, and Linda, whose last names I never learned, despite the fact that during my time in treatment I spent more time talking to them over the telephone than any of my closest friends. As many of my readers will discover, it's the people you deal with daily—in the sonogram room and in the blood lab and at the reception desk—who (as much as or more than the doctors) can make infertility treatment either a repeating nightmare or a bearable reality. In my case, due to the people I've named, it was most definitely the latter case.

INTRODUCTION

What This Book Is About

Having babies is the simplest thing in the world—or so it seems when you're young and unready for parenthood. Think back to when you were in high school and your mother and your gym teacher talked to you about pregnancy. They made it sound as if a girl could get pregnant at any time of the month, from doing just about anything with a boy. Well, they weren't *exactly* lying, since in your teenage years (when you probably were terrified of the prospect of having a baby) your ability to conceive was at its peak. It's when you are older, settled down, and longing to share your home and your future with children that you find out that the union of egg and sperm does not come about quite so easily as you were led to believe at age fourteen.

You may try to conceive for some months, or even a few years, before concluding that you have a problem with your fertility. And then you begin to think about seeking medical help.

Finding out about medical treatments for infertility is easy enough. Information is everywhere. Every other day, it seems, newspapers, magazines, and TV shows are talking about some miraculous new technique doctors have discovered to get childless couples to conceive. They're making babies in test tubes, they're making babies for postmenopausal women, they've even made it possible for a grandmother to give birth to her own grandchildren on behalf of her daughter who was born without a womb!

After hearing story after story of babies born through the wonders of technology, it's easy to start thinking that if doctors can do all these impossible things for other couples, surely it won't be any problem for them to fix what's wrong with *us*. You might imagine that all you'll need to do is take a pill for a while—something like a birth control pill in reverse—and presto! you'll be pregnant.

Well, if you are thinking along those lines, you are going to be shocked by what you find out when you begin to investigate the subject in any depth. Those of you who have already looked into treatment, or maybe have already started seeing a doctor, know only too well that

15

nothing in the field of human fertility is so easy—nothing is ever guaranteed.

Now, if you are reading this without any preconceived notions of what treatment will be like (or if you perhaps have already suspected that reversing your infertility could be difficult), let me just touch on what a few of the more common hurdles are:

• Despite all the advances made, much about conception is still poorly understood. Doctors can't figure out what is wrong in all cases, and in some cases, even when they *can* figure out what the problem is, they can't fix it.

• Doctors often disagree about diagnosis and treatment. To see how common such disagreement is, just take out two or three different doctors' books on infertility from your library and compare texts on any given topic. The first book will define Condition X as a major cause of infertility and state that it must be corrected surgically. The second book calls the same condition unimportant, and says that in most cases it's best left untreated. The third book says that Condition X by itself is not a problem, except when it is accompanied by Condition Y, and then it's serious and should be treated with drugs. Now whom should you believe?

• Even the treatments rated most effective can't ensure or even dependably predict a "favorable outcome" (fertility specialists' term for a baby).

• Fertility treatment is *unbelievably expensive,* and few insurance companies cover it fully. A large number of companies actually exclude fertility from their policies altogether.

• It can be difficult for the ordinary consumer to choose a clinic that provides a level of care worth the thousands of dollars such care will often cost. It takes some facility with statistics just to be able to analyze the data each clinic will show you as you are shopping around. Quacks abound, as do honest doctors who simply lack the level of skill needed to produce good success rates. Furthermore, some doctors are highly skilled at certain aspects of treatment but not so proficient at others. How do you know you have chosen the doctor who's best for *you?*

The point of this list of difficulties is not to discourage you from going any further. After all, this book is about being a *successful* fertility patient. The point is to get you to start out with a realistic appraisal of what's involved in being a patient.

Let's back up one step before that, however, and address the question of how you tell whether you really need to become a patient at all. Is there any way to find out, *before you spend a lot of money on doctors,* if you have given yourself enough time to try to become pregnant naturally? Is there any way you can find out on your own if a problem definitely exists? This book includes some simple tests you can give yourself at home that will alert you to certain types of fertility problems you may have. You just may discover that there is nothing in your background to indicate a possible problem, in which case you might want to keep trying on your own a little longer. The first chapter contains a list of things you can do right away to maximize your chance each month to get pregnant. It could be that this information is all you need to be successful in your quest to have a baby.

For those of you who *should* go on to seek medical advice, you will unquestionably be better equipped to cope with the frustrations, and the cost, and the physical side effects, and the uncertainties and all the other negative factors that are part and parcel of being a fertility patient, if you go in armed with knowledge about the field. Among the things you need to know are what tests are commonly used to diagnose patients, what treatments are generally available and what controversies exist about those treatments, and how clinics dress up their success rates. You will certainly find it a less daunting chore to pick the right doctor if you know how to talk with confidence to jargon-spouting specialists, how to ask the right questions, and how to decode the answers.

That's what I intend for this book to help you to do.

This is a *patient's* book. It's not by a doctor; it's by someone like you who wanted more than anything to have a baby. I had my first fertility consulation with a specialist in March 1988. I went through a full battery of tests, and then began trying different drug combinations over a period of months. Along the way I often felt downhearted and full of qualms; I argued with doctors; I often wished I had just had some inkling of what treatment was going to be like, so I could have avoided some painful mistakes (tests I really didn't need, uncomfortable treatments I might have been able to forgo). I was lucky, though. Eleven months later I conceived and after an uneventful pregnancy I gave birth to a beautiful baby girl.

Shortly after my daughter's first birthday I went back to my fertility doctor and asked for help in trying to have a second child. But this time I was far more self-assured in my dealings with my doctor. I knew exactly which drug I wanted to try first, and for how long. When I did not conceive after six months on the mild drug I had requested, I moved on (with my doctor's encouragement) to the far more potent drug that had produced my first pregnancy. This time the drug worked on the very first attempt—but then, sadly, I lost the pregnancy in the eighth week. A few months went by before I was ready, both physically and emotionally, to try again. I went back to the same drug regimen that had worked before, and yet again conceived on the first cycle. Today I am thrilled to be the mother of two adorable little girls. Now, having spent a total of three and a half years of my life as either a fertility patient or a high-risk obstetrical patient, I feel well qualified to advise other patients about coping with the infertility experience.

I have not written *How to Be a Successful Fertility Patient* to promise that if you follow what I say you will end up as I did. I have written this book in part to warn couples away from doctors who make too many promises and deliver too little.

I do firmly believe, however, that the patient who knows what to expect and what to be wary of, who doesn't blindly follow the doctor's orders but knows that it is ultimately the patient, not the doctor, that must make the big decisions—it is this patient that has the best chance of finding the right solution to her or his problem of infertility.

Patients Sometimes Know More Than Their Doctors

How can an ordinary person hope to become knowledgeable enough, quickly enough, to make the right choices at the right time, in the highly specialized and jargon-filled field of fertility, without blindly relying on doctors and other experts? By listening to other patients who have been there before you. It isn't possible, of course, for you to meet and talk directly to couples from all parts of the country, and thereby hear of the widest possible variety of experiences in treatment. Hence the reason for this book.

I have conducted extensive interviews with dozens of patients, both female and male, and their spouses, who taken all together represent just about every type of infertility and means of treatment available today. In my talks with couples I paid particular attention to their complaints about their treatment, and I asked them for their suggestions for things patients could do to receive more effective or more compassionate care.

In addition to these face-to-face interviews, I also conducted a survey by mail of ninety-two couples from all over the United States (plus one from Canada). A detailed questionnaire elicited comments on every aspect of fertility care from the first meeting with the doctor to the final outcome of treatment. The interviews and the survey responses gave me confidence that my descriptions of medical events are true to the patient's experience—even if those descriptions don't exactly match the emotionless language of the medical texts.

Keep in mind, though, that my limited survey does not constitute a scientific study. You should not expect to be able to reach an informed conclusion about the efficacy of one drug over another based on a few anecdotes from this book. Nor is it my purpose to explain *how* a particular drug causes ovulation, or exactly what a surgeon is doing during an operation to remove endometriosis. There are already a good number of books that delve into the medical facts, and if you are interested in finding out the technical hows and whys of infertility treatment, then you may check the Suggested Reading List at the back of this book for titles.

What the patients' stories and survey results *will* tell you is what it *feels* like to undergo this or that test, or stay on this or that drug regimen. Reading about the choices other couples have made—about seeking help in the first place, about selecting a clinic, about which tests to undergo, about what a particular procedure was like, about alternatives to that procedure that the doctor never even mentioned until the opportunity to try them had passed—should help you with some of the tough decisions you face from the moment you first decide to seek medical help through the conclusion of your time as a fertility patient.

Throughout this book you will be reminded of a few things that many doctors don't like to admit:

- that it's *your* reproductive system, and the choices to be made about tests and treatments ultimately must be yours
- that in most cases there is not one right way to solve problems—only ways that might work better than others for someone like you
- that not all patients are equally well suited to tolerate difficult forms of treatment, and that a patient's attitudes toward discomfort and risk are as important to consider as his or her physical suitability for the treatment
- that not all fertility doctors are equally skilled at their profession—that though most fall somewhere in the range between merely adequate to truly excellent, there are doctors who seem to remain in

practice, despite their low success rates or outright incompetence in the field
- that only *you* can judge your own depth of desire to have a baby and evaluate its importance against other factors (such as the desire to avoid pain or the difficulty of paying for treatment), as you decide how long to keep trying
- that the whole tortuous process of infertility diagnosis and treatment creates enormous stress, and that many couples will need help from an outside counselor to cope with the effects
- that not everyone can be helped medically
- that when the patient feels confident and in control of what is happening to his or her own body, treatment is less stressful, the patient is less likely to give up too soon, and the overall odds of success are improved

Research bears out that those couples who become *active participants* in the quest to end their infertility do indeed conceive and carry babies to term at higher rates than those who are more passive about their care.* Premised on this fact, *How to Be a Successful Fertility Patient* can help you to have the best odds possible to have a baby through medical intervention.

WORDS FROM A WELL-PREPARED PATIENT

Interview question: Was your fertility treatment easier or more difficult than you had expected?

Answer: It was exactly what I expected. I was *expecting* it to be uncomfortable, expensive, and inconvenient . . . and it was.

Jane from California

How to Use This Book

This isn't a novel, so don't feel you must start at Chapter One and read it straight through.

*Results of a study of forty-eight couples in the Boston area, as reported on the *CBS Evening News*, March 23, 1992.

But do begin there if you are not *sure* that you have a fertility problem and want to find out how to take some simple, at-home tests to start to check yourself out, before you schedule a consultation with an expensive specialist.

Those of you who have already been trying to get pregnant long enough to feel sure that there is a problem but still have not seen a doctor should start at Chapter Two, which covers the basics of smart doctor-shopping (and just as important, smart health-insurance-policy shopping). Also discussed are the pros and cons of working with the different subspecialties in the fertility field (reproductive endocrinologist, OB-GYN, urologist, and others), how to evaluate the success statistics of clinics, and what to make of advertising by doctors and clinics.

Those who have already chosen a doctor or clinic but have not yet been diagnosed with a particular problem can jump right into Chapter Three, which contains descriptions of the most commonly performed tests and what former patients have to say about each.

After you have been told that a particular problem exists, turn to Chapter Four for a discussion of what the diagnosis means in layman's terms. This chapter also covers controversies about certain diagnoses, and how your personal history, your age, and your attitude affect your prognosis for cure.

Once your doctor has determined what is wrong, he will probably recommend a particular course of treatment. Here's where patients really need help! You need to know whether what's being offered as treatment is the only option available, or if there are any alternatives that might suit your needs better. You need to know what questions you should ask your doctor about whatever treatment you are considering. You need to know how the different treatment options each might affect your life-style, your long-term health, and your relationship with your spouse or partner. All this is covered in three chapters: Chapter Five, which contains a patient questionnaire to help you determine whether a conservative, moderate, or aggressive approach to treatment would work best for you; Chapter Six, which describes the drug regimens commonly prescribed for a variety of female and male forms of infertility (a section also gives an overview of infertility surgeries); and Chapter Seven, which covers the higher-technology options, called ARTs ("assisted reproductive technologies"—that is, in vitro fertilization and its variants).

After you've been in treatment for a while and are beginning to get frustrated that you still haven't had a baby, turn to Chapter Eight for some help in deciding when to switch treatment methods, switch doctors or clinics, take a break from treatment, or give up on medical intervention altogether and seek some other resolution to your infertility.

Chapter Nine is all about the stress of infertility treatment—and it might just be a good idea for a patient at any phase of treatment to read this chapter first, before the stress gets out of hand. Former patients talk about strategies that have helped to keep them going, and discuss the pros and cons of keeping their treatment a secret. Also included are discussions of three nonmedical alternatives for couples: adoption, the child-free life-style, and "partial parenting" (the latter two terms are explained beginning on page 358 and page 361, respectively).

You will want to go right to Chapter Ten if you don't fit the traditional husband/wife role that doctors are most used to dealing with or if you face other social hurdles. Single women, unmarried heterosexual couples, Lesbian or gay male couples, postmenopausal women, couples coping with a serious illness or disability, and couples whose options are restricted by the teachings of their religious faith may all want children just as much as anyone else—and they have a right to be helped! This chapter tells how to find open-minded doctors who will give you the treatment that is right for your special situation. Chapter Ten also deals with couples who already have a child and are having difficulties conceiving another (what doctors call "secondary infertility").

Save Chapter Eleven to read should you get pregnant, and then find out about the special considerations that ex–fertility patients should keep in mind when choosing an obstetrician. Also discussed are coping with the critical first three months when your sense of vulnerability to miscarriage is most intense, and parenting after infertility.

You will note that throughout the book, certain terms appear in boldface. These terms, which are medically oriented or specific to the infertility field, are defined in the Glossary in the end matter of the book. Two other sections appear in the end matter: a Suggested Reading List of books recommended for their coverage of certain topics only briefly discussed here; and a Resource Guide listing organizations that distribute information on various aspects of infertility—but I will name the most important of these organizations now, because it's one that every infertile couple should be aware of as soon as possible.

It's called RESOLVE, Inc., and it's a nationwide network linking some fifty-four local chapters, made up of volunteers and members who are all in some way united by the experience of infertility and its treatment. Infertile couples can attend monthly meetings for the exchange of information and ideas, to find emotional support, and to benefit from a variety of lectures, seminars, and literature about all kinds of topics of interest, from azoospermia to ZIFT. You will notice as you read more of this book that there are references to RESOLVE and its services in almost every chapter, and that is because the programs run by RESOLVE are so useful and so comprehensive. If you are not already a member, my first piece of advice is join today! Call the national business office number, (617) 623-1156, for information on the chapter nearest you. RESOLVE also maintains a helpline, at (617) 623-0744, that you can call during regular working hours to get answers to specific questions. I have always found the RESOLVE staff members to be knowledgeable and easy to deal with, and I am confident that you will discover the same.

Good luck to you as you start your quest to make your family complete!

A NOTE ON GENDER TERMS AND NAMES USED

It runs counter to my belief in the equality of the sexes to refer to all doctors with the pronoun *he,* or to use the pronoun *she* for all nurses and other medical support staff, yet it runs counter to my instincts as a writer to keep using the cumbersome phrase *he or she* or worse, the computerese *s/he.*

Still, a book needs pronouns, so there's got to be a determination of usage made one way or the other. To solve the dilemma I have based my usage decision on the gender proportions I have found to hold true in the field, according to my research. About 85 percent of my interviewees, I discovered, were seeing male doctors, so roughly 85 percent of the time in the text that I use a pronoun for a doctor, I will say *he;* the other 15 percent of the time I will say *she.* I found that virtually all of the nurses and support staff that my respondents dealt with were female, so I will always use *she* when referring to nonphysician staff.

For those readers who would argue that it would be better to alternate using *he* and *she* equally to remind ourselves that in a fairer world *she* would be equally as expected in the fertility specialist's role as *he*— let me respond this way: Much that was negative about the infertility treatment experience as my respondents described it came from dealings with arrogant and insensitive *male* doctors; much of the positive side of the experience came from dealings with sympathetic, compassionate female support staff. So when I use male pronouns most of the time for doctors I am in no way implying that males are in any way better suited to be infertility doctors. If anything, the opposite appears to be the case—but female fertility specialists *are* harder to find. Until such time that half the doctors are women, male pronouns will remain the norm.

About the patients' names used in this book: To protect my respondents' privacy I have assigned made-up names to the very real people quoted in these pages—the one exception being for those former patients who also deal with infertility on a professional basis (as clinical psychologists or social workers) and who specifically requested credit for their written or spoken comments on infertility.

HOW TO BE
A SUCCESSFUL
FERTILITY PATIENT

CHAPTER ONE

IF YOU THINK
YOU MIGHT BE INFERTILE . . .

If you think you might be infertile and you've done any reading at all or spoken to any experts on the subject, you've probably heard this rule:

"You are infertile if you have had unprotected intercourse for one year without conception."

Some doctors add: "If you are a woman over thirty-five and have been having unprotected intercourse for six months without result, it may be worthwhile to begin investigating your fertility potential now."

But I am looking at this problem not from the doctor's rule book but from the perspective of all of the infertility patients I have interviewed, and here's what experienced couples have to say:

"Why wait a year or even six months when you could begin looking into your fertility right away? Then, if you discover any of the indicators of a problem, you can bring your findings to a doctor and have a head start on getting the right treatment."

A woman usually has only between eleven and thirteen chances per year to try to get pregnant, and there is no sense wasting any of them—which is what will happen if you have an easily detectable problem but you don't know it. It's neither difficult nor expensive for you to begin checking out the workings of your own reproductive system. You can learn a great deal about your own fertility potential *right away* by following this four-step program:

1. Take your own medical and reproductive history
2. Give yourself a physical exam
3. Chart your BBT (basal body temperature) for 2 to 3 months
4. Test your ovulation with an LH (luteinizing hormone) home testing kit for 2 to 3 months

Instructions for completing each of these four steps follow, section by section.

TAKE YOUR OWN MEDICAL AND REPRODUCTIVE HISTORY

The first and simplest thing to do is to investigate your own past and your partner's past for any possible indicators of the origins of a fertility problem. The questionnaire that follows is similar to one you would fill out if you went to see a fertility specialist. Commentary on your answers follows in the next section, including whether a yes answer to any question indicates a problem that you should discuss with a doctor without delay.

MEDICAL AND REPRODUCTIVE HISTORY QUESTIONNAIRE

Female

1. *Basic Information*
   How old are you? What is your weight and height?
2. *Pregnancy History*
   Have you ever been pregnant? How many times? Dates of pregnancy or pregnancies. Outcomes: Live births? Stillbirths? Miscarriages (spontaneous abortion)? Medically induced abortions? Ectopic pregnancies?
3. *Menstrual History*
   Age at time of first menstrual period? Usual number of days of menstrual period? Usual number of days between menstrual periods? Are periods regular? How would you characterize menstrual flow: light, moderate, or heavy? Do you experience pain or cramping with your period? If so, light, moderate, or severe? Do you sometimes or frequently experience cramping or pain about at the midpoint between periods? Have you experienced any marked change in the flow or crampiness of your period over the years? Do you sometimes experience spotting or bleeding between periods? Have you ever suffered from **Premenstrual Syndrome (PMS)**, a collection of symptoms usually starting about a week before the onset of the menstrual period, including bloating, depression, fatigue, breast soreness or lumpiness, and irritability?
4. *Contraceptive History*
   Have you ever used a method of birth control? If so, which one(s)? Dates and duration for each method used. If IUD (intra-uterine

device), what type and brand (e.g., Dalkon Shield, Copper 7)? If birth control pills, what brand and dosage? Have you ever had any problems with the method you used (vaginitis or other side effects, pain, cramping, excessively heavy menstrual periods, etc.)?

5. *Sexual History*
   How often on average do you and your partner have sexual intercourse? Do you have (or have you ever had) pain with intercourse? Do you regularly use a commercially available lubricant? If so, what brand? What position do you most often use for intercourse? Do you practice or have you practiced anal intercourse? Do you currently have any sex partners besides your spouse or partner? Have you had sex with any bisexual or homosexual men? Do you have reason to believe that any past sexual partner carried a sexually transmitted disease (such as chlamydia, gonorrhea, syphilis, herpes, or AIDS)? Do you regularly or occasionally douche after intercourse?

6. *General Physical Condition*
   What was the date of your last complete physical, including a pelvic exam and Pap smear? Are you currently taking any medications? If so, what? What dosage, frequency, and duration (how long do you expect to take the medication)? Do you smoke? Do you drink alcoholic beverages? If so, what kind, how much, and how often? Do you use or have you used illicit drugs such as marijuana, cocaine, LSD, barbiturates, amphetamines, steroids, and so forth? About how many hours of sleep do you get a night? Do you exercise regularly, and if so, what type of exercise, how long is each workout, and how many workouts per week? How would you characterize your diet: generally well balanced? very low or very high fat? very low or very high protein?

7. *Family History*
   Do you know if your parents had any difficulties with fertility either before or after you were born? Do you know if your mother was ever prescribed the drug DES (generally taken to prevent miscarriage) during her pregnancy with you? Do you have any brothers or sisters? Older or younger? Age of both parents when you were born. Are you adopted? If so, do you have available a complete medical history of your genetic parents?

8. *Operations, Illnesses, and Conditions*
   Have you ever had any operations? If so, what for, when, and with what outcome? Do you have or have you ever had allergies (if so, to what)? headaches or migraines? blurriness of vision or double vision? fainting spells? epilepsy? thyroid problems? rubella

(German measles)? multiple sclerosis? lupus? diabetes? heart problems? asthma or lung problems? kidney problems? gout? gastrointestinal problems or ulcers? eating disorders such as anorexia nervosa or bulimia? giardia, salmonella, botulism or other systemic infections? back pain? persistent vaginal infections such as yeast (*Candida albicans*) infection or trichomoniasis? fibroid tumors or fibrocystic breast disease? exposure to radiation, lead, mercury, or any other environmental toxins? For each illness or condition, note date, how treated, and outcome.

Male

1. *Basic Information*
   How old are you? What is your weight and height?
2. *History of Partner Pregnancies*
   Have you ever caused your current or past partner(s) to become pregnant? How many times? Dates of pregnancies. Outcomes: Live births? Stillbirths? Miscarriages (spontaneous abortions)? Medically induced abortions? Ectopic pregnancies?
3. *Sexual History*
   How often on average do you and your partner have sexual intercourse? Do you always ejaculate? Do you sometimes or regularly have difficulty getting or maintaining an erection? Do you regularly use a commercially available lubricant? If so, what brand? What position do you most often use for intercourse? Do you practice or have you practiced anal intercourse? Do you currently have any sex partners besides your spouse or partner? Have you ever had sex with another male? Do you have any reason to believe that any past sexual partner carried a sexually transmitted disease (such as chlamydia, gonorrhea, syphilis, herpes, or AIDS)?
4. *General Physical Condition*
   What was the date of your last complete physical? Are you currently taking any medications? If so, what? What dosage, frequency, and duration (how long do you expect to take the medication)? Do you smoke? Do you drink alcoholic beverages? If so, what kind, how much, and how often? Do you use or have you used illicit drugs such as marijuana, cocaine, LSD, barbiturates, amphetamines, steroids, and so forth? About how many hours of sleep do you get a night? Do you exercise regularly, and if so, what type of exercise, how long is each workout, and how many workouts per week? How would you characterize your diet: generally

well balanced? very low or very high fat? very low or very high protein?

5. *Family History*

Do you know if your parents had any difficulties with fertility either before or after you were born? Do you know if your mother was ever prescribed the drug DES (usually taken to prevent miscarriage) during her pregnancy with you? Do you have any brothers or sisters? Older or younger? Age of both parents when you were born. Are you adopted? If so, do you have available a complete medical history of your genetic parents?

6. *Operations, Illnesses, and Conditions*

Have you ever had any operations? If so, what for, when, and with what outcome? Do you have or have you ever had allergies (if so, to what)? headaches or migraines? blurriness of vision or double vision? epilepsy? cancer? mumps after puberty? diabetes? heart problems? asthma or lung problems? kidney problems? gout? gastrointestinal problems or ulcers? fainting spells? giardia, salmonella, botulism or other systemic infections? back pain? urinary-tract infections or tinea cruris ("jock itch")? an injury to the scrotum (whether or not you saw a doctor for it)? exposure to radiation, lead, mercury, or any other environmental toxins? For each illness or condition, note date, how treated, and outcome.

UNDERSTANDING YOUR ANSWERS

Female

1. Basic information

Age: If you are thirty-five or over you may well have what's known as "age-related subfertility." Being subfertile doesn't mean you can't conceive; it means that, statistically, you are considerably less likely to conceive each month than a woman whose ovaries have not been working for quite so many years. However, age alone is not an indicator of fertility in any *individual* case, and many women of thirty-five or even forty and older can still conceive as easily as younger women—so you should not instantly conclude that you will need medical help if you are over thirty-five. It's simply that, on average, you are more *likely* to need medical help.

Height and weight: Get hold of a chart listing the appropriate weight range for your height (your insurance agent should be able to provide you with a currently accepted weight-height chart). If you are more than about 10 percent *under* the recommended weight, your production of hormones associated with body fat could be adversely affected. On the other hand, obesity may be an indicator of a particular form of infertility called **polycystic ovarian disease** or **PCO** (see Chapter Four for description of other symptoms of this disease).

2. Pregnancy History

If you've ever been pregnant, even if it ended in a miscarriage or an ectopic pregnancy, that's a very good sign. You *can* conceive. If you already have given birth and you have been unable to conceive again after a full year of trying, then you are considered to have **secondary infertility** (discussed on page 389 of this book). If you have suffered two or more miscarriages, you may want to turn to page 163 to read about **recurrent miscarriage.**

If you have ever had a medically induced abortion followed by complications such as excessive bleeding, infection, or incomplete expulsion of fetal tissue, you should certainly see a gynecologist (*not* the same one who performed the abortion) to discuss the complications you suffered and to be tested to see if any damage was done to your reproductive organs.

If you have ever suffered an ectopic pregnancy, you should contact the doctor who treated you at the time and ask whether it is likely that one of your **fallopian tubes** could be scarred or blocked.

3. Menstrual History

A very late age of first menstruation (seventeen or older) is sometimes an indication of a hormonal problem, as is the absence or irregularity of menstrual periods, or periods that are closer together than every twenty-five days or farther apart than every thirty-one days. If your menstrual history fits any of these descriptions, you should see your gynecologist to begin investigation into your hormonal production right away. If your periods are excessively long (more than seven days) or short (less than three days) or if menstrual flow is so light as to be hardly more than spotting, or if it seems abnormally heavy, a consultation with your gynecologist is also advisable. Severe cramping or pain with menstruation can sometimes be an indicator of endometriosis, a relatively common condition often accompanied by problems of fertility. However, some cramping or pain at about the midway point between periods is just the opposite—it generally is an indicator that ovulation has occurred, and that tends to mean that your reproductive system is working as it should. Any marked changes in your menstrual pattern over the years (whether an increase or decrease in the menstrual flow or in the crampiness you experience) could also be an indicator of a fertility problem. Increased flow could result from the presence of a **fibroid tumor** in your uterus; increased crampiness could be a sign that endometriosis is developing or has developed; greatly diminished flow could mean that your hormonal output has decreased; when menstrual flow varies greatly from cycle to cycle (heavier than normal one cycle, very light the next), that could be a symptom of the onset of menopause. Any bleeding or spotting between periods should be checked out without delay, as some serious medical conditions first manifest themselves through nonmenstrual vaginal bleeding.

Premenstrual Syndrome (**PMS**), though often a subject for debate in medical literature, is believed by many doctors to be due to imbalances in the production of hormones during the last two weeks of the menstrual cycle. If you suffer from PMS you should not only have a talk with your doctor about it (mentioning, of course, that you are also trying to get pregnant), but you might also want to do some independent reading on the subject. See the Suggested Reading List at the end of this book for recommended titles.

4. Contraceptive History

Most methods of birth control are safe, with few serious side effects; however, some have been associated with certain kinds of infertility, especially the IUD called the Dalkon Shield, made by A. H. Robins Company (now bankrupt due to lawsuits). That device caused **pelvic inflammatory disease** (**PID**) in thousands of women who used it, and it was finally withdrawn from the market. Other types of IUDs still on the market have also been linked to higher than normal rates of PID and infertility. It is for this reason that fertility specialists advise against using any form of IUD for women who have not yet had all the children they want. If you have ever worn any form of IUD, it would be worthwhile for you to call your gynecologist and discuss testing for fallopian tube scarring, infection, or other damage that could have occurred.

The "pill," or oral contraceptive, works by inhibiting ovulation. It does this by means of a synthetic hormone called progestin. Because some women retain progestins longer in their systems than others, if you have used the pill in the past year you may still be "protected" from

THE IUD AND INFERTILITY

One Patient's Story

*E*ighteen months after my IUD was inserted I began having pain, bloating, and an increasing feeling of sickness in my abdomen. I went to the gynecologist who inserted it, and he just brushed it off as a "cyst." I was told to go home and take aspirin. By the next month I was in horrible, doubling-over pain and bleeding heavily. I went back to the doctor and was hospitalized that day. A **laparoscopy** revealed severe **pelvic inflammatory disease.** I did not know it then but I was completely infertile because my tubes had been scarred shut. . . . My whole experience in treatment [she had had tubal surgery, and then tried IVF, without success] was a nightmare I could have avoided completely if only my OB-GYN had told me "There is a *chance* that the IUD can cause infertility." I would have *never considered* putting it in my body.

*M*onica from Ohio

pregnancy, even though you stopped taking it several months before. Begin charting your **basal body temperature (BBT)** and **ovulation,** as described later on in this chapter, and if you find no evidence of ovulation, call your doctor and ask how long it would be reasonable to wait for ovulation to return and at what point a consultation would be necessary.

Obviously, if you suffered any significant side effects (pain, cramping, excessively heavy menstrual periods) because of the contraceptive method you used, there could be damage to your reproductive system. If you didn't discuss your symptoms with your doctor at the time, you should certainly make an appointment right away to see if you have suffered any lasting injury to your ovaries, fallopian tubes, or uterus.

5. Sexual History

If you have intercourse less than twice a week on average, the answer to your infertility may simply be that you're not "doing it" enough! If you have experienced pain with intercourse, you may have one of the symptoms of endometriosis—see your doctor. If you frequently use a commercially available lubricant, such as K-Y jelly, it is possible that the thick substance is interfering with the transit of sperm to your **cervix**. (Yes, I know it says on the box that K-Y is *not* a contraceptive—but all that really means is that couples mustn't depend on it to block sperm, though it sometimes does.)

Position during intercourse *can* make a difference, especially if you usually end up in a vertical (standing up) position. Gravity causes the semen to flow downward, so fewer sperm are placed at the opening of the cervix at the top of the vaginal canal (which is the optimal spot for the ejaculate to go). One notable fertility expert, Dr. Sherman J. Silber, author of *How to Get Pregnant* (Warner Books, 1980), discourages the use of any sexual position other than the traditional one of man on top by the couple hoping to maximize the chance of conception. That position, he asserts, "allows the greatest contact of the semen with the cervical mucus" (p. 115). If the couple should prefer to have intercourse with the woman on top, then he suggests that the woman roll onto her back after intercourse and raise her knees so that gravity will assist the flow of sperm toward the opening of her cervix.

Anal intercourse is *not* a good idea for couples who are trying to conceive. "Wasting sperm" isn't the problem; a fertile man has enough to spare. But the practice can all too easily spread harmful bacteria from the anus to the vagina, causing an infection that could—though symptomless—be destructive of the woman's reproductive tract. If anal intercourse is an important component of your sexual relationship, you don't have to give it up—but you *do* have to use a condom. Handle and dispose of the used condom extremely carefully. Your husband should wash his hands and penis afterward with antibacterial soap.

If you ever practiced anal intercourse with a past partner, you should have yourself tested—even though you may have no symptoms of any illness—for a variety of infections and sexually transmitted diseases. See a doctor you trust enough to discuss your sex life with, and she will tell you what tests you should undergo.

If you answered "yes" to the question about having sex with partners outside of your relationship, you are well advised to protect your system from any potentially fertility-damaging germs by use of a condom. You may also wish to consider that secret sexual activity frequently brings emotional turmoil with it—the stress of divided loyalties—as well as sexual exhaustion that can interfere with your having intercourse with your spouse at the right time of the month. If you were to consult a professional counselor (and that is probably a good idea in your situation), you would probably be asked why you want to start a family when your commitment to your child's father is so shaky—and that's a worthwhile question for you to ponder.

For those who have had past sexual contact with a homosexual or bisexual man, the main concern is whether you have been exposed to the AIDS virus. A simple blood test will provide the answer, and you should have it done before continuing to try to conceive.

For those who have had past sexual contact with *anyone* without complete assurance of that person's sexual health at the time, it may be worthwhile having yourself tested for a variety of sexually transmitted diseases that can impair reproductive functioning—especially since many of the women who are infected experience few or no symptoms of the disease. If it should turn out that you have been suffering unknowingly from an infection contracted long ago, it's important not to get tied up by feelings of guilt, or to feel that your infertility is somehow a punishment for your "promiscuous" past. Such thinking is depressing, unproductive, and *untrue*. Millions of adults who came of age in the pre-AIDS days of the sixties and seventies and had dozens of partners still have gone on to become parents without difficulty, while plenty of other couples who lived "chaste and pure" lives still are infertile. Nature has a baffling way of distributing illnesses without regard to the moral qualifications of the victim. The main thing is to find a doctor you can trust not to be judgmental, and to get you started with the appropriate treatment. Keep in mind that most doctors these days have heard just about everything, and they *really don't care* how you've chosen to run your personal life.

Douching after intercourse is to be avoided by women who wish to conceive. The douche washes out sperm (the short-term effect) and it can also alter the level of acidity in the vagina for weeks afterward, making it a less hospitable environment for sperm (the long-term effect).

6. General Physical Condition

If it has been more than a year since your last physical and Pap smear, attend to that first. Let your internist know of your concerns about your fertility and he will pay special attention as he performs a pelvic exam, looking for any obvious abnormalities in your ovaries, uterus, and cervix.

If you are currently on any medication, whether prescription or over-the-counter, call your doctor and ask if the medication could possibly be interfering with your ability to conceive—or if you do conceive, if it could have a harmful effect on the development of the embryo. So many medications do have adverse effects that it is impossible for reasons of space to list them all here. If you want to have a home reference book on the effects of medication, consider purchasing a copy of the *Physician's Drug Handbook* or look for the layman-oriented *Essential Guide to Prescription and Over-the-Counter Drugs* (see the Suggested Reading List for further information).

If you smoke, you already know that it's bad for your long-term health. But did you also know that smokers on average conceive with much greater difficulty than nonsmokers, and that they miscarry at significantly higher rates?

Drinking alcohol in moderation has not been shown to have any adverse effects on fertility, but binge drinking is associated with a wide variety of bodily ills. Don't forget that drunkenness could lead you to forget what day of your cycle it is, and you could miss an opportunity to have intercourse at the optimal time.

Nearly all of the illicit drugs can have deadly effects on the developing embryo, so if you even occasionally indulge, you should quit, but especially during the last two weeks of your cycle before your menstrual period, when you could be pregnant and not know it. Steroids, taken by some women athletes to build up muscle tissue, will definitely harm your reproductive system (though if treated promptly, damage can often be reversed). Past use of LSD, even very long ago, has been implicated in chromosomal abnormalities in children born to users, so you might want to consult a geneticist before you attempt to conceive.

Adequate sleep—at least seven hours for most adults—at regular hours has been shown to help the body in maintaining normal rhythms and cycles, including the menstrual cycle; so if you have been keeping odd hours, for the sake of your reproductive health consider changing your routine.

We all know that regular exercise contributes to overall health, but it is also true that taken to extremes, exercise can impair fertility. What is extreme? Studies do not show clearly how much exercise a woman has to do to cause her **estrogen** production to fall to infertile levels; on the other hand data is clear on what level of exercise will *not* impair fertility: a half hour at a time, no more than twice a week. If you are doing more than that, and are set on continuing, you might want to have your estrogen level tested to see if it is still normal.

When you are trying to have a baby, it is not the time to take up any fad diets or make any major changes in your eating routine. A well-balanced diet is always a good idea, but if like most Americans you're still eating too much fat and sugar, you needn't worry. With fertility, it's the extremely *low-fat* diet that is especially suspect—though extremes of any other kind are best avoided, too.

7. Family History

Infertility is not an inherited trait. After all, your parents did have you, didn't they? However, it *is* possible that you could have inherited a tendency to low hormone production or imperfectly shaped reproductive organs that could make it more difficult for you to conceive. If you are adopted and can't ask your biological parents about their reproductive history, you might still be able to see their medical histories to look for evidence of genetically transmissable characteristics. Ask your adoptive parents to help you find the information you need.

If your parents are alive (and you are willing to discuss this very personal subject with them) you might find it worthwhile to ask them about their reproductive history. Did they have any trouble conceiving you or other children? Has your mother ever been told she had a uterine, ovarian, or hormonal problem that could affect her ability to conceive? If your mother says yes to this question, then you should be sure to tell your doctor of this aspect of your history during your initial consultation for infertility.

Many mothers who had children during the 1950s were given a drug called DES by their doctors to prevent miscarriage. It was not until the first generation of "DES daughters" born to these mothers reached the age of puberty that the harmful and serious side effects of the drug on children were discovered. "DES daughters" can be affected by a wide variety of reproductive-tract problems, including vaginal cancer, wombs of abnormal size, shape, or position, and poor or absent ovulation. If you were born during the fifties you should ask your mother if she ever took *any* drug to prevent miscarriage (she may not remember the exact name of the drug she took). If the answer is yes, you should certainly bring up this fact in your first consultation with a fertility specialist—and you probably ought to see one soon.

8. Operations, Illnesses, and Conditions

Some operations have an obvious connection to fertility. If you have ever had **fibroid tumors** removed from your uterus, you were told at the time that your future fertility could be affected. Of course if you ever had a tubal ligation (female sterilization) you know you have been rendered infertile by the procedure. A past **D and C (dilatation and**

curettage) possibly could have had complications that have affected your fertility. However, some of the operations women undergo can affect their fertility without their awareness of the fact. An operation to reduce an overactive thyroid gland or to remove tumors on the pituitary gland in the brain are two examples. If you have any doubts about side effects of any operation you may have had (no matter how many years ago), you could get peace of mind either by contacting your surgeon and asking specifically about any possible impact on your fertility, or you may just want to go to a medical library and look for a book or journal article that describes your operation and all its possible side effects.

The long list of diseases and conditions (and it is by no means comprehensive) are all subjects of concern for the fertility patient. In some cases drugs to cure the disease or alleviate the condition can impair fertility; in other cases drugs that must be taken on a regular basis can interfere with the developing embryo, should a pregnancy occur. Oftentimes there is controversy within the medical community as to whether a condition or illness, or the drugs used to treat it, can have harmful effects on the reproductive system or on a recently created embryo within it. So to be on the safe side, if you answered yes to *anything* on the list, be sure to bring up the matter the first time you have a consultation with any professional about your fertility. And if you are taking a drug for any ongoing problem, be sure to remind the doctor of that fact once more, before you begin to take any medication prescribed for your infertility. Doctors frequently forget to review patients' histories before they write prescriptions, causing inadvertent though sometimes serious drug interactions for the patient.

If you have had cancer or heart, kidney, or lung disease, or suffered any injury or illness that has left you disabled, be sure to read the section in Chapter Ten, "For the Couple Coping with Serious Illness or Disability."

Male

1. Basic Information

Age: Male fertility does not usually decline until after fifty, but if you are that age or older you should probably make arrangements to have your sperm analyzed soon.

Height and weight: Get hold of a chart listing the appropriate weight range for your height (your insurance agent should be able to provide you with a currently accepted weight-height chart). If you are more than 20 percent *under* the recommended weight, your production of hormones associated with body fat could be adversely affected. If the weight chart places you in the obese range, it is possible that there is some other problem related to your weight (such as diabetes) that could also be associated with certain fertility problems (such as **retrograde ejaculation**).

2. History of Partner Pregnancies

If you know that you have ever caused a woman to be pregnant, you should be encouraged. You *can* father a child. Unless you have undergone some physical changes due to illness or injury, your sperm should remain fertile. However, if your wife or partner has suffered repeated very early miscarriages (before six weeks), it is possible that chromosomal defects in your sperm could be a problem.

3. Sexual History

See Sexual History for females for commentary on frequency of intercourse.

Of course a man must ejaculate if he is to impregnate a woman in the normal way. A man must also be able to get and maintain an erection (though occasional problems with arousal are something every man experiences and are no cause for concern). But don't think it's hopeless if due to some physical or psychological problem you are unable to complete the sexual act. Artificial insemination of your wife or partner with your sperm could be the answer—but you should definitely consult a doctor to discuss your options.

See Sexual History for females for information on the significance of use of lubricants, position in intercourse, the practice of anal intercourse, homosexual activity, extramarital affairs, and past contacts with partners whose sexual histories are unknown to you.

4. General Physical Condition

If it has been more than a year since your last complete physical, it's time for you to have a checkup. Be sure to tell your internist that you and your wife or partner are trying to have a baby.

If you are currently taking any drugs, whether prescription or over-

SMOKING AND MEN

I smoked cigarettes for twenty years. When my wife and I had our consultation at the fertility clinic, the people there were adamant that I stop smoking. I did, and my sperm count became normal—but I also had had **varicocele** surgery. I'll never know which was the most influential, but I urge patients who smoke to stop. Prior to going to —— Clinic, none of our physicians had ever focused on smoking as an issue.

*S*tan from New York

the-counter, ask your prescribing doctor if there could be any impact on your production of sperm.

If you smoke, you should know that smokers have malformed sperm in greater numbers than nonsmokers.

If you drink alcohol in moderation, you need not be concerned; however, if you are prone to binge drinking, you should keep in mind that alcohol in large quantities generally interferes with a man's ability to complete the sexual act—and if you binge too often, you could easily end up unable to perform at the time of the month when your wife's fertility is at its peak.

Illicit drugs are associated with a variety of impairments to male fertility: marijuana, for example, has been linked to excess production of female hormones in men who smoke regularly; LSD has been shown to cause chromosomal damage; and steroids taken by athletes may make them look more "manly" even as they cause complete sterility.

Regular sleep, at least seven hours a night, has been shown to be beneficial to most of the body's systems, including the reproductive system.

Regular exercise is also a good thing for one's overall health—but not right before having sex. Intensive workouts, especially running, rowing, bicycling, and other activities usually done in nylon shorts or pants, can build up heat in the testicles, which can lead to poor sperm production.

Fad dieting, especially any diet based heavily on only one form of nutrition (ultrahigh protein, for example, or ultrahigh carbohydrate), can throw all kinds of processes in your body out of whack, including your reproductive processes.

5. Family History

See Family History for females for the significance of finding out about your parents' reproductive histories. Even though males born to mothers who took the drug DES during pregnancy do not seem to suffer the same destructive consequences to their reproductive systems that females do, there nevertheless is some limited evidence that some males were affected. If your mother informs you that she was given DES during her pregnancy with you (or any other drug for miscarriage, whether she remembers the name or not), you should definitely discuss this information with your doctor and decide whether you want to be tested for a fertility problem right away.

6. Operations, Illnesses, and Conditions

See Operations, Illnesses, and Conditions for females for a discussion of why it's important to inform your doctor of any past operations, even those you may not think could have any impact on your reproductive system. If you were operated on in childhood to correct an undescended testicle, you should probably make an appointment with a urologist to find out if the corrective surgery has affected your reproductive capability.

The list of illnesses and conditions on this questionnaire (though it is by no means comprehensive) are all subjects of concern for the fertility patient. In some cases the drugs commonly used to cure the disease or alleviate the condition can impair male fertility; in other cases doctors may be in disagreement as to the impact of the disease or its treatment on the male reproductive system. In either case, if you answered yes to anything on this list, it would be worth bringing the subject up the first time you have a consultation with any professional about your fertility. And if you are taking a drug for any ongoing problem, be sure to remind the doctor of that fact once more, especially before you start taking any medication prescribed specifically for your infertility. Doctors often forget to review patients' histories before they write prescriptions, causing inadvertent though sometimes serious drug interactions in the patient.

If you have had cancer or heart, kidney, or lung disease, or suffered any injury or illness that has left you disabled, be sure to read the section in Chapter Ten, "For the Couple Coping with Serious Illness or Disability."

GIVE YOURSELF A PHYSICAL EXAM

I am not talking about a medical examination here, but just about giving your body a basic once-over to see if you can find any obvious physical anomalies that you should have a doctor take a look at.

Let's start with the man:

Undress completely and stand in front of a full-length mirror in good lighting. Look closely at your penis and testicles. Do they look normal (do you look more or less like the rest of the guys you see in the locker room)? Be sure there is no swelling or shriveling of the testicles. No unusual bumps or lumps anywhere? No part that is painful or unusually tender to the touch? Is the skin color the same as it always was?

Now take a look at the rest of your body. Do you have a normal amount of body hair (taking into account the general level of body hair of members of your race or ethnic group)? No sudden hair loss anywhere? And you've experienced no sudden weight loss or gain?

Now think about your sexual functioning. Are you able to arouse yourself easily when you want to? The next time you ejaculate, examine your semen. Is it the same milky-colored fluid that it's always been? Would you say that there is at least a teaspoon worth of volume?

If you answered anything other than "normal" to all these questions, go ahead and schedule an appointment with your regular doctor, or if you prefer, with a urologist (a specialist in the male reproductive and urinary tracts) or an andrologist (a specialist in male fertility).

Now let's talk about the woman:

You have undressed completely and are looking at yourself in a full-length mirror in good lighting. Does your figure look normal to you, with no sudden weight loss or gain? Look closely at your body hair, especially any dark or coarse hair on your face, on your belly, on your arms, on your big toes, or encircling the dark part of your nipples. Many normally fertile women have some hair in these locations, but you may be concerned if you have recently experienced an increase in body hair growth, or if you believe you have considerably more hair than most of the other women you have seen without their clothes on. Such hair growth could indicate that you are producing an overabundance of **androgens,** or male hormones, that could be interfering with your reproductive functioning.

Now look carefully at your breasts. It doesn't matter if they are smaller than average or bigger; size is no index of fertility—unless you have no breast development whatsoever (in which case you most likely have some other signs of incomplete sexual development as well, such as absence of menstrual periods). Now squeeze your nipples. Does any sort of fluid (whether milky white, yellowish or clear) come out? (If so, you very likely have an excessive level of the hormone **prolactin** in your system, and you should see your gynecologist.)

Now sit down on the bed or floor and hold a mirror so that you can look at the external parts of your genitals. Does everything look more or less as it always has? No obvious swelling, shriveling, irritation, or discoloration? No unusual or odorous discharge present?

Now, with clean hands, insert a finger or two inside your vagina and feel your vaginal walls. You should be able to do this without any sensation of burning, dryness, or discomfort. There should be no obvious lumps or abrasions, although your finger may hit a rubbery feeling object at the end of the vaginal canal—but relax, that's just your cervix.

If you find anything during this once-over that troubles you or seems to you to be different or abnormal, then make an appointment with your gynecologist and let an expert take a look.

Now for a very important part of your self-exam: you should learn to watch out for and understand the changes that take place each month in your *cervical mucus*. What is cervical mucus? You have probably noticed it: a whitish, clear, or yellowy discharge that appears at various intervals of your cycle. The color, consistency, and amount of the discharge can tell you something very valuable about your fertility during each phase of your cycle. For most women, right after menstruation there is little mucus present, or the mucus appears white, thick, and dry-feeling. Moving toward midcycle (toward the normal time for ovulation) the mucus changes, becoming more abundant and more slippery, a colorless fluid with a consistency rather like that of raw egg white. When you remove a bit of this midcycle mucus from your vagina, you find that it feels stretchy, and you are able to draw out a long thin string of it between your thumb and forefinger (see page 47). A German doctor gave this stretchy quality a name—**spinnbarkeit**—and when your cervical mucus has the quality, the mucus has become the optimum medium for sperm to swim through. When your mucus shows spinnbarkeit, you can also be fairly confident that you will ovulate within the next few days.

After ovulation is over, the cervical mucus changes again, becoming

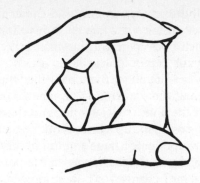

less plentiful and again thick and difficult for sperm to penetrate. The mucus may be white again, or white with a yellowish tinge, or truly yellow.

To familiarize yourself with the patterns of your own mucus, during at least one bathroom break a day you should insert a finger and extract a bit of mucus from your vagina, examine it in the light, and note its color and consistency and when it appeared in your cycle. With a little practice you should be able to recognize at a glance the different types of mucus you produce, and even if your menstrual periods are not regular, you should be able to tell when ovulation is a few days away.

This next part of the woman's self-exam is not for everyone, but if you are the sort of woman who likes to have as much information as you can about your own body, read on. You can learn to examine your own cervix, the organ at the end of your vaginal canal that is normally seen only by your gynecologist when you have a pelvic exam. First you need a **speculum,** a device that will hold your vaginal walls apart to allow a look inside. You can buy a plastic, presterilized one sealed in a bag from a medical supply house at low cost (a few dollars at most).

Take off your clothes from the waist down and have close by a flashlight and a hand mirror. Lubricate the speculum well with K-Y jelly, then slowly and gently insert it into your vagina as deeply as it will go (a squatting position may be most comfortable for this, or sitting in a reclining chair). Pull—gently!—on the lever that causes the speculum to open up and separate your vaginal walls. (You should probably practice getting the speculum to open up and lock a few times before you try inserting it.) Now hold the mirror in front of the opening of the speculum and direct the flashlight beam so that you can see inside your vagina. Your view inside will be of a pinkish or reddish body part with a small hole at the center. You now know what your cervix looks like.

The size of the hole that you see (which is called the *os,* or mouth of the cervix) will vary somewhat depending on where you are in your menstrual cycle. Most of the time it will look tiny and closed. Around the time that you ovulate, the os opens up a bit—though you may find it difficult to see this if you are producing a large amount of cervical mucus.

You will also want to look for changes in the position of your cervix in the vaginal canal and changes in how it looks and feels. Right after menstruation the cervix is normally rather low in the vaginal canal (if you insert your finger, you will probably be able to feel it). Around the time of ovulation, however, it rises up to its highest point (now it may be too far up to reach with your finger). At this time it also feels softer to the touch than at other times in your cycle.

Medical students are taught an acronym to help them remember the qualities that the cervix is supposed to exhibit at the time of ovulation. It is SHOW: *s*oft, *h*igh, *o*pen, and *w*et. If you examine your cervix at the right time of the month and see the signs of SHOW, you can have some confidence that you do indeed ovulate.

On the other hand, if you examine your cervix every few days for an entire cycle, and every time the cervix seems low down in your vagina, looks dry, and the os looks closed tight, you have some fairly conclusive evidence that you are not ovulating, and you should see a fertility doctor.

ABOUT BASAL BODY TEMPERATURE (BBT)

If nothing in your medical history or your limited self-exam leads you to make a doctor's appointment right away, then on to the next step. Women, you will gain invaluable insight into your reproductive health (and your doctor will be impressed at your level of knowledge) if you chart your basal body temperature (BBT) for two or three months.

What is BBT? It is your body temperature (usually taken orally) upon waking up first thing in the morning. Why is it important? Because BBT fluctuates according to a regular pattern during the normal menstrual cycle as different events occur. When a woman's ovary is preparing an egg to be released (ovulation), the hormone estrogen is produced and

BBT is usually low (for most women, between 97.0°F and 97.8°F). A day or two before ovulation, **luteinizing hormone (LH)** is released, and BBT may dip by 0.2° or 0.3°. After the egg has been released, the spent egg follicle converts into what is called the **corpus luteum** (Latin for "yellow body"), which produces the hormone **progesterone** to provide a nourishing lining for the uterus for the fertilized egg (if conception should occur). Progesterone in turn causes BBT to rise—in most cases at least 0.5° after ovulation is over—and to stay elevated at around the same level for twelve to fourteen days. When BBT drops to preovulation levels, it nearly always means that menstruation is imminent.

If BBT remains elevated for more than a day or two beyond the day that the period is expected (assuming you have a regular cycle), then you may well be pregnant. (Either that, or you are running a fever.)

As you can see, the changes in BBT reveal something about every phase of the menstrual cycle. If your BBT follows the pattern described above (a pattern that your doctor will call "biphasic," meaning having two phases, one of low temperature followed by one of high), you can feel fairly confident that you ovulate normally, producing the necessary hormones in the proper sequence. However, if your BBT remains at the elevated level for less than ten days, you are probably producing an insufficient amount of progesterone, and have what is known as a **luteal-phase defect.*** If you have no rise in temperature but readings remain within 0.5° of each other, regardless of the number of days after menstruation, then you probably do not ovulate, or at least, did not ovulate during that particular cycle.

Taking BBT

Many things can affect the temperature inside your mouth first thing in the morning, so it's very important to follow some consistent rules:

- Take your BBT on first waking, without getting out of bed. Keep your thermometer on your nightstand so that you can grab it when you're still half asleep.
- Keep regular hours. Lack of sleep, interrupted sleep, or significant changes in your daily routine can affect your BBT.
- Don't put anything else in your mouth for at least a half hour before you insert the thermometer. If you need to go to the bathroom

---

*The days prior to ovulation are known as the **follicular phase**; and the days following ovulation but prior to menstruation are called the **luteal phase**.

early in the morning before your normal temperature-taking time, be sure not to drink a glass of water or smoke a cigarette while you're up. If you think you might not go right back to sleep, then take your temperature immediately. You are probably better off taking your temperature a bit too early than taking it after you've been awake for a while.

- As near as possible, take your temperature at the exact same time every morning. If you think you might sleep late one day, set an alarm for the usual time, take your temperature, put the thermometer back on the table, and go back to sleep.

TIP!

$\mathcal{G}$et a clock with a four- or five-minute snooze alarm. That way you can stick the thermometer in your mouth the moment the alarm first rings, fall back to sleep for just the right amount of time, and be awakened to read your correct BBT.

- Use only a special BBT thermometer, one specially calibrated to ensure accuracy and capable of registering to the tenth of a degree. Ovulindex, Marshall, and B-D are widely available brands at well-stocked pharmacies. Also acceptable is a high-quality digital thermometer that records to the tenth of a degree. Don't use fever strips that you put on your forehead, or conventional fever thermometers that register only every 0.2°—they will not give you the precision that BBT requires.

Graphing BBT

Buy ordinary graph paper and enter your daily temperature on it as shown on the examples on the next page.

If you have already decided to see a fertility specialist, then don't make your own forms for graphing BBT but call the doctor's office and ask for a few blank BBT graph forms to be mailed to you. Doctors generally prefer to read BBT charts done on their own forms.

Graph for at least two months—three to four months is even better. Even very fertile women occasionally fail to ovulate and so may have

BTT CHART — NORMAL BIPHASIC

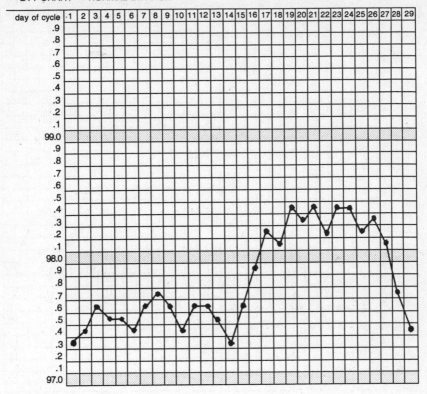

an abnormal-looking chart. The more months you graph, the more clearly you can see any patterns that could indicate trouble.

It's important to number the days of your cycle correctly. The first day of bleeding of your menstrual period is called Day One. If your period begins late in the evening, count the following day as Day One. You do not need to begin taking and recording your temperature until bleeding has stopped (for most women that's Day Five or Day Six). You can mark down the days of bleeding with an X on your chart. Continue taking and recording your temperature every morning until your next period starts (mark that event on your chart with an X). Use a fresh sheet of graph paper for the next month's chart.

You should also record other data on your monthly temperature charts. If you are also examining yourself for signs of cervical mucus (as described in the section above), note on your chart those days when your mucus is clear, stretchy, and copious. If you are performing an ovulation dipstick test (covered in the section immediately following

BBT CHART—LUTEAL-PHASE DEFECT

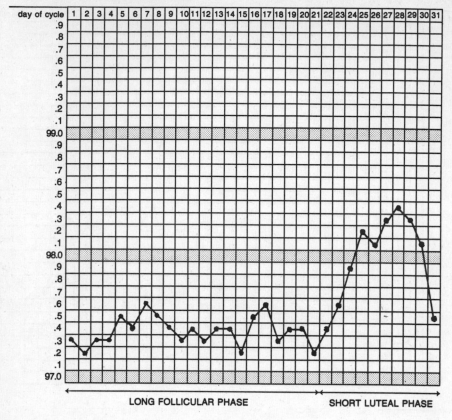

LONG FOLLICULAR PHASE   SHORT LUTEAL PHASE

this one), record a minus sign (−) for those days on which you tested negative and a plus sign (+) on the day you test positive for the ovulation hormone. Also record with a check mark the days when you and your partner have sexual intercourse (if you are doing this according to a doctor's instructions, you may be told to use the letter *c* (for "coitus") to mark days of intercourse.

Add notes to the bottom of your chart to explain any anomalies in your record. If you forgot to take your temperature one morning, note that fact. If you woke up much later than usual, had a sleepless night, traveled across time zones, caught a cold or flu, had a glass of water early in the morning, or did anything else that you believe has altered your normal BBT for the day, jot down an explanation at the bottom of the chart. Your completed chart may look something like the graph on page 54.

BBT CHART—IRREGULAR CYCLE, NO INDICATION OF OVULATION

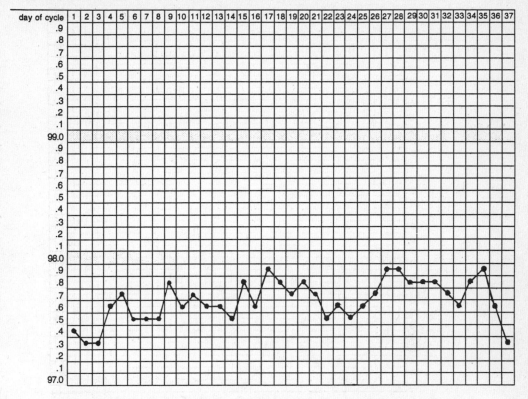

PATIENT'S TIP

Take Your BBTs to Someone Who Knows How to Read Them!

I did *years* of monthly temperature charts. My regular doctor always said they were fine. When I saw Dr. T. [a fertility specialist], he looked at them and said he could tell right away what was wrong—that I probably only had four ovulations over the last several years. Dr. T.'s prediction of my infertility problem was hormonal imbalance (nothing at the right level at the right time) and he quickly confirmed it through some pretty routine blood tests. From there we were able to decide on a course of action.

*S*arah from Louisiana

BBT CHART WITH USEFUL ADDITIONAL DATA AND PATIENT'S NOTES

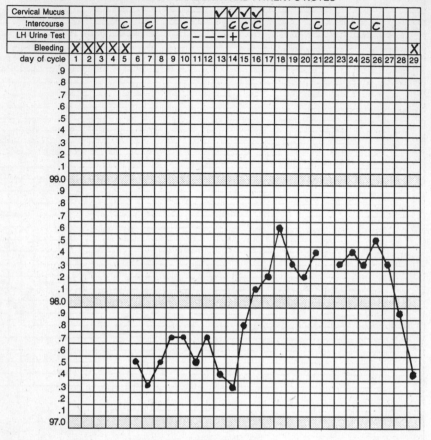

Day 18: Took temperature 5 min. after waking

Day 22: Forgot to take temp.

OVULATION TEST KITS

Charting your BBT will give you useful information about your body's reproductive capabilities throughout your cycle, but for information specifically about your ovulation, you should buy an ovulation test kit, which will enable you to test your first morning urine for the presence of LH, the hormone that is produced about thirty-six hours prior to the release of the mature egg. Testing your urine is a relatively simple mat-

Gadget Alert!

You probably have come across health-care-product catalogs advertising certain gadgets that promise to make charting your BBT easier and error-free. You may be tempted to spend up to $300 for an "ovulation computer"—but is it worth it?

Let's take a look at a few of these items and see what they do:

- *Woman's Biomonitor,* Self-Care Catalog, (800)345-3371, $289—A combination alarm clock, digital thermometer, and automatic recording device in a box that measures five by five and a half inches. The alarm beeps every morning at the time that you set, reminding you to insert the thermometer in your mouth; it beeps again when the temperature is taken; then it automatically enters the temperature into memory and displays a graph of the month on a tiny viewscreen. Since it does not print the graph for you, you still have to laboriously enter the data on graph paper to make a permanent record to bring to your doctor. *My recommendation:* Get a $10 alarm clock, a $12 thermometer, and a $2 pack of graph paper and save the rest of the money to pay for something you *really* need.
- *Rabbit Ovulation Computer,* Fortune's Almanac Catalog, (800)331-2300, $169—Essentially the same sort of device as the Biomonitor above, though somewhat smaller (five and three-quarters by three inches) and cheaper—but still no better than your own thermometer and alarm clock. *My recommendation:* Stick to the old-fashioned way.
- *Ovudate Urinary Thermometers,* Franklin Diagnostics, (201)285-1135, $30—This is a set of urine collection cups. When you go to the bathroom first thing in the morning, you urinate in the cup and a set of heat-sensitive dots on the bottom of the cup registers your BBT to the nearest 0.2°. Because urinary temperature is not affected by cold air in the room, by body movements, or by drinking a cup of water, many women will find it easier to get a valid reading using this method of BBT measurement. The kit includes twenty-eight cups and a graph form to record temperature. *My recommendation:* Once you have charted your temperature for at least two months with a thermometer that is accurate to a tenth of a degree, you might want to switch to the Ovudate method, but *only* for those days of your cycle that you expect your temperature to remain relatively stable—for example, the week following menstruation, and the week preceding your next period. Around the time you expect ovulation to occur, it is extremely important to get maximum precision in your temperature taking. *This advice is valid only for those whose first two months of charting shows a predictable pattern to BBT.*

ter, so even if you did poorly in high school chemistry class, don't worry: it will be hard to mess this test up. The instructions that come with the test will tell you what day of your cycle to begin testing, how to collect your urine, what to do with it once you've got it, and how to interpret the results.

Most big drugstores will carry several brands, so which one do you choose? The chart on pages 58–59 can help you to decide what features you want from your ovulation test kit.

A word of advice: If you are already a patient at a fertility clinic, you may be steered toward the purchase of kits sold directly by the clinic that may be more expensive (though no more accurate) than those sold in any drugstore. This was the experience of former Washington, D.C., patient Anne, who paid $64 for a 10-day kit her doctor sold her, when she could have gone to a nearby drugstore and bought two 5-day kits of a different brand for $26 each. Clinics whose doctors push you to buy their products could be more interested in their own financial health than in your reproductive health.

You may think $30 or $40 is a lot of money to pay each month for a kit that you use only for a few days in a row. But when you consider the cost that the average fertility doctor charges for a short consultation, the cost of the kit will actually seem quite low. Once you become a patient, you are undoubtedly going to be instructed to start testing yourself, so you might as well get a head start on the process—and who knows, if you time your intercourse to coincide with your ovulation as predicted by the test, you just might get pregnant this month, and save all the money you would have spent seeing a fertility specialist!

Now suppose you have followed this advice and spent good money for a kit, and you have tested yourself according to the instructions but have found no evidence of ovulation at any time in the month. What should you do? Your two best choices are (1) test yourself for another month or two months, or (2) make an appointment to see a fertility specialist right away. I would advise you to take the first course if you are aware of some event in your life (such as multi-time-zone travel or a bad case of the flu) that could have thrown off your ovulation as a one-time occurrence; but if you are anxious to start working on your fertility problem as soon as possible, then by all means call for an appointment with a specialist now. And don't forget to bring all your ovulation test kit data with you when you go!

FORTY SIMPLE THINGS
YOU CAN DO *RIGHT NOW*

Below is a list of forty simple things that you can do right now, with little or no expense, to boost your chances of conception.

FOR WOMEN

1. *If you smoke, quit!* Studies have consistently shown that smokers have lower fertility and higher miscarriage rates than nonsmokers.
2. *Cut out caffeine.* A 1989 study by the National Institutes of Health showed that women who drank more than a cup of coffee a day (or consumed a comparable amount of caffeine from other sources) were "consistently less likely" to conceive than women who refrained from caffeine consumption.
3. *If you are too thin, gain weight.* Women who are more than 10 percent underweight are far more likely to experience irregular ovulation and menstruation patterns than women who are of average weight or are slightly overweight for their height (according to an article by Rose E. Frisch in the March 1988 issue of *Scientific American*).
4. *If you engage in strenuous exercise more than twice a week, cut back.* A Harvard study published in February 1988 followed 2,622 women athletes and showed that those who trained more than twice a week at sports such as hockey, tennis, swimming, gymnastics, and running had reduced levels of the estrogen needed to maintain normal ovulation. Light exercise had no harmful impact on fertility, but the researchers concluded, "If you are a marathoner or an Olympian and you want a baby, you are going to have to stop."
5. *Keep regular hours and get adequate sleep.* When trying to conceive, you want your body's internal clock to work as smoothly as possible, so that you will more easily be able to predict the time of your ovulation. Maintaining a regular schedule, including at least seven hours of sleep each night, has been shown to help bring about hormonal regularity.
6. *Avoid plane trips to far-flung places.* Traveling across many time zones can disrupt the monthly cycle of even the most regular of

OVULATION TEST KITS—
A COMPARISON

Brand Name	Number of Steps	Total Test Time	How Performed	Positive Indicator	Remarks
Ovu-quick*	7	6 min.	Use dropper to draw urine from collection cup. Dispense 6 drops on test pad. Add 3 drops of Liquid A to pad. Add 6 drops of Liquid B to pad. Wait 1 min. Add 6 drops of Liquid C to pad. Wait 3 min. Add 6 drops of Liquid D to pad. Read result.	Bottom dot will appear as dark or darker blue than top dot.	This is the only brand that does not use first A.M. urine. Very convenient to do in P.M., instead of in rush before getting to work. One of the liquids used during the testing week must be prepared in advance and kept refrigerated between cycles. Claims to be the #1 recommended brand by fertility specialists. Was most expensive of brands I purchased for testing: $70 for 9-day kit.
Clearplan Easy	1	5 min.	Urinate on end of test stick. Wait 5 min. Read result.	Blue line in lower test window will be darker than line in upper test window.	Easiest to use, very easy to read results. Biggest drawback: if you accidentally

(continued)

Brand Name	Number of Steps	Total Test Time	How Performed	Positive Indicator	Remarks
					splash some urine on the test window, you have ruined that day's test stick.
First Response**	5	5 min.	Use dropper to draw urine from collection cup, add to vial. Wait 3 min. Pour in test well. Add chemical from tube. Read result.	Pink dot in test well is positive. If dot is white or faint pink, result is negative.	Most difficult results to interpret. No "control" spot for color comparison, so how can you be sure if a light pink result on your first day of testing is positive or negative?
QTest	6	35 min.	Use dropper to draw urine from collection cup, add to vial #1. Wait 5 min. Put test stick in vial #1, wait 20 min. Rinse stick in cold water. Put in other vial, let stand 10 min. Remove, blot, read results.	Bottom pad on end of stick will be darker blue than top pad.	Complicated to perform, easy to miss a step. Requires longest wait of all the brands I tested.

*Similar version by same manufacturer is marketed under the brand name Ovugen.
**Identical version by same manufacturer is marketed under the brand name Answer.

women. If you'd love to fly away to some exotic spot for your next vacation, try flying north or south rather than east or west.

7. *Use an ovulation test kit every month.* The preceding section describes why and how the results of your ovulation testing can help you to maximize your chances of conceiving.

8. *Keep a basal body temperature (BBT) chart to keep track of your ovulation.* How to do this and why it's important are explained in the section beginning on page 48.

9. *Check your cervical mucus daily as your fertile time of the month is approaching.* The section beginning on page 45 explains how recognition of the different types of cervical mucus in your vagina can help you to identify the best time of the month to try to conceive.

10. *After making love, lie on your back with your hips slightly elevated for about a half hour.* This will tilt your vaginal canal so that the ejaculate will be forced by gravity to flow toward your cervix, giving your partner's sperm a better chance of getting into your uterus (and from there, into your fallopian tubes). Putting a pillow or two under your hips is a comfortable way to achieve the right degree of tilt.

11. *Have any vaginal infection, such as yeast* (Candida albicans) *or trichomoniasis, treated promptly.* The discharge that accompanies most forms of vaginitis will interfere with the ability of sperm to reach your uterus—besides which the itching and burning of the infection will probably make you feel like refraining from sex!

12. *Don't douche!* Not even during the nonfertile part of your cycle. Douching can change the normal pH balance of the vagina (pH is the way acidity is measured), and even a slight change in this balance can create a hostile environment for sperm (they really are pretty delicate creatures). You don't know how long it could take for the pH to return to normal, so why do anything to change it in the first place?

13. *Drink lots of fluids.* Drinking six to eight glasses of water a day is helpful to your reproductive system in a variety of ways. It increases your ability to become naturally lubricated during sex, without the use of artificial jellies; it helps your vagina to maintain the proper pH; and it may aid the buildup of nutrients in the lining of your uterus that nourishes the fertilized egg after it implants.

14. *Take vitamins.* The evidence is far from conclusive on the efficacy of vitamins, but if we're not sure they help, we *are* sure that they

don't hurt. Vitamin E, the B complex vitamins, and vitamin C have all been touted at one time or another as beneficial to the functioning of the woman's reproductive system. However, fat-soluble vitamins—such as vitamin E—should not be taken in megadoses.

15. *Distract yourself during the last two weeks of your cycle.* During the time between your ovulation and the start of your next period it's easy to become overanxious about whether "it worked" this month or not. But this type of stress is just what you don't need. Now's the time to put away the calendar and try to take your mind off your monthly cycle. If you can keep yourself busy or focused on some other date (a planned celebration or some other positive expectation), you'll be less likely to feel pressure as the anticipated date of your period approaches—and that can only be good for your reproductive system as well as for your peace of mind.

FOR MEN

16. *Stay out of Jacuzzis, hot tubs, and saunas, and don't take prolonged hot showers.* Even if you've been told that you have a good sperm count, you'll want to avoid heating up your genitals. The testicles are extremely sensitive to heat, and any single prolonged exposure could severely reduce their ability to produce healthy sperm for an unknown length of time.

17. *Don't wear tight jeans.* This is for the same reason you want to stay out of the hot tub: tight jeans let heat build up in your testicles, killing sperm.

18. *Wear loose, clean underwear made only of natural fibers.* Nylon or polyester-blend fabrics hold in more heat than does cotton, which "breathes" and allows air circulation and absorption of sweat. In other words, cotton helps keep your genitals cool (which you need to do for the reason stated above) and free from microorganisms that breed in hot, moist places and can cause infection (which you need to prevent for the reasons stated below).

19. *Have "jock itch" and urinary-tract infections treated promptly.* Even if these microorganisms don't interfere with your sperm production, they can be transmitted to your partner, causing her to develop a discharge that can block the transit of sperm to her uterus. Besides, you probably won't feel like making love if you have the itching and burning of an infection in your crotch.

20. *Don't use cocaine or marijuana, even in small amounts.* Cocaine has been shown to reduce sperm production; marijuana has been linked to increased levels of female hormones in men.

21. *Avoid strenuous exercise before lovemaking.* Bicycling, jogging long distances, rowing, and other forms of strenuous exercise have been shown to decrease sperm production if undertaken a few hours before intercourse. Again, the buildup of excessive heat is the suspected cause. Swimming, however, does not allow heat to build up and so has no negative impact on sperm.

22. *If you are too thin, gain weight.* Men who are more than 25 percent underweight have been found to have reduced levels of prostate fluids and shorter-lived, less-motile sperm.

23. *Avoid exposure to lead.* Lead is in car batteries, paints, and other building materials. While lead exposure is a well-known hazard to women who are already pregnant, male workers exposed to lead, according to the federal Occupational Safety and Health Administration, may also suffer a variety of ills, including decreased sex drive, impotence, and decreased ability to produce healthy sperm.

24. *If you work at a job that requires you to spend most of your time in one position, try to switch jobs or try to get more exercise during your day.* Whether you spend most of the day sitting down or standing, staying in the same position for hours at a time is harmful, and not just to your circulatory system: apparently it can also decrease the efficiency of your reproductive system (reported in an article, "Causes of Infertility," by Jerry Carroll in the *San Francisco Chronicle,* March 5, 1990).

25. *Take the Recommended Daily Allowance (RDA) of vitamin E.* Some nutritionists have suggested that vitamin E aids in the production of healthy sperm, though there is no scientific study to confirm this. But it certainly would not hurt you to try it, as long as you do not take megadoses of the vitamin.

FOR THE COUPLE

26. *Pay attention to your business travel schedule.* If either one of you works at a job that requires you to travel frequently without your spouse/partner, check the schedule against the woman's approximate date of ovulation, so that you won't be apart during the fertile time of the month. If you think you might be, try to reschedule the trip or find a substitute to go for you.

27. *Plan your next vacation to include the fertile time of the month.* Stress doesn't *cause* infertility, but there's no doubt that added stress will contribute to the problem. A vacation is a great way to cut down on stress, and you're also more likely to make love more frequently when you both are away from the pressures of everyday life. The ideal time for frequent lovemaking is around the time that the woman's ovulation is expected to occur.

28. *Make love* every day *during your fertile period.* You may have heard somewhere that you should make love only every other day during the fertile time of the month, to allow for the man's body to "recharge" and produce sufficient new sperm. New evidence suggests that this notion is just a myth. The most active, potent sperm are contained in the first few drops of semen, and these sperm are just as likely to be present in a man who has recently had intercourse as in one who has abstained for the last forty-eight hours. In addition, when a woman is not especially fertile, it may be because her egg does not live very long after ovulation (it may have only six hours of life, instead of twelve or more). So her best chance to conceive may be to have sperm in her reproductive tract *before, during, and after* the day she is most likely to ovulate. Of course, anything she does to pin down the time of ovulation (by keeping an accurate BBT chart or using an ovulation test kit) will be helpful.

29. *Just prior to and during ejaculation, the man should try to penetrate deeply.* According to Dr. Joseph Bellina, coauthor (with Josleen Wilson) of *You Can Have a Baby* (Bantam Books, 1985), "The very first drop of fluid [semen] may contain 80 percent of the sperm in the total ejaculate" (p. 66). If the penis is deep in the vagina, right near the cervix at the moment of ejaculation when that first sperm-laden drop emerges, the sperm will have less distance to travel to reach the uterus and will be more likely to retain their vigor until they reach their destination, the fallopian tube through which the egg is traveling.

30. *Don't use a thick lubricant like K-Y jelly before lovemaking.* Sperm can't swim through it easily. If you feel you need extra lubrication, use saliva or a small amount of vegetable oil.

31. *Keep your lovemaking special.* After months of keeping track of the woman's fertility cycles, some couples find themselves suffering from "calendaritis"—a loss of interest in sex just at the time when they know they "have to do it." If you think you've been affected by this bug, or you want to prevent it from entering your love life, then do something different this time. Come home from work

in the middle of the day, or meet at a romantic little inn somewhere, or deck yourselves out in sexy, fantasy clothing, or watch an erotic movie together. Use your imagination and have fun!

32. *Avoid all toxins.* Both male and female reproductive organs can be adversely affected by a wide variety of toxins, including nearly all pesticides, many solvents, cleaning chemicals, and paints. Read all labels carefully before use. If warned about breathing the substance or letting it come into contact with your skin, you can automatically assume that getting it into your system won't do your reproductive tract any good either, and it may well do some harm.

33. *Avoid people with colds, flu, and other contagious illnesses.* If one of you catches something during the fertile time of the month, there goes your lovemaking for that month, most likely. Also, the elevated heat of a fever can destroy male sperm and reduce a woman's chances of producing a healthy egg.

34. *Avoid certain over-the-counter drugs.* Decongestants and allergy relief medications are especially suspect because they work to reduce the production of a variety of bodily fluids in addition to those in your chest and nose. In women the production of vital cervical mucus may be affected; in men the volume of seminal fluid could be decreased. So if you can do without the drug, by all means avoid it during the fertile time of the month.

35. *Check with your doctor before taking any prescription drugs.* Tagamet, an ulcer medication, and digitalis, for heart disease, and certain antibiotics have been shown to affect either male or female fertility. Before you leave your doctor's office with that prescription, make sure he knows that you are trying to have a baby. If the drug does have any known negative impact on the reproductive system—or just as importantly, if it could interfere with the early development of a fetus—the doctor will perhaps be able to substitute a drug that doesn't have the harmful side effects, or he can at least warn you not to "try" that month.

36. *Be more safety-conscious than ever.* Accidents can not only bruise you or break your bones, but they can sure wreck your love life, too! So be extra careful when you drive or use sharp tools or engage in any kind of sport or activity requiring your full attention. And when you're out in the sun, use plenty of sunscreen, because making love with a painful sunburn won't be easy!

37. *Now is not the time for you to remodel your house, move, or change jobs*—unless you absolutely cannot avoid it. These activities rate

high on the list of stressful situations for couples, and there's no doubt that added stress decreases the chance of conception.

38. *Don't make any sudden, radical changes in your diet or life-style.* Even if you've been told you ought to gain or lose weight to improve your fertility, don't do anything extreme, like going on a fast or signing up for one of those liquid protein plans. Introduce any needed changes in a slow, sensible manner, and if you have any doubts about the changes on your reproductive system, be sure to ask your doctor.

39. *Keep track of all news about fertility research.* Pay attention when there's a report on TV or an article in the newspaper or in a magazine about fertility. You might just learn something that could help you right away to increase your odds of conception. If you get the Lifetime cable channel, watch for a show called *Obstetrics and Gynecology Update:* fertility is a frequent topic of discussion of this half-hour, doctor-hosted program. You might also consider subscribing to *Fertility and Sterility,* the magazine of the American Fertility Society (see Resource Guide at the back of this book for information). Advances are being made all the time, and you never know when something will be discovered that will be just what you need to overcome your problem.

40. *Join RESOLVE, the national infertility support network.* Any couple trying to have a baby, whether currently under a doctor's care or still trying on their own, can benefit from the information provided in RESOLVE's regular newsletter, and many will find strength and comfort in attending the small group meetings sponsored by their local RESOLVE chapter, where they can share their feelings and learn from other couples who have experienced the same problems. Call (617) 623-1156 for information on membership, or write to RESOLVE, Inc., 1310 Broadway, Somerville, MA 02144-1731.

CHAPTER TWO

FINDING THE RIGHT MEDICAL CARE

(and the Insurance to Pay for It)

ABOUT INSURANCE AND INFERTILITY

You are now fairly sure that you have a fertility problem and you may also have some idea (or even a very definite idea) where your problem lies. You have furthermore come to the conclusion that your difficulty in conceiving can't be fixed simply—by rearranging your travel schedules (for example) so that you and your spouse can have intercourse more frequently at your fertile time of the month.

It's now time to see a doctor.

Now we'll be talking about *serious* money, so even before the discussion of doctor shopping begins, let's talk about how you're going to pay for the fees. Keep in mind that some couples who end up needing very high-tech treatments, such as **in vitro fertilization (IVF)**, **gamete intrafallopian transfer (GIFT)**, or **zygote intrafallopian transfer (ZIFT)**, can easily end up spending $10,000 *per month* for medical care. And even the very simplest, low-tech treatments, like taking Clomid, will cost you about $7 *per pill*.

Most health insurance policies won't cover any part of this*—but you just might be able to get a policy that will accept some or much of the expense. But you must act now, *before* you are diagnosed. One type of exclusion found in nearly all policies is that for a "pre-existing condition." In other words, if you know ahead of time that you're going to be running up big medical bills for treatment of your health problem, then that problem is automatically not covered.

*In a *New York Times* article titled "Insurance and the Cost of Infertility" (March 5, 1989) reporter Julie Johnson noted that fewer than *half* of the for-profit insurance carriers offer complete coverage for infertility services.

Why is infertility excluded so often from health insurance? Some company officials answer that the treatment for it is "experimental" and that health insurance is only for "standard care"—but that explanation makes no sense when you consider that IVF has been practiced successfully since 1977, and drugs like Clomid and Pergonal have been in use longer than two decades. You may be told that correcting faults in the reproductive system is "optional," and that your health does not depend on having a child. And yet the same health insurance carrier will offer at no extra charge full coverage for contraceptive devices or prescriptions for the woman who makes the choice *not* to have a child, and will extend full maternity benefits for the woman whose reproductive system is healthy enough to allow her to choose to have her baby at a time that suits her. It's the couple with the medical difficulty impeding free choice who are faulted for wanting benefits in exchange for their premiums.

Faced with the obvious unfairness of this situation, infertile couples from many states around the United States are in revolt. Led by RESOLVE, they have mounted lobbying campaigns in state legislatures to try to enact laws mandating that any company offering insurance to cover medical problems must include coverage for problems of the reproductive tract. As of this writing, ten states already have laws on the books requiring coverage of varying degrees for different types of treatment. These states are Maryland, Illinois, California, Connecticut, Arkansas, Hawaii, Mississippi, New York, Texas, and Rhode Island— and if you live in any of them, you are lucky! Of course, you may still have to argue with your company about what specifically is covered, and fight on a bill-by-bill basis to get it to pay, but at least you have some legal basis when you file a claim (advice on how to fight for coverage follows on page 76).

About twenty more states have legislation under consideration. Call your local RESOLVE chapter to find out if your state is one of them. If a bill is pending, the best thing you can do right now for your future financial health is to join the lobbying effort and see if you can get your state to mandate coverage to pay for your treatment before you start running up big bills.

What about the rest of us who live in states where insurance companies are free to ignore infertility as a health problem? Suppose you want to get started on treatment right now—what should you do?

That depends on whether you have a current health insurance policy or not. If you are not covered at all by a policy from your place of employment, or if you aren't employed, you will need to start looking into buying your own private health insurance policy *now*. Though the cost of an individually purchased policy will seem exorbitant, you need to keep in mind that for most patients it will still be far cheaper than the out-of-pocket costs of treatment (especially if your treatment ends up involving any surgery or high-tech procedures). Sell the car and use public transportation, or move to a smaller, cheaper place, if that's what it takes for you to find the money to be covered. Your sacrifices to pay for premiums today may make it possible for you to afford the kind of treatment that will help you tomorrow. But without any kind of health insurance, only the very richest Americans will be able to consider the full range of treatment options. Besides, if you *do* get pregnant, you will need the maternity benefits of health insurance, and it will be too late to buy a policy that will cover you (see "pre-existing condition," above, for the reason for exclusion).

Finding Out What Your Current Policy Will Pay For

Let's say you already have health insurance through your job. You need to find out just what your policy will pay for and what it won't. You need to get accurate answers to all the questions about infertility coverage that you come up with. Unfortunately, finding someone who knows what he's talking about may not be so easy. Infertile couples have told me that when they start calling company officials with questions, more often than not they hear different things depending on who happens to pick up the phone. Lynn's experience with her insurance company in Virginia was typical: "I spoke to one person who told me that most procedures for infertility would be covered. A couple days later I called back and asked someone else the same question. This time I was told that only diagnostic procedures would be covered—you know, just tests. The third time I called, someone else said that *nothing* was covered. It was so frustrating."

The lesson for Lynn and others is this: regardless of what you hear over the telephone, *get it in writing*. The company undoubtedly has a pamphlet or brochure spelling out what items are covered and what items are excluded. Get hold of that and read through the whole thing carefully. Find out exactly what it says about

- reimbursement for office visits for infertility
- reimbursement for all tests (see Chapter Three for names of tests to ask about)
- reimbursement for fertility drugs, including injectable drugs and

suppositories (see Chapter Six for names of drugs to ask about)
- coverage for surgery (ask: "Are only those procedures requiring overnight hospital stays included, or are in-doctor's-office procedures and one-day surgeries covered, too?")
- reimbursement for multiple ovarian sonograms and blood tests (required when a patient takes certain powerful fertility drugs)
- coverage for the **assisted reproductive technologies** (**ARTs**), such as IVF, GIFT, and ZIFT (and if covered, ask: "Is there a limit on how many 'tries' the insurance company will support?")
- any minimum waiting period before coverage takes effect (for example, a policy might require a couple to try to have a child naturally for five years before treatment would be covered)

If some or all of the major infertility services are covered, does the coverage only begin after a deductible is met (and if so, what is it)? Will the insurance company pay in full, or must the patient make copayments (and if so, what percentage of the total bill must be paid)?

The brochure may not have specific answers to all these questions (it probably won't), so your next step should be to write a letter to the insurance company asking for an answer in writing to all those things you still need to know. Don't worry too much about whether the letter from the insurance company is accurate in its answers. Even if the insurance company's reply letter to you contains false information, the company is responsible for making good on any promises made to you in writing. Of course you must save the letter to use in case of a dispute.

Another approach to the problem of what your current policy provides is to assume, unless a medical procedure is excluded by a specific reference in the insurance company's informational literature, that it is in fact covered. Be warned, however, that taking this attitude could lead you into conflict over bills, and you must be prepared to fight. You do have the law on your side: courts have consistently found that companies must cover you for all health claims except those they have explicitly written out of their policies, and that the exclusion must be found not in the fine print of the contract that you sign, but in the more readable layman's language of the company's pamphlets or brochures. Conflicts crop up because your interpretation of the policy's language and the insurance company's interpretation are two different things. (For more about how to handle conflicts, see page 76.) Those with a cautious nature are better advised to hunt for a policy that affirmatively says it provides coverage for most or all infertility tests and treatments.

INFERTILITY COVERAGE AND THE COURTS
Three Important Cases

*D*oes the name Christine Craft ring a bell? She's the woman who lost her job as a newscaster at a Kansas City TV station for "not being deferential to men." She filed an employment discrimination case against her ex-employer and in 1981 won a whopping judgment from the jury. Clearly, she's not a woman to mess around with. A few years later, when her health insurance company refused to pay for her IVF treatment on the grounds that IVF is not a "cure" for infertility, she was back in the courts, making legal history again, this time on behalf of insurance consumers. She lost in the lower-court round of her case but did not give up. Her lawyer took the case to the Connecticut Court of Appeals, arguing that IVF is now widely accepted as a standard treatment and is therefore covered by her policy, which had no specific exclusion for infertility care. When the Court of Appeals ruled in her favor, Ms. Craft—and thousands of others like her who then could cite *Craft* v. *Connecticut General*—recouped the money spent for the expensive procedure.

A similar case in the California court system was filed as a class action suit by five thousand women members of the Kaiser Foundation Health Plan, which had refused to pay for IVF, although there was no specific exclusion of the treatment in their health insurance contracts. The judge in the case not only ordered reimbursement for the patients but also ordered the defendant to pay plaintiffs' attorneys' fees to the tune of $770,000. (When seeking a lawyer to take your own insurance case to court, you might mention this California judgment as reason for your case to be handled on a contingency basis.)

A case in Iowa brought forth a ruling on the validity of artificial insemination as a medical treatment of infertility. The employer-operated health insurance plan had turned down the members' claims, saying that artificial insemination is not performed "because of an illness or injury of the patient"—but the Iowa Supreme Court disagreed, 5–0. Infertility is an illness, at least in Iowa.

Shopping for Better Insurance Coverage

Okay, now you've found out that your current health insurance policy is not so good. You're ready to start shopping around for something better. Basically, there are five possibilities to look into: (1) upgrading your present coverage at your or your spouse's job; (2) you or your spouse switching jobs and going to work for a company whose health insurance plan includes coverage for treatment of infertility; (3) moving to a state that mandates infertility-treatment coverage; (4) buying insurance on your own; and (5) joining a health maintenance organization (HMO).

UPGRADING YOUR PRESENT COVERAGE

Many employers offer several plans or levels of coverage for their employees. It is mainly a matter of contacting the person or department in your company that handles benefits and finding out what other possibilities there are.

You might also want to look into buying a special rider to cover your infertility expenses. If the health package offered through your place of employment does not include infertility, contact your company benefits officer to find out whether it is possible for you to pay extra out of your own pocket to get coverage for the full range of infertility tests and treatments. A rider, if available, will usually seem very expensive, and it may still contain a good many limitations (waiting times until coverage begins, restrictions on the number of cycles that will be covered, and so forth), but for most couples it will still be a worthwhile choice.

It should be noted that many employers allow you to change your health benefits only at certain set times of the year, called "open seasons." Sometimes it is the health insurance carrier, not the employer, that imposes this limitation on when a new policy may be issued. Policies bought outside the open season may include restrictions about payment for some medical problems, including infertility, that are waived for policies bought within the open season. Since few insurance companies advertise when these consumer-friendly open seasons occur, you will have to ask the agent about them before you sign up.

When an employer doesn't offer any insurance benefit package covering infertility, there may yet be another approach. If you work for a firm that insures its own employees out of an internally raised fund, or if it only offers one health insurance policy that completely excludes infertility, you may be able to negotiate your way around your employer's benefit limitations. This strategy works best for those who are sure of their own value to their employer. If you know that you are irreplaceable, or at least very difficult to replace, then go to your employer and ask for a better insurance deal—or you will leave. The employer could permit you to join a different health insurance plan than the other employees, or could even consider switching the entire firm over to a different health insurance company that offers broader coverage. I attended one RESOLVE meeting on insurance at which a member reported that his employer had agreed to extend him coverage for his infertility treatment, "on the condition that I keep it a secret from my coworkers. My boss was afraid if everyone found that the company was paying my bills, they'd all come asking for special deals."

SWITCH JOBS

If it comes down to a choice between your stable current job that does not give you the needed coverage and an uncertain new job that *will* cover you adequately, which do you choose? If after thinking it all through carefully, you'd rather risk a period of financial uncertainty than a lifetime of childlessness, move on! When interviewing for new jobs, be sure to ask plenty of detailed questions about health insurance coverage—but don't limit yourself to questions about infertility or you might alert your potential employer to the fact that you have an expensive medical problem. Ask about the full range of coverage, including maternity care, catastrophic illness coverage, home nursing during convalescence, dental coverage and anything else you can think of. To protect your privacy you should not (and by law cannot be required to) answer questions about your marital status, your lack of children, or your plans for having any children in the future. Nor would you be comfortable working for a company that considers your personal family choices to be any of its business.

MOVE TO ANOTHER STATE

Yes, it seems extreme, but it isn't so farfetched a solution for those who live within an hour's drive of a state that has mandated coverage for infertility treatment. Change your residence, accept a longer commute to work, and become eligible for the kind of coverage you just couldn't find in your old hometown. Those who do not live close to a state with mandatory insurance could still find relocation a plausible solution, especially if one spouse or the other has a highly marketable job skill that makes it relatively easy to get job offers from employers in states with good insurance laws. And look at it this way: if you succeed in having a child, you'll probably need a bigger house—so why not make the move now and get the insurance advantage that goes along with a new house in one of the states with fair-coverage laws?

BUYING INSURANCE ON YOUR OWN

Here are two important tips on shopping for an insurance policy:

1. Get reliable answers to your questions about infertility coverage *before* you give the insurance agent your name and address.
2. Ask your questions about infertility coverage mixed in with questions about maternity benefits, psychiatric care, home convalescent care, and a range of other health coverage issues.

Following these two tips, you will not alert insurance company officials to the fact that you are a potential customer who could easily run up bigger reimbursable expenses than your premiums will bring in. You do not want to run the risk that the company will refuse to write a policy in your case. (Lest you start to feel that you are trying to hoodwink the insurance company into striking a bad deal by insuring you, keep in mind that over the long haul, a reasonably healthy person is still more likely to pay much more in premiums than the cost of that person's reimbursable medical expenses.)

What questions should you ask? Basically, the same ones you asked when checking out your current insurance policy (see the preceding section for list). If the agent you first contact can't answer your questions, ask him or her to find out the answers and call back (now you will have to give your name, but that can't be avoided).

Call as many health insurance companies as you have the time and energy to get to. Don't be surprised if you have to call more than a dozen to find one that covers, let's say, just four IVF attempts. Volunteers from the Washington, D.C., chapter of RESOLVE checked out every major health insurance company in the metropolitan Washington area and here's what they found: out of *nineteen* different insurance companies contacted, only two offered any reimbursement at all for IVF, GIFT, or ZIFT attempts. Nine companies reimbursed for artificial inseminations. Fourteen offered coverage limited to consultations and tests related to the diagnosis of infertility. Two would only partially cover the diagnostic phase, and one company totally excluded *any* medical expense related to infertility from its coverage. (These figures add up to more than nineteen because of overlapping categories.) In my interviews with couples I have also heard of a great many other rules and regulations that seem designed primarily to frustrate and confuse the couple in need of medical care (see "Rules, Rules, Rules," page 82).

As you can see, insurance for infertility is a thorny jungle full of obstacles and traps. Stumble onto the right path and you may make it out with your shirt still on your back. Take a wrong step and you could easily fall into the quicksand of debt. But here are a couple of pointers that might help you along the way:

- If you already have a fairly good idea what sort of treatment you will need, and if that treatment is likely to be a single surgical procedure (such as the correction of a man's varicocele, or the opening of a woman's blocked fallopian tubes), then don't go crazy looking for the most complete insurance package. Just look until you find one that takes care of the procedure you believe you must undergo.
- Choose "high option" over "low" or "standard option" if available. A policy that will pay for your office visits and prescription drugs will nearly always be a better deal for infertile couples, since both diagnosis and treatment will involve repeated trips to see a specialist. The higher cost of "high option" will still be lower than your specialist's bills, believe me!

And here are a couple of traps to watch out for:

- *The phrase "usual and customary."* You may encounter it in a sentence like this: "Insurance Company X will pay all physicians' *usual and customary* fees." What that means to you in practical terms is that you will wind up paying a big portion of your doctor's bills, since your doctor undoubtedly charges double what the insurance company has determined to be the "usual and customary" fee for that service. Take office visits: they will probably cost you around $100 each, while your insurance company says what is "usual and customary" is $55 per visit—and that's all of the tab the company will pick up.
- *Restrictions on where you may buy drugs; requirements to purchase generic rather than brand-name drugs.* Some fertility clinics supply the patient with expensive drugs such as Pergonal or Metrodin as part of their overall treatment package. You apply to your insurance

company for reimbursement of that part of the bill, only to find out that your policy specifically excludes all drugs purchased through the doctor's office. Then you go to your local drugstore to fill your progesterone prescription, but when you present your insurance card to have the company make its copayment, the pharmacist tells you, "This prescription is for natural progesterone, but your insurance will only pay for progestin, a synthetic substitute." You call your doctor about the switch only to hear her react with horror: "You can't take a progestin—it's not the same, and if you do get pregnant, it could cause deformities in your fetus." (This dialogue supplied from experience by former patient Margaret of Washington, D.C.) So, before you sign up for that "all prescriptions free" policy, find out if it really means what it says.

Once you have located the policy you want, you may have to do one of two things:

- *Drop out of the health plan offered through your employment and buy full coverage independently*. You should only do this if you will get some money put back into your paycheck for dropping your employer-linked coverage. If your job automatically includes health benefits, without regard to your take-home pay, then you are better off choosing the next option.
- *Carry double insurance.* Remain a member of your employer-provided health plan but also pay independently for a policy that will cover infertility. After you get pregnant, you can drop this second policy and have your maternity-care bills picked up by your regular insurance company.

THE HMO AND FERTILITY TREATMENT

For the potential fertility patient, an HMO (health maintenance organization) has both pluses and minuses. The biggest plus is not having to deal with all the paperwork, the filing of claims after every doctor's appointment or lab procedure (and when you're in treatment you may well be in your doctor's office *every day* for a week to ten days of each month!). The biggest minus is the lack of choice. The way most HMOs are set up, you must first see your regular internist or family doctor to be diagnosed. After that doctor stipulates that you have a problem with your fertility, you will be directed to a specialist—and you must see the one your regular doctor picks for you (whether you like him or not).

You do not have the option to shop around for the fertility clinic that has the best success rates. However, this limitation may work in your favor. If you find an HMO affiliated with a major hospital that has a fertility program (for example, the George Washington University Hospital HMO in Washington, D.C., or the Johns Hopkins University Hospital HMO in Baltimore), you will undoubtedly be referred for treatment to the doctors in that program, and you can feel confident that you are receiving the same high level of care as other patients who are paying top rates out of pocket to see your doctor.

HMOs also tend to be limited in the types of fertility treatments they will cover—though I have heard of a few that will pay for a set number of IVF or GIFT attempts.

Disputes over Coverage

For those of you who are tied to a company that gives you less than complete infertility coverage, there will come a time when one of the bills you have submitted that you were *sure* would be reimbursed comes back with this stamp in big, red letters: REJECTED. Is there anything you can do?

Yes. You can fight! It's an old cliché, but in the insurance world it's certainly true: nothing ventured, nothing gained. The following strategies may work, at least in part, to get you the coverage you thought your premiums would provide.

INFERTILITY AND THE HMO

A Sampling of Patient Experiences

*M*y HMO said they wouldn't cover my infertility treatment because I hadn't been trying for two years. And when I reached that point they *still* wouldn't cover me.

*P*olly from Illinois

*M*y HMO assigned me to an OB-GYN. They wouldn't let me see an infertility specialist. I had five or six doctors. Doctors would leave or move from one center to another. I battled the HMO for three

---

(continued)

years (my husband's whole office is on the HMO, so we couldn't switch insurance companies). I finally went outside the HMO to see a fertility specialist at a full-service clinic on my own (my parents helped to pay the fees). My first cycle I got pregnant with twins!

Becky from Virginia

I had to pay the fertility clinic myself because my HMO required one year's treatment with an OB-GYN before allowing me to see a specialist.

Leigh from California

In order for our HMO to cover the cost of a specialist, I had to be referred by my doctor. My husband and I went to talk to my doctor about this. He immediately became defensive, saying I did not need a specialist. We decided to go ahead and see the specialist anyway, but kept working on getting my doctor to give me a referral. After my first visit with Dr. T. [the specialist they paid for out of pocket], I went back to my first doctor again to try go get him to refer me. He was still defensive and said he could do anything a specialist could, and if I insisted, he could put me on Clomid. Never did he mention doing a single blood test to collect any information. Luckily for us, we were able to change insurance companies at this time, which allowed us to go to Dr. T. without a referral. We were finally headed somewhere!

Sarah from Louisiana
(who went on to have
two children through ZIFT)

I've switched jobs but am continuing my medical coverage from my old job and paying for it myself to protect my benefits. My new employer pays for an HMO, but anything I would do would be "pre-existing" and thus not covered. Also, the HMO would require me to go to a different clinic than the one I am currently using (and like). They would make me go to a public hospital infertility clinic that is like a mill, in my opinion. So my major costs so far have not been for treatment but for the continued private insurance, which covers me 80%/20%. It's cheap at any price!

Rose from Washington

Write letters

Phone calls generally are handled by low-level employees who are trained to give one canned response: "Sorry, not covered." Letters, on the other hand, tend to be taken more seriously, if only because they leave a "paper trail" for state insurance regulators to follow. In most states an insurance company is not allowed to ignore complaints in writing, but must give the complainer some kind of response within a set number of days.

To be most effective, letters should have your policy number right at the start, as well as the reference numbers (or invoice numbers) of all disputed bills. You should give the full name of the doctor you saw, the date(s) that you saw him, and the correct name of the medical procedure performed on the date(s) listed. Then, as clearly and concisely as possible, tell why you believe your policy should pay for the bill.

It may help matters if you can find out the "procedure codes" that your insurance company assigns to various medical treatments and tests. Using the codes and terminology that the insurance company itself has devised for the items it covers should help to convince company officials that your bills should be reimbursed. The sample letter on the next page provides a general format you can use in your disputes.

Don't expect to win your case with a single letter. You will probably receive a computer-drafted (and possibly unintelligible) letter in response. It is important to write back, refuting any incorrect statements contained in the insurance company's letter to you. You may end up carrying on a correspondence with a computer for months, but remember, *persistence often pays off*. The insurance company ultimately could decide it's too much of a nuisance to have to keep writing to you and just pick up your bills to put an end to the matter. You may not ever receive formal acknowledgment that your claim had merit—but one day the red REJECTED stamp just disappears. (That is how it went for several former patients I interviewed.)

Enlist your doctor's support

First, find out exactly what infertility services your insurance company will cover, and by what terms (or better yet, code numbers) those tests and procedures are known. Then ask your doctor to describe, using exclusively the terms your insurance company uses and accepts, any

SAMPLE LETTER TO
HEALTH INSURANCE COMPANY

Your name
Your address
Your city, state, ZIP code

Today's date

Name of insurance company president
[or name of claims supervisor]
Insurance company address
City, state, ZIP code

Re: Your policy number
      Claim number[s]

Dear ———:

On [date] I submitted a claim for [fill in name of medical treatment] performed by Dr. [fill in name] at [location] on [date]. On [date] I received your form rejecting my claim on the grounds that [restate the reason for rejection found on the form that the insurance company sent you].

I have reviewed my insurance plan and I believe my claim should have been fully covered under the plan's rules. Please cite for me the specific wording in my policy that is the basis for your denial of my claim.

I am looking forward to a speedy review and response to this matter. If I do not receive a reply in writing from your office within [date no more than two weeks away], I will contact the [name of insurance regulatory agency for your state].

Thank you for your prompt attention to this letter.

Sincerely,

Your name

cc: Employer's benefits officer
    [if your place of employment has one]

tests and procedures you undergo. All too often patients are denied coverage merely because their doctor has used a word that the insurance company associates with a noncovered item, instead of another, perfectly accurate term for the same diagnosis or treatment. For example, your doctor diagnoses your lack of ovulation as being caused by an excess production of male hormones in your ovaries. He writes "anovulation" on your bill—but that is a term your insurance company has defined as a form of infertility, a noncovered condition, and the company won't pay. However, if he had written the bill to reflect the underlying cause of the ovulatory problem, polycystic ovarian disease (PCO), then he would have been using a term that is on the insurance company's list of covered illnesses, and your bills would have been paid as a matter of course.

Doctors sometimes may need to write their own letters or submit notes to your insurance company backing up your claims. If a doctor consistently refuses to help you deal with your insurance company, you should find a doctor who *will* help. Caring doctors realize that most patients can't pursue treatment without insurance reimbursement, and that insurance companies often give patients a hard time. When choosing a doctor, be sure to discuss how his office deals with insurance problems, so you know in advance what kind of help, if any, you can expect (more on this subject in the section on choosing a doctor, which follows).

Get a hired gun

After you've spent hours on the phone driving yourself nuts in circular conversations with different insurance company employees, and after you've spent months firing off letters of complaint and receiving garbled, computer-generated replies, you may not have the strength to go on fighting anymore. But you don't have to surrender—just find someone to carry on the fight on your behalf. Someone who's a professional, who has done this hundreds of times, and who knows far better than you how to get the job done. There are two good choices for this role: a professional claims advocate, or a lawyer.

The professional claims advocate is a consultant (often an ex–insurance company employee) who takes complaint cases, usually on an hourly rate basis, and shepherds the complaint through the insurance company's internal appeals process, perhaps taking it on to the state's insurance commission or insurance appeals board. Advocates generally write better letters than you could do on your own, and they are better acquainted with the rules—and the loopholes—of your policy contract.

They also know which insurance company employees to talk to, and which to avoid. One big drawback, however, is the cost. Hiring a professional claims advocate could get expensive, and might be worth doing only if the total dollar amount to be recouped is at least twice as much as the claims advocate's estimate of her or his final bill. To go about finding a professional claims advocate, try asking for recommendations from your state insurance commission or call a consumers' rights organization, if there is one in your city or town. Your local RESOLVE chapter might also be able to give you a reference.

Some lawyers specialize in insurance claims and appeals—but lawyers are even more expensive than claims advocates. Fees can be anywhere from $150 an hour on up. When the total dollar amount of your disputed claims is up in the tens of thousands, however, the few thousand you spend to get good legal advice may be more than worth it. Sometimes a sharply worded letter from a well-known attorney can produce fast results; it proves to your insurance company that you are serious about pursuing your claim. I spoke to one patient who was offered an acceptable settlement—partial payment of her infertility expenses—after just one such letter was sent out.

APPEAL THROUGH THE STATE

Insurance is a regulated industry, and your state will have some form of insurance commission or appeals board to hear cases brought by unhappy consumers. Call your state government's general information line to find out the exact name of the board and its office telephone number. Call to find out what you need to do, step by step, to file an appeal. If you pay careful attention to all the paperwork requirements, you should be able to prepare your appeal without an attorney's help— although it may well be worth the price of an hour's consultation to have an experienced lawyer look over your appeal and advise you as to any needed improvements in language on your forms.

USE THE RESOURCES OF RESOLVE

RESOLVE's volunteers can give you valuable advice on a wide range of insurance difficulties. Contact your local chapter—you may even find that it has a committee set up specifically to work on insurance problems. If there isn't a special committee, then attend the general membership meetings, where you'll be sure to run into members who have encountered (and possibly overcome) problems like yours. If there is no local chapter near you, then write to the national office and request RESOLVE's brochure called *Understanding Health Insurance Coverage.* Or call the national helpline—(617) 623-0744—with your questions.

TAKE IT TO SMALL CLAIMS COURT

If the amount in dispute is less than the maximum for claims under your state's rules for small claims court, then this could be the best route for you to take. You don't need a lawyer to file or argue in small claims court—indeed, in some states, lawyers are prohibited from representing small claims court plaintiffs—but you do need to understand your policy contract and have all your facts in order. You will be at an advantage if you are also a strong, confident, and *brief* public speaker. Sometimes insurance companies will not even bother to send a representative to court, and so plaintiffs win by default. If you are not all that confident about your ability to prepare and present a good case, then consider spending a couple hundred dollars to have a lawyer give you an hour or so of advice about your courtroom appearance. And remember, too, that filing in small claims court just could be all you need to do to push your insurance company into offering you an acceptable out-of-court settlement.

RULES, RULES, RULES

Patients Talk About the Frustrations of Dealing with Health Insurance Companies

Prior to Massachusetts' mandatory coverage bill in July 1988, we had constant hassles over insurance payments. If my doctor had only written "ovarian cysts" instead of "infertility" on the bills, I would have had coverage.

Joan from Massachusetts

I had to appeal my insurance company's decision on several occasions. I had my doctor write a letter . . . and I won!

Laura from Maryland

(continued)

When our insurance company refused to pay for inseminations, we questioned them and were told they do not pay for "out of body experiences"! We ended up spending over $10,000 in infertility bills out of our own pocket.

Diane from Indiana

My insurance company stated that IVF, GIFT, and ZIFT are considered "experimental" and thus exempt from coverage. They did not seem to understand that paying for one or two GIFT cycles could eliminate the need for endless subsequent blood tests and ultrasounds that produced no result.

Marcia from New Jersey

My doctor has disguised procedures so I have not had any problems with insurance.

Rhonda from Connecticut

We got full coverage for the diagnostic workup and partial coverage for treatment for a while, but the insurance refused to pay for the treatment once they realized what was happening.

Sally from Virginia

My insurance company will cover drugs such as Pergonal, but *not* if they are connected with an IVF or artificial insemination attempt.

Kathleen from Delaware

(Author's note: This is the most nonsensical rule I have ever heard of! The insurance company agrees to pay for an ultraexpensive drug—but only if it's not used as part of a treatment designed to maximize its effectiveness!)

My insurance company has been slow to pay . . . but they *do* pay. Since my clinic participates in their program, I've had to pay relatively small amounts out of pocket. Record-keeping, however, has been a *nightmare*.

Allison from Maryland

(continued)

Our PPO (Preferred Provider Organization) covers 80 percent of the bills after copayments and 100 percent after a $1,200 coinsurance level has been met. It doesn't cover artificial insemination or IVF at all.

Jeanette from Texas

I had four sonograms done at $330 apiece. The insurance company dubbed them "unnecessary testing." They've hired "price-choppers" solely to find areas to cut payments on bills. . . . I've found the best policy with insurance companies is to tell them as little as possible. Don't make objections over small amounts they don't pay when they should. Only rock the boat over the big stuff—$75 or more.

Joan from Massachusetts

Our insurance will not cover IVF, even though Hawaii has mandated coverage. I [Alex] am in the military and the military is exempt from mandated coverage. There is a new military facility in Texas that provides IVF, but we do not meet the criteria for it.

Alex and Vera from Hawaii

Our insurance covered the blood tests but didn't pay for anything else involved in our two IVF attempts. We pay these expensive premiums and they don't do *anything* for it!

Tina from California

The insurance company does not cover "injectable medications"—so nothing for Pergonal, Lupron, hCG.

Many patients

I had IVF during a diagnostic laparoscopy. The doctor wrote it up as two separate bills, one for the laparoscopy, which was a covered surgery, and one for the lab procedures for IVF (not covered). I simply did not submit the noncovered bills to the insurance company and so most of that IVF cycle was reimbursed.

Polly from Illinois

(continued)

*M*y insurance company has paid as a matter of course because the doctors have always put the diagnosis as "endometriosis" rather than "infertility." The insurance will not pay anything for infertility charges.

*C*arla from Texas

*T*o get compensated we had to term the aspiration of eggs "aspiration of ovarian cysts."

*L*orraine from Louisiana

I was one of the fortunate few—my husband's insurance company covered everything. Of course, they often knocked off part of the amount because the doctor's bill was "above the customary charge" for such treatment.

*B*etsy from New Jersey

*O*nce I had an insurance man ask me what these drugs were used for, and I informed him "pelvic pain due to cysts" . . . which is true, to a degree. . . . My advice to patients: never use the word "infertility" and never send in anything that you know they won't cover.

*J*ulie from California

*O*ur insurance paid 100 percent of the hospital's charges for GIFT, but the doctor's fee was not covered.

*G*wen from South Carolina

*O*ur insurance covers only blood tests, ultrasounds, and surgery.

*A*lice from Arizona

*T*he cruel irony: My choice to be a stay-at-home mother [of her first child conceived without any medical intervention] has resulted in my unemployment—thus no employer's group health plan under which I would have coverage for our state's mandatory coverage of one IVF attempt. Only if I leave my child to go back to work will I get the health care I need to have another one.

*V*era from Hawaii

(continued)

I bought an individual policy with a two-year "pre-existing" clause. Then I heard of a competing company with only a one-year waiting period. We're now one year into payments, waiting to begin an IVF cycle that will be $12,000, with 80 percent covered. But now we've learned the policy does not cover medications!

*R*uth from California

When Coverage Cannot Be Obtained

Now you've looked into all the ways to try to get insurance coverage, but for one reason or another, none of them will work for you. So it looks like you are stuck paying for all or most of your treatment costs out of pocket. Now you could use a few ideas to help you handle the financial burden.

1. *Order your fertility drugs directly from a discount pharmacy.* Here are three that advertise low prices for two ultraexpensive but commonly prescribed drugs, Pergonal and Metrodin. All three pharmacies will ship by next-day air.

    Park Avenue Chemists (New York), (800) 842-6600. Have doctor fax prescription in to (800) 637-8153. Pay by credit card.

    Eveready Drugs (New York), (800) 424-3378. Have doctor call with prescription. Must pay UPS/COD.

    The Medicine Shop (New York), (800) 578-7294. Have doctor call with prescription. Pay by check or credit card.

2. *Offer the doctor a deal.* Try talking to your doctor about your payment problems to see what you can work out. Some clinics are prepared to help patients by allowing a long-term schedule of payments (of course, you *could* end up paying for your child's conception till he or she is in the third grade). Even if your doctor does not offer you this option, nothing is lost by asking if he'd be willing to consider it. If that doesn't work, perhaps you could sug-

gest an equitable barter arrangement: Let's say you're in the plumbing business and you agree to do over the doctor's bathroom in exchange for four IVF cycles. (When working such arrangements out, be careful to stay on the right side of the IRS!) Most doctors who view their practices as something more than a money-making enterprise will go to some lengths to ensure that their patients are able to get the treatment they need, especially if they appear to be the sort of people who believe in making good on their debts.

3. *Borrow money.* Naturally you will feel somewhat hesitant to go into debt over something so open-ended and uncertain of outcome as fertility treatment. It will seem a bit like mortgaging your house to buy lottery tickets. But if you and your doctor both conclude that you have a very good shot at having a child through a certain expensive procedure, and you don't mind taking a risk, then ask yourself these questions: Is my salary likely to increase enough to cover the repayment of the debt over time, as well as the added expense of raising a child? If medical intervention should fail, would I at least take comfort in the idea that the money went to give me the best possible chance to have a baby? Will I be able to qualify for a loan from a lender with reasonable rates of interest? If you answered yes to all these questions, then perhaps a loan is for you. Those who have a warm and intimate relationship with parents or grandparents of some means might also wish to consider asking within the family for the loan. Occasionally, parents desiring intensely to become grandparents will pay for treatment outright as a gift. Of course there is a trade-off, as the couple loses the option of keeping their infertility a private affair. On the other hand, the bond between grandparents and grandchild may become stronger when the grandparents look upon the child their generosity helped to bring into the world.

4. *Pinch pennies.* Sometimes couples are too quick to conclude that they can't afford infertility treatment. I've talked to more than a few couples who thought long and hard about where the money would come from, and then decided, no matter what they had to do to get it, that they would come up with the money to pay for the treatment that would bring a child into their lives (see box, page 89, for examples). Here are some things you might consider scrimping on to help save money for treatment: (1) vacations (well, you'll need to get away, so you should still go somewhere, but just don't make it to Venice *this* year; go camping in a nearby national park instead); (2) trans-

portation (do you really need that late-model car when you could just as well commute by bus or by bicycle?); (3) gifts (this is the year to make your own Christmas and birthday presents for the gang—and they'll appreciate the effort so much more than if you bought them the usual, overpriced stuff from a store); (4) clothing (most couples will look just fine wearing last year's styles—but if you really need to replace your old coat, try shopping at used-clothing and consignment stores).

5. *Talk to RESOLVE members to get some good money ideas.* There really is no end to the number of tips you can pick up from others who have been there before you. Be willing to bring up the subject of money at meetings and you will be surprised at how open everyone is about the subject, and how much useful advice you will get. RESOLVE fund-raising functions can also be a source of bargains for couples seeking treatment. My local chapter once put on an auction and sold doctor-donated IVF and GIFT treatment cycles to the highest bidders—couples who paid between $2,000 and $3,600 for medical services that would otherwise have cost them $8,000. If your local RESOLVE chapter has not considered this method of raising money, you might want to suggest it.

Nearly all the couples I interviewed found their infertility financially draining, and were strapped for money nearly the whole time they were in treatment. But with a little creative budgetry (and a few good yard sales, too), just about everyone managed to end up with their credit ratings intact.

One final thought about the sacrifices you must make to afford infertility treatment: If you do get pregnant and have a baby, you're going to be strapped for money for the next twenty-some years as bills come in for diapers, toys, food, clothing, and ultimately, that (projected) $300,000 bill for college tuition. So you might as well get used to being broke now!

FINDING THE RIGHT MEDICAL CARE

Infertility is getting to be a crowded field. The number of medical specialities laying claim to expertise keeps growing—as does the confusion for the prospective patient. There are OB-GYNs, reproductive endocrinologists (REs), urologists, and even some internists and general prac-

WHAT I DID FOR LOVE

Or, How I Got the Money to Pay for Treatment Despite Lack of Insurance Coverage

*W*e lived at my brother's house to be near the clinic. One year in an eight-by-ten room, all our stuff in boxes. We were *broke*! No vacations, nothing.

*J*oan from Massachusetts

*W*e got a bank loan to pay for the IVF, and we've put off buying a new car.

*C*arla from Texas

I'm staying in a job I hate because it pays well and offers good insurance coverage.

*B*renda from New Jersey

Interview question: Have you had to forgo any optional expenditures, such as a vacation or a new car, to pay for treatment?
Answer: What's a vacation? What's a new car?

*N*ina from Ohio

I received a discount for being one of the first to try the new GIFT program set up at a hospital near my home (I had been going to a clinic about 100 miles away).

*D*iane from Indiana

*W*hen we were at ———— Clinic, they had a patient bulletin board for the exchange of information, etc. Someone from Syracuse had posted a note that they were coming in for IVF treatment and needed a place to stay for two weeks. Finances were a significant issue for them, and they were looking for a situation with modest rental—a house swap, house-sitting, etc. We called them and they stayed at our house. We had a wonderful bonding and they were lucky to become pregnant on the first cycle. They continue to tell us they

(continued)

really believe it was so much a factor that we took them into our home and helped them; otherwise, they might not have been able to come for treatment.

Buffy from New York

We put off buying any furniture or doing any landscaping. My in-laws gave us $1,000 toward IVF, and my parents gave us $4,000, which we're going to use toward a GIFT procedure.

Marcia from New Jersey

We feel like we can't spend any extra money we may have because what if we need to do IVF? You see something you want—a new TV—and try to figure out how much more treatment you could buy if you didn't buy the TV.

Alice from Arizona

We've postponed trips to Asia and Australia at least three times. We share one car. No new furniture, no carpeting, no microwave. No airplane trips to visit family and see my sister's baby.

Vera from Hawaii

As a way to save money on drugs, the nurse at my clinic recommended getting Metrodin driven in from Mexico. It's $65 a shot here [in San Francisco] but $25 a shot from Mexico. We arranged it, but the person bringing the drugs in didn't come in on time and we had to delay a cycle of treatment.

Tina from California

My grandparents have given us $40,000 so far to pay for our infertility bills.

Laura from Maryland

titioners who hold themselves out as able to diagnose and treat the infertile with a wide variety of techniques. There are big treatment centers operated out of major hospitals as well as smaller, independent clinics; there are group practices in which one or some or all of the doctors will handle fertility cases; and there are solo practitioners, who tend to be more limited in the types of treatments they can provide.

No doubt about it, infertility is big business ($2 *billion* a year, according to the *Wall Street Journal*), and the competition for the patient's dollar is fierce. Just take a look at any upscale magazine these days to see the glossy ads put in by clinics to bring in new patients (for more about advertising, see page 98). When you consider how steep most doctors' fees are for the higher technology treatments (such as IVF and GIFT, which can run anywhere from $6,000 to $12,000 per cycle), it's no wonder that doctors go to such lengths to sell their services. But how do you know you are seeing someone who's worth what he charges? Or put it the reverse way: how do you know you aren't wasting your money on some quack who will string you along for months, piling up charge after charge, as your womb remains unfilled? This is no idle concern—see the section about the Cecil Jacobson case (page 306) for the most notorious example of a quack in practice.

Beyond getting someone who's competent and honest, for treatment involving the most intimate details of your lives, you will also want your doctor to be sensitive, accessible, and good at explaining what's going on—not to mention charming, brilliant, witty, and good-looking. A tall order—and one that no patient or ex-patient I interviewed would say his or her fertility specialist filled very well. All the couples I talked to (including those who said they were very satisfied with their treatment) had at least one bad thing to say about their doctor. The most commonly used adjective of criticism was "arrogant" followed closely by "insensitive," "difficult to reach," "too busy to keep track of his patients" and "unresponsive to our concerns."

Is there a reason why these terms crop up so often to describe fertility doctors? Here is what I have concluded: While still in medical school the students who are most likely to be drawn to this specialty are the ones who are attracted to the idea that they can create life in a test tube. It takes a certain amount of ego, or if you prefer, arrogance, to see yourself in that God-like role. But in order to complete the very rigorous training required to become a fertility specialist, the student or intern will need to spend months or years of his life locked up in the lab, working with rat embryos in experiment after experiment. That tends to be of interest to the more plodding, methodical personality with a deficiency of social skills. The would-be fertility doctor also has to believe he could spend much of his time telling desperate would-be parents that their treatment has once again failed, without himself becoming depressed or self-doubting. That aspect of the job tends to foster a certain air of detachment.

It is perhaps not so surprising, assuming these conjectures to be true, that fertility patients so often find their doctors to be less than ideal personalities. But when looking back on treatment from a few years' perspective, many of those who were most critical of their doctor's manner also commented that in the end that was something that really didn't matter all that much. Far more important was whether the doctor was good enough at what he did to get the diagnosis right the first time, and choose the treatment that had the best chance of success. Those who found doctors who were able to make it possible for them to have babies were willing to forgive almost any conduct, even outright boorishness, because of the outcome of their treatment.

I also discovered through my interviews (also not so surprising) that different patients have different levels of tolerance for insensitivity in their doctors. Some patients very much need a good hand-holder; others don't need or expect sympathy, but they do need clear and concise explanations of medical events in layman's terms. For still others the doctor's personal qualities are not at issue; what they're looking for is the very highest level of surgical or laboratory skill. And then there are patients whose number one priority will be to find a competent doctor whose fees they can afford (or whose charges will be covered by their insurance).

Because of these differences in what patients want and need, it's not possible to draw up a simple list of qualities to tell you to seek out when choosing your fertility doctor. Only *you* can know what priority you wish to assign to the various traits a doctor may exhibit. Before you begin seeking recommendations, you should sit down with your partner and talk about what you really want:

Is a good "bedside manner" something you can't do without?

Is cost a determining factor?

Is the doctor's success rate (for cases comparable to yours) your number one concern?

Does the doctor's sex, age, or background make a difference to you?

You will also find it easier to know what kind of doctor could help you best if you have some advance idea of the kind of help you will need:

Do you think you have a problem that could require surgical correction?

Is there a likelihood that you will need high-tech treatments such as IVF or GIFT?

Do you already know (or strongly suspect) that the infertility is a female problem, a male problem, or a combination of male and female?

Once you have identified some of the basic requirements that you have, you are ready to begin your search for candidates who fit your bill of particulars. Let's take an example:

Lisa and Joe are fairly certain that their trouble in conceiving has something to do with Lisa's irregular ovulation (she's tested her urine for a few cycles in a row and has yet to get a positive result)—but they'd prefer to go to a clinic that could check out the fertility of both sexes, rather than seek help separately (Lisa to a gynecologist, and Joe to a urologist). They are both more interested in where the doctor went to medical school than in what sort of personality he has. Cost is not important to them, as they had wisely switched insurance several months earlier to a high-option policy that covers IVF and GIFT. Lisa says she thinks she would feel more comfortable with a woman doctor, more or less her own age (late thirties), and Joe says the doctor's age and sex are not important to him.

Now Lisa and Joe have already narrowed down their search field quite a bit. They have ruled out solo practitioners and group OB-GYN practices in favor of one of the bigger, well-established (though expensive) fertility clinics. In their mid-sized city there are only two clinics that are on the approved list put out by the American Fertility Society. They check out the medical backgrounds of all the doctors at those clinics and find that one doctor is a thirty-seven-year-old graduate of the Harvard Medical School who specializes in ovulatory dysfunction. They make an appointment for a consultation for her first available date.

WHAT TYPE OF DOCTOR SHOULD YOU SEE?
A Pro/Con Table

	Pro	Con
Internist/ family doctor	Has known you for years; you know you will feel comfortable discussing intimate problems	Treatment options very limited; you will need referral to specialist for anything other than very low-tech treatments
OB-GYN	Can handle many forms of female infertility; may be less expensive than fertility specialist or clinic	Will have to share waiting room with many pregnant women; unable to diagnose and treat male problems, if any
Urologist	Can handle many forms of male infertility; may be less expensive than fertility specialist or clinic	Unable to diagnose and treat female problems, if any. May be difficult to coordinate male treatment with female's
Solo practitioner	Has smaller patient load; may develop better personal relationship with patient	Usually limited in treatment options; will need to see unknown doctor while your doctor is on vacation; emergency and off-hours contact may be a problem
Group practice	If your doctor is unavailable can see other member of group; likely to have a doctor on call for emergencies and off-hours needs	In large, busy group practice you may feel like a number, may be seen by other doctors who don't know your case history— or even your name
Fertility Clinic	Able to offer complete range of fertility services; usually coverage for weekends, holidays (good emergency access); usually offers convenient hours for	Usually more expensive than nonspecialist doctors; at large clinics you are very likely to feel like a number sometimes; will probably have much of test and treatment

(continued)

	Pro	Con
	tests; since practice is limited to fertility, you have some assurance that doctors will be current and experienced	information relayed to you through nurses; may have a waiting period for initial consultation; may have limits on who will be accepted as a patient
Hospital-affiliated fertility program	Able to offer complete range of fertility services; usually excellent emergency response, and coverage for weekends and holidays; can perform all tests and procedures, including surgeries; may be first in area to try experimental techniques	Location and parking for many big-city hospitals can be difficult; may have to go to other departments of the hospital for blood tests and sonograms; waiting period for tests may be lengthy; in big hospital program, very easy to end up feeling like a number

Getting Recommendations

Now that you have at least a general idea of the sort of doctor you'd like to see, you next need to know how to get names to check out to see if they fit the bill. The following will probably be useful sources of recommendations:

1. *Your family doctor or internist.* Call or go in to see your regular doctor and discuss your desire for medical help in conceiving. Mention all the qualities you are looking for in a fertility specialist and ask your doctor to suggest two or three doctors who might suit your needs. But what if your regular doctor should tell you that you don't need a specialist and suggest that you let him handle your infertility problem himself? That might be a good starting point for the couple with what turns out to be a very easy-to-correct hormonal imbalance. But if pregnancy does not result after the first few cycles of treatment, it's time to seek out someone who is specifically a fertility expert—and a good internist would agree.
2. *Other couples who have been in treatment.* Former patients can almost certainly give you a more complete sense of what it will be like to work with a particular doctor than another doctor can. They may not be able to tell you a lot about the doctor's medical training and

background, but they will tell you things you may find just as useful (or more), such as whether the doctor returns phone calls promptly; whether she remembers patients' names and histories; whether you have to wait an hour beyond your appointment time to be seen; and whether your questions get brushed aside or given careful, intelligible answers.

3. *RESOLVE.* If you do not already know couples who have been in treatment, join RESOLVE and meet some. Your local RESOLVE chapter may also have compiled data on the doctors its members have most often complained about and/or the doctors its members would most highly recommend. If there is no local chapter in your area, you can call the national office for advice about finding a reputable doctor who meets your criteria.

4. *Informational seminars sponsored by fertility clinics or hospital-affiliated fertility programs.* You may see ads in magazines or newspapers inviting attendance at free lectures by fertility specialists. By all means go and listen, collect the free brochures, and ask all the questions you have about infertility treatment—bearing in mind all the while that these free seminars are really just an elaborate form of advertisng. Clinics put them on specifically to attract new patients and make more money. Still, it is possible to get a general idea of how well the program is run, and what sort of doctors and staff are in it, by going to the informational seminar. Just don't sign up as a patient on the spot. Investigate the clinic's success rates and check out what former patients have had to say about the place before you decide.

5. *SART's annual survey findings.* The Society for Assisted Reproductive Technologies regularly publishes reliable data on the success rates of doctors and clinics that are members of the American Fertility Society. Information on ordering the survey is provided in the Resource Guide at the back of this book.

Your Initial Consultation; or,
Getting the Most Out of Your "Look-See" Visit

At this point you should have the names of at least two doctors or clinics that seem to fit your most important requirements. Call each office you are seriously considering and schedule an appointment. Yes, it's more expensive to check out clinics this way, but the money you spend up front meeting doctors could well keep you from wasting

What's the Number One Recommendation of Former Fertility Patients?

With every interview I conducted, and on every mail survey I sent out, I asked this question: If you had just one piece of advice to give to a person who has recently discovered a fertility problem, what would it be?

By far the number one answer was: *see a fertility specialist.*

I heard story after story from patients who said they'd wasted precious time in treatment by internists and OB-GYNs who were not experts in the fertility field. Tests that would have been routine for a reproductive endocrinologist were never performed or even mentioned, and misdiagnosis was frequent. Fortunately, most of these stories eventually had happy endings, as patients went on to find doctors able to give them the level of care they needed to conceive.

thousands on a doctor who ultimately could turn out to be all wrong for your case. If you should absolutely be won over by the staff at the first clinic you check out, then go ahead and call the other places and cancel your appointments. When you've made all the "look-see" visits you feel you need, you should have a good basis for comparison and can feel confident that you have made an informed choice, whichever clinic you pick.

Even before your appointment date comes up, you should be getting some sense of how well the practice is run. Is the person who schedules the appointments polite? Were you able to get an appointment date within a reasonable period of time? Were you told anything in advance about how you would be billed for your consultation? Were you told what medical records, personal data, or insurance information you needed to bring? If your phone call was put on hold, did someone get back to you relatively promptly? If the answer to all these questions was yes, proceed with a feeling of confidence to the doctor's office.

While you are in the waiting room, check it out (if you become a regular patient, you're going to be spending *a lot* of time in the place). Is it cramped or depressing? Are the chairs uncomfortable? Are the magazines months out of date? Is it too hot or too cold? Do the other waiting patients seem irritated, angry, or upset? If the answer to all these questions is no, that's another good sign.

ABOUT ADVERTISING
The Lure of the Adorable

*O*pen any upscale magazine these days and you may see something like this:

EVERY BABY IS A MIRACLE.

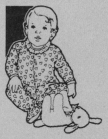

At the Center for Advanced Reproductive Technologies Miracles Are Happening Every Day.

For the infertile couple the miracle of life doesn't just happen on its own. It often needs help from medical science to come about. We at the Center for Advanced Reproductive Technologies are dedicated to providing couples with state-of-the-art techniques for the diagnosis and treatment of all forms of infertility. Our highly skilled physicians and embryologists have a success rate that is unsurpassed in the metropolitan area. Call today (800-555-4IVF) to arrange a tour of our modern, conveniently located facilities.

FIND OUT WHAT WE CAN DO TO HELP MAKE A MIRACLE FOR YOU!

Ads have quotes from happy couples; ads feature babies who are heartbreakingly cute; ads show doctors who are compassionate and

(continued)

wise; ads tell of success at the cutting edge of technology; ads make the whole prospect of fertility treatment sound like a fascinating and always rewarding adventure. If you haven't yet been through the real thing, you might not suspect that *it just ain't gonna be the way the ads show it.*

Of course, when we see ads for shampoos and deodorants full of rosy pictures of happy families at play, we know we are not being told anything of consequence about the product. Just as the non-brand-name shampoo can be as good as or better than a heavily advertised brand, so can unadvertised fertility clinics be as good as or better than those that do advertise.

Does this mean that you should just ignore the ads you see? Not necessarily. If you are just beginning to search, and you haven't yet heard any names in the field, ads may give you a place to start. But you need to check out the clinic that runs attractive ads with the same caution and thoroughness you would apply to a clinic you heard about from any other source. You'll ask your regular doctor for her opinion of the place; you'll find out what RESOLVE members who have been there have to say; you'll call or visit and see how the place stacks up against your list of requirements; then you'll decide.

While you're checking and looking, you might want to keep these two facts always in your mind: (1) that the attractiveness of the ad tells you far more about the doctor's ability to pick a good ad agency than about his skill at making babies; and (2) that part of what you pay him will go to pay for his advertising.

One more thing: If you decide after reading this that you would only go to a clinic that does *not* advertise, remember that doctors who don't advertise are not necessarily more skillful or less profit-driven than those who do. There is no substitute for the investigation that patients must do to assure themselves that they will be receiving high-quality care.

Now you have been led back to the doctor's private office. Take a close look at the certificates and diplomas on the wall to see where the doctor has been at all the different stages of his professional life. Look for any awards or commendations. Look especially for an indication that the doctor is either *board certified* or *board eligible* in one of the fertility subspecialties—meaning that the doctor has passed (or will soon take) a very difficult examination on medical treatment of infertility, graded by other top experts in the field. If you do not know the answer to this question before you actually meet the doctor, *this should be one of the first things to find out*. Although it is quite possible to get decent fertility care from a doctor who is not board certified, you will have some very solid assurance that you are not seeing a quack if you know that at least one of the doctors in the practice or clinic has been accorded this level of professional qualification.

Now the doctor has arrived and you have the opportunity to ask your questions. It may help you not to forget anything important if you bring along a notebook with your questions written down in advance. That way you will also be able to take notes to help you remember the doctor's answers.

The following are some of the things about the doctor's practice or clinic's operations that you will want to find out:

- *Track record.* Ask for a handout, if the doctor has one available, showing the number of patients treated for various conditions (including yours, if you already know what your fertility problem is) who have gone on to have live births. (For some tips about reading doctors' statistics, see section on page 105.) Also of value: How long has the doctor or clinic been operating? Before specializing in infertility, did the doctor practice any other specialty, and if so, what? Is the doctor a member of the American Fertility Society or any of its subgroups (the Society for Assisted Reproductive Technologies, the Society of Reproductive Endocrinologists, or Society of Reproductive Surgeons)?

- *Years of experience.* Ask your doctor, "How long have you specialized in infertility?" Preferably, the doctor will answer five years or more. However, if the doctor is young, an answer of less than five years will be acceptable, provided that there is a more experienced doctor as a partner in the same practice. Younger doctors are somewhat more likely to be trained in the latest techniques. Couples are advised to be cautious of the older doctor who has recently switched from general obstetrics and gynecology to infertility. With its promise of high fees and its lack of calls for 2 A.M. deliveries, infertility easily attracts some OB-GYNs mainly interested in making more money for less work, who have not undergone the rigorous training needed to master the delicate and complex tasks involved.

- *Hours of operation.* When is the clinic or practice fully staffed? Are there times when it is partly open, such as half-day Saturdays? Is the blood lab and **sonogram** room open on weekend mornings or open on some government holidays? This latter question is especially important if you end up using powerful fertility drugs that require seven-day-a-week **monitoring** (described in detail on page 232) by a trained sonographer and laboratory analyst. For those not able to take much time off from work, a clinic with early-morning or late-evening hours will offer an advantage.

- *Medical emergencies.* Is a doctor on call twenty-four hours a day in case of an emergency, such as severe pain from an ectopic pregnancy or profuse bleeding of a threatened miscarriage? What hospital emergency room will the patient be directed to use? Will a doctor from the clinic or practice go to the hospital to speed the admissions process and oversee the patient's care? If a patient has an urgent question off-hours that is not a true emergency, is there a number to call to talk to a doctor?

- *Range of medical services available.* Does the practice or clinic treat patients for problems other than infertility? For example, if the doctor is an OB-GYN, does she see normally fertile pregnant women, too? (If the answer to this question is yes, you may want to ask yourself, "Will I find it too stressful to sit in the waiting room looking at all these other women's pregnant bellies day after day?") If the practice is limited to certain types of infertility care, such as female systems only, will you be given a referral to a doctor who can handle the necessary male testing? If it turns out that surgery is indicated in your case, is the doctor qualified to perform the operation, or will you need a referral? Are there any new technologies or procedures the clinic or practice is not equipped to perform (such as micromanipulation of sperm, **cryopreservation** of embryos, or **host uterus**)? And if it turns out that you could benefit by one of these technologies, would you be referred to a clinic where you could be helped?

- *Convenience.* If you're going to be visiting the clinic frequently, and perhaps even daily for up to seven or eight days in a row, then it's important that the clinic be close enough to home or work for you to get there and back within a reasonable period of time. If you will be driving, you also need to know whether there's a place to park, and whether you'll have to pay extra for parking each time you go. What's the travel time like at rush hour? Can you get there by public transportation?

- *Support staff and services.* Who else works there? How many nurses are there, and are they specially trained to advise fertility patients about some aspects of care when the doctor is not available? Are there enough receptionists to answer the phone so that you don't end up on hold for ten minutes each time you call? Does the clinic or practice handle its own lab work? If not, where do blood and semen samples go for analysis? How long does it take to get results back? What about sonograms? If they're not done in the same building, where must you go and how long does it take to get there? What about a pharmacy? Are drugs dispensed through the clinic or practice, or can they be purchased in the same building, or can patients choose their own pharmacy to fill prescriptions for fertility drugs?

• *Criteria for patient acceptance.* Will the doctor attempt to help anyone who is trying to conceive to do so? Or are there some established criteria that patients must meet, such as age (some clinics will not accept women over forty) or marital status (many will only work with married couples) or length of time spent trying naturally to achieve a pregnancy (some doctors still advise couples not to start testing until they have tried for at least a year to have a baby without success)? If you are looking into IVF, GIFT, or ZIFT, must you have first tried other low-technology methods (and for how long) without success?

• *Scheduling.* How easy is it to get an appointment at a time convenient to the patient? About how long does a patient usually wait beyond the scheduled appointment time to see the doctor? For IVF, GIFT, and ZIFT, is there a waiting time to get into the program? Are new patients accepted only at certain intervals? Is there a regular time to call the doctor with questions or to report problems or receive medication instructions?

• *Billing.* Will bills be sent directly to the patient's insurance company, or does the patient do all the claim filing? Will the doctor or office staff support the patient's claim in the event of a dispute with the insurance company over coverage? Must payment be made on a per-service basis, or can one be billed monthly? For IVF or other high-tech, high-cost procedures, is payment required upfront in a lump sum, or can payment be stretched out over a long period of time?

• *Emotional support.* Does the clinic or practice have a counselor on staff to help the patient cope with the emotional stresses of treatment? If not, does the office refer patients to a professional familiar with the emotional fallout of infertility?

This list is by no means comprehensive. If there are certain areas of special concern to you not covered here, by all means ask the doctor about them!

If you find you do not get a chance to ask all the questions on your list because the doctor dominates your first meeting, doing all the talking and question-asking, that's a bad sign. He probably will not listen very well to your concerns once you become his regular patient. However, if he provides an overview of his practice that answers nearly all of your questions before you have had a chance to ask them, then don't worry too much about his dominating your initial meeting: by anticipating your questions, he has made it clear that he is concerned with providing patients the information they need to make an informed choice.

If you do ask your questions and the doctor can't give you answers in terms you can understand, then this doctor is not for you, and you should keep looking till you find a doctor who can communicate better. (If you interview several doctors and you can't understand much of what any of them have to say, then perhaps you need to brush up on your biology vocabulary. See the section beginning on page 109 for help in that regard.)

In addition to getting answers to your questions, in your initial meeting you should also be trying to pick up clues to the doctor's personal style. Does he come across as paternal? Professorial? Or perhaps patronizing? Does he seem interested in you and your spouse as a couple or as a case? Does he seem fidgety and intense or cool and composed? If he strikes you as both knowledgeable and concerned, that's encouraging. If he leaves you feeling ill at ease (even if you can't quite put your finger on the reason), keep looking. But if the doctor gives off no particular vibes, good or bad, then don't worry too much about it. Make your decision based solely on the objective facts about the practice that you have been able to gather. Getting a gut feeling about whether you will be happy working with this doctor is a plus, but you may not be able to tell that much about him from a single visit.

Keep in mind: you are *not* marrying this person. You can *always switch* if you feel for whatever reason that the doctor-patient relationship is not working out. You don't need to make excuses or apologize, either. Just ask for your records and go (more on the hows and whys of doctor-switching in Chapter Eight).

While the main purpose of your look-see visit is to get a sense of what the doctor is like, it will also be important for you to give the doctor the correct impression of the sort of people you and your spouse are, and the role you expect to play in your own treatment. Your initial consultation is your opportunity to set the tone you want, to let the doctor know that you are intelligent, informed people who expect to be treated as full partners in the decision-making process about your own bodies (if that is indeed how you view your role; those who are content to be more passive and leave the big decisions up to the doctor should also be sure to convey the extent of the trust you'll be placing in him). You should also make him aware of any personal situations, quirks, or traits that are relevant to the doctor-patient relationship: for instance, that you are extremely squeamish about having blood drawn, or that your religion forbids you to have intercourse on religious holidays. If it is important to you to be addressed in a particular way—whether as Mr. and Mrs. Lastname or by your full first name instead of a nickname—let the doctor know that too. It is always a good idea to begin as you wish to proceed.

The doctor should also be given whatever information you already have about the functioning of your reproductive system(s). If the woman has been doing BBT charts or ovulation tests, she should be sure to bring her data along. If your regular doctor has already done one or two simple tests, be sure to have those test results sent along in advance of your first consultation with a specialist. Be sure to mention anything in your medical history or anything you have observed about your body or its cycles that you think *might* have bearing on your fertility—even if the connection seems farfetched. Let the doctor be the one to say what's medically relevant and what isn't.

As you describe your own medical detective work to the doctor, pay careful attention to his reaction. If he appreciates the groundwork you have done, that's a good sign. But if he dismisses your own impressions of your reproductive health and makes it seem as if only he can tell you what's really going on inside your body, take that as an indication of how he will react in the future. This could well be a doctor who, after you call to report the painful side effects you are having from the fertility drug you're on, will tell you bluntly that you are imagining the symptoms, and that that drug could not possibly be causing the effects you described. (I heard stories about doctors like this from at least three former patients.)

When you have visited all the doctors' offices and clinics under consideration, sit down with your spouse or partner and evaluate your findings. Here's a suggestion from a couple, Ann and Tom, about how to reach the decision in a logical, systematic way. They assigned point values to each of the features they most wanted in their fertility program. Then they rated the two best clinics they had seen in each of the categories they had created. Their ratings chart looked like this:

ANN AND TOM'S COMPARISON OF TWO FERTILITY CLINICS

(POINT SCALE IS 1 TO 10; 10 = HIGHEST)

	Independent Fertility Clinic, Inc.		Famous University Hospital Clinic	
	Ann's rating	Tom's rating	Ann's rating	Tom's rating
Track record	10	10	8	7
Impression of doctors	6	7	6	7
Impression of other staff	9	7	5	6
Range of services offered	9	9	10	10
Convenience	8	8	5	6
Billing/handling of insurance claims	$\frac{3}{45}$ +	$\frac{4}{45}$ =	$\frac{5}{39}$ +	$\frac{5}{41}$ =
		90 points		80 points

Ann and Tom choose Independent Fertility Clinic, Inc. because it ranks 10 points higher overall on their combined ratings scale.

You may not want to go about selecting your clinic so methodically, but just by talking over the various points of each clinic you have investigated, you and your partner should not find it too difficult to identify which of the choices you think would work best for you.

About Statistics
(And Other Bendable Objects)

*Y*ou don't have to be a math or science whiz to understand the statistics of doctors' success rates—but it sure helps! Since a great success rate is one of the main reasons for a couple to select a clinic,

(continued)

and since clinics with poor performance can sometimes manage to look good by manipulating their data, it's important to understand at least a few elementary facts about how fertility statistics are gathered and what they mean.

To understand what a clinic's success rate really means, the single most important question you have to be able to answer is: What's the *basis*? "Basis" means the whole from which all subsequent percentages will be taken. An example would be as follows: You read that of one hundred women who began a ZIFT cycle in April at Clinic A, 16 percent went on to give birth to a live baby; but at Clinic B, of one hundred women who began a ZIFT cycle in April, 23 percent went on to give birth to a live baby. Well, you think, Clinic B must be better at ZIFT than Clinic A, so I'll go there. But you would be fooled by not having compared the *basis* of A's statistics to the *basis* of B's. Yes, both used a hundred women as the starting figure—but the hundred that Clinic B used for statistical purposes all happened to be women under the age of thirty-five, with both ovaries working properly, whose husbands had normal sperm—while Clinic A's one hundred women included some in their early to mid forties, some who only had one working ovary, and some whose husbands had abnormal sperm or borderline sperm counts. Clinic A accordingly had a much more difficult basis to work with. If the two *bases* had in fact been equal, then Clinic B's success rate would have been far inferior to Clinic A's. Lesson: *Always find out what the basis consists of.*

Clinics that juggle their statistics will sometimes shift the basis around within the same study group. The following is an example: One hundred women enter the IVF program at Clinic C. Five percent drop out early before they have completed their course of prescribed medication; 17 percent will not undergo egg retrieval because their ovaries did not respond effectively to the drug they were given; 23 percent had eggs retrieved that failed to fertilize when combined with their husband's sperm; and 36 percent had embryos develop from the combination of egg and sperm, with the embryo failing to implant in the woman's uterus. As for its "success rate," the clinic reports a live birth rate of 31 percent from the embryos created in its IVF lab.

That 31 percent looks pretty good, you think, when compared with success rates of 14 percent and 16 percent of the two other IVF clinics you have investigated. But not when you realize that the basis for each round of statistics keeps shifting. The way this clinic has

(continued)

worked it, after the first 5 percent dropped out, the basis became 95 women. When 17 percent of the 95 did not make it to the next stage of the process, the basis was lowered again; now it's 79. After another 23 percent of that 79-woman group dropped out at the egg-retrieval stage, the basis became 61. Then 36 percent of the group of 61 didn't have any embryos created, leaving only 39 women as the basis from which the final live birth rate has been calculated. And 31 percent of 39 is just 12, and 12 of the original hundred equals an overall success rate of 12 percent—a rate that is actually *below* that of the average clinic. The couple who knows enough about statistics to ask about the basis can then go on looking for a clinic with a higher rate.

A more obvious problem turns on what the success rate is actually a measure of. A few clinics will lay claim to achieving high "fertility rates," but what does the term actually mean? Is it the percentage of the couples treated who have produced an embryo? Is it the percentage of couples who have had a pregnancy that can be confirmed by ultrasound? Or is it a percentage of couples treated who go on to have a live birth? Only the last category will be a statistic of importance to you. It is far easier to rack up an impressive number if what you count as "success" is only part of the process—and it is far easier to get an egg to fertilize in a lab dish than it is to get it to grow into a fully formed baby. But it's a baby you want, not a two-celled organism, so the "take-home baby rate" (as some clinics have labeled it) is what you want to make sure you are getting when you check the clinic out.

LOOKING FOR DR. RIGHT

Former Patients Give Some Pointers

Before I started treatment I guess I had a subconscious image that my fertility doctor would be a "Marcus Welby" type. He would pore over my history and rack his brains for ways to help me. I thought that he would really make a personal crusade out of my infertility.

(continued)

What I found out was that doctors, while caring, are *incredibly* busy people, who are only thinking of you when you're right there in front of them, paying for an office visit. . . . They always had to look through my chart to remember my name and history. And phone calls? You had to be persistent to get anything accomplished by phone. If the clinic has one of those voice mail systems, where you have to push buttons and leave messages, pretend that you have a rotary phone and hang on. That way you'll get to talk to a real live person!

Betsy from New Jersey

Author's note: I think Betsy is right on the mark about most doctors. And great idea about getting past that voice mail gauntlet!

*In*fertility should *never* be treated by solo practitioners. The doctor cannot be available twenty-four hours a day, seven days a week. I felt that I was "out of sight, out of mind" in between appointments. He had a wonderful bedside manner, but his facilities and techniques needed updating.

Marcia from New Jersey

Here's a couple who really did their homework:

We ordered the American Fertility Society's publication on all the IVF clinics and reviewed it carefully. We requested brochures from no less than thirty clinics in the U.S. and reviewed every one. We spoke to doctors, reviewed success rates, and also read several general books. We attended ———— Hospital's seminar on IVF, which was *excellent* (and free). We also joined RESOLVE and read the national and local RESOLVE newsletters, as well as almost all of the publications they'd ever done. In short, we became as educated as possible about infertility. . . . In the final analysis, we narrowed down our choice to one clinic in San Francisco and one in New York. We finally chose the one in New York because it was closer to home. It turned out that the clinic had a waiting list of several months. While we waited we decided to try a few more Clomid cycles with our regular doctor. On the second try we became pregnant and today have a beautiful baby girl.

Barbara and James from New Jersey

(continued)

*F*ind out who normally returns phone calls, the doctor or the nurse. In many practices the doctors hardly ever speak to the patients directly. All messages are relayed through nurses, and not always completely accurately. Sometimes you ask questions of the nurses and they tell you one thing, and when your doctor finally calls you, he tells you something completely different. I think it's wisest to find out before you sign up what the policy is on returning calls. If you don't like it, find an office that handles calls differently.

*A*nne from Washington, D.C.

I liked the first doctor we consulted a lot more than my wife did. But she's the one who has to go to all these appointments, so I respected her decision to keep looking for someone else. She switched a few times before she found someone she could feel comfortable with. Part of me wanted to tell her just to stay put, but I knew in the end it had to be her decision.

*F*rank from Washington, D.C.

I found it was easier for my husband to get answers to questions than it was for me. He could be more pushy. It took some of the responsibility off me and it made him the persistent one—not me, the patient. There's a role the patient plays. The doctor sees you differently from a well person.

*J*ane from California

I always write down my questions for the doctor. My doctor is so used to my list that he always asks me, "How many questions today?"

*L*aura from Maryland

BIOLOGY REFRESHER COURSE: HOW HUMAN REPRODUCTION WORKS

Now you have decided on a doctor and you *think* she'll be good at explaining what she's doing in terms you can understand—but suppose it turns out that she's far better at helping couples have babies than she is at telling them what she's doing to try to make it happen?

If you have forgotten all those names of anatomical parts and processes that you memorized during your tenth-grade biology course, you could be in trouble. So for those of you who could use a brief tutorial, the following account ought to be of help.*

Remember that all boldfaced terms in the text are also defined in the Glossary at the back of this book.

Let's start with the female.
You've seen diagrams like the one below.

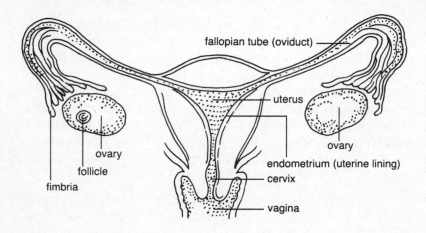

To be honest, the woman's insides in real life don't look very much like this neat little line drawing. The **fallopian tubes** are long, stringy things that can twist around in weird directions, and the ovaries are gooey, oddly shaped lumps; but the configuration still is more or less as shown here.

In a normally fertile female past the age of **menarche** (first menstruation), the following cycle runs at about twenty-eight-day intervals (a few days more or less is also normal).

At Day One of the cycle, the lining of the uterus, thickened with blood and nutrients that would have fostered the growth of an embryo (had the woman become pregnant during the previous cycle), is shed during the three-to-seven-day period called menses, or menstruation.

At this time one of the two ovaries is just beginning to work at preparing a new egg (or *ovum*) to be released mid-cycle (about two weeks from Day One). A **follicle,** or sac that contains the egg, will grow

*Those who are interested in a more detailed and scientific account of how the reproductive system works should consult the Suggested Reading List at the back of the book for titles.

in size as the egg matures over the next fourteen days. This time period is called (logically enough) the **follicular phase** of the cycle. Hormones such as estrogens and **follicle-stimulating hormone (FSH)** are produced in varying quantities as the egg ripens. A day or two before the egg is ready to be released, the level of another hormone called **luteinizing hormone (LH)** suddenly surges, after which the mature egg is expelled by the follicle from the ovary. This moment is called **ovulation.**

The ends of the fallopian tubes contain little finger-like structures called **fimbria** that sweep out and catch the ovulated egg and carry it into the fallopian tube.

If the woman has recently had sexual intercourse with a fertile man, there will be live sperm present in the fallopian tube (they got there by swimming up from her vagina through the opening in the cervix, then up her uterus and into the tubes). If sperm aren't already present, and she has intercourse with a fertile man during the next day or night, while the egg is still traveling down her fallopian tube toward her uterus, conception will still be possible.

Fertile sperm are attracted to a fertile egg by a chemical it produces (what this chemical is and how it works is just now the subject of research). Thousands of sperm beat against the tough outer layer of the egg (called the **zona pellucida**). Ultimately only one sperm will penetrate, and fertilization occurs. (If two eggs happen to be released that cycle, and each is fertilized by a sperm cell, then fraternal twins will be the result.)

The fertilized egg begins dividing as it travels down the fallopian tube toward the uterus. It is now called the pre-embryo, or **zygote.**

Meanwhile, the spent follicle undergoes a change and begins to produce the hormone **progesterone** (once it starts making progesterone it is called the **corpus luteum,** which is Latin for "yellow body"). This hormone thickens and nourishes the lining of the uterus (also called the **endometrium**) to prepare it to receive the **implantation** of the pre-embryo.

After it attaches itself to (or implants in) the wall of the uterus, the multicelled organism is called an embryo.

Doctors now believe that sperm and egg will quite often combine but will not develop beyond a few cell divisions, or else will not implant—meaning that many infertile women do in fact become "pregnant" but only for a few days, or even a few hours of the cycle. A normal or perhaps heavier than normal period begins as the fertilized egg that did not implant is washed out with the flow of menstrual blood. Loss of the fertilized egg is not called a miscarriage or a spontaneous abortion, but a "missed conception."

Occasionally a fertilized egg will implant itself in a place other than the uterus, most likely in the fallopian tube. Such a pregnancy is called **ectopic** (meaning "out of place") and is a serious condition requiring corrective surgery.

If the fertilized egg does successfully implant in the uterus, the woman's body continues to produce progesterone, and she also begins to produce a hormone called **human chorionic gonadotropin (hCG)**. This hormone can be detected in small amounts in the woman's blood sometimes as early as ten days after fertilization, and in her urine about fourteen or fifteen days afterward.

For what happens to the successfully implanted egg after pregnancy has been confirmed by a blood or urine test, you need to buy a pregnancy book (although Chapter Eleven will cover some aspects of pregnancy after infertility).

Now for the male side of the story.

Within the normally fertile man's scrotum are two testicles. Each one carries out two important functions: (1) producing **testosterone**, the hormone responsible for giving the man his male appearance and sex drive; and (2) producing sperm. Inside the testicle are *seminiferous tubules* containing the "mother cells" that manufacture the primitive cells called *spermatocytes*. These will eventually develop into mature sperm.

To aid in the production of sperm, the pituitary gland in the brain causes the release of FSH (yes, the exact same chemical that the woman's body produces to stimulate egg production). FSH acts upon the *Sertoli cells* (also found in the seminiferous tubules in the testicle) to nourish the developing sperm to near-maturity. The pituitary gland also releases LH, the same chemical that in the female causes the mature egg to ovulate, to stimulate the *Leydig cells* in the testicles to make testosterone.

When almost fully mature, the sperm leave the seminiferous tubules and are passed on to the **epididymis**, a long, coiled tube attached to the back of the testicles. At this point the sperm should have an oval head and a long, beating tail, and be able to swim (this swimming ability is called **motility**). It takes about seventy-two days from the time the first primitive cells are formed to the time the sperm are fully mature and ready and able to impregnate an egg.

When the man ejaculates, the sperm rush out of the epididymis and through the **vas deferens**, or sperm ducts, along the way combining with several fluids (one produced by the man's Cowper's gland, one produced in the prostate gland, and one produced in the seminal vesicles—see diagram below for location). The resulting mix of fluids and sperm is called semen.

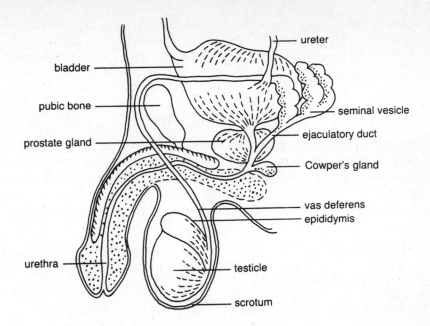

The semen is ultimately ejaculated through the urethra out the opening at the tip of the penis. If the penis happens to be inside the vagina of an ovulating woman at the time of ejaculation, then the sperm—about two hundred million of them—will find themselves in a very friendly environment. They will swim easily in all directions in the woman's abundant cervical mucus. Some of those millions will find their way through the opening in her cervix and up through the uterus to her fallopian tubes, though many more millions will die. Only a small percentage of the ejaculated sperm will survive long enough to reach the egg. Once found, the egg will be surrounded, the sperm beating against its outer layer, but only one will ultimately penetrate and cause conception to occur.

Sperm ejaculated into the vagina of a nonovulating woman will encounter a hostile environment. The woman's cervical mucus will be thick and impenetrable and the opening to her cervix will be closed. This does not mean, however, that the sperm have no chance to fertilize an egg. Healthy sperm may live as long as seventy-two hours if kept warm enough and wet enough (and if the wetness has the proper pH balance). If the woman is close enough to the time of ovulation to begin producing the proper cervical mucus, a few of the millions might still be alive when the egg appears, and so fertilization is still possible.

Of course, if the man has a lower-than-normal sperm count, with sperm of poor shape (**morphology**) or poor motility, the chances of any of his sperm surviving to cause impregnation are greatly reduced. It would be especially important for him to try to achieve optimum timing of intercourse with his partner's day of ovulation.

What Can Go Wrong

We've seen how it's supposed to work, but we've also seen that there are a great many opportunities for things to happen that can prevent conception, or for things that are supposed to happen to somehow not happen.

The following list shows the most common problems in women:

Hormones are not produced in proper synchrony, or in sufficient quantity (when the deficit occurs after ovulation, it is known as a **luteal-phase defect**).

The fallopian tubes are blocked.

There are problems with the egg (eggs are produced but not ovulated, or eggs are ovulated but are of poor quality and cannot be fertilized).

There are problems with the uterus: it is too small, or divided into two chambers (**bicornuate**), or has only one side (**unicornuate**), or has a partial divide (**septate**), or is badly positioned (prolapsed or retrograde).

There is an overgrowth of endometrial tissue outside the uterus (**endometriosis**).

The ovaries are filled with cysts and produce too many male hormones (**polycystic ovarian disease**, or **PCO**).

The woman is producing **antisperm antibodies** vaginally or systemically.

The cervical mucus is a hostile environment for sperm (too acidic or of poor consistency).

The thyroid gland in the throat that influences the production of hormones is not functioning properly.

The pituitary gland in the brain that directs the release of hormones is not functioning properly.

The most common problems in men are as follows:

There are too few sperm (**oligospermia**) or no sperm (**azoospermia**) or the sperm are defectively shaped or have poor swimming ability (poor morphology or motility).

The epididymis is infected or damaged by disease (**epididymitis**).

There is a varicose vein in the testicle (**varicocele**).

There is a blockage (**occlusion**) somewhere along the normal path sperm follow during ejaculation.

The semen is not ejaculated out the penis but is instead ejaculated into the bladder (**retrograde ejaculation**).

The man has problems becoming aroused or remaining aroused and is unable to complete the sexual act.

These lists are by no means comprehensive. They can't be, because doctors do not completely understand human reproduction (though there are very few fertility specialists who will tell you this) and therefore can't be sure they have identified every infertility-related problem that exists. Many couples, after months of testing, will still be told they have **unexplained infertility,** meaning no specific problem has been uncovered—though they still do not conceive.

For a more detailed description of the problems listed here, see Chapter Four on understanding your diagnosis.

CHAPTER THREE

TESTS

You have chosen a doctor and you *think* you've got someone who's good. The doctor came well recommended and you were impressed by his manner, his medical background, and the running of his office. You are all set to go to work.

The first thing he tells you is that he will start doing some tests to find out where your problem lies. He tells you (the woman) that in the next several months you will undergo

- a blood workup
- a pelvic ultrasound
- a hysterosalpingogram
- an endometrial biopsy
- a postcoital test
- a hysteroscopy or
- a laparoscopy

and your husband will have

- a complete semen analysis and
- a chlamydia test.

Your head is spinning. What are all these tests? What do they reveal? How are they done? Does the doctor do each one or will we need referrals to someone else? Where are they performed? When during the menstrual cycle will each be done? Is each one really necessary? Will any test need to be repeated? Will they hurt? Could there be complications? Will it be necessary to take time off from work? Will I need to do any special preparations before each test? How will we feel afterward?

If you have found a doctor who's good at communicating, he will be able to answer all these questions in terms you can understand. He may even have handouts to give you that will cover most of what you want to know. But not all doctors give their patients the opportunity to ask all the questions they'd like, and among those doctors who do, some are not very good at giving clear answers (a point that more than a few patients raised during interviews). To aid those whose doctors turn out to be less than ideal in this department, for each of the major tests that women and men undergo, I have asked each of the questions raised in the paragraph above, and provided answers based solely on reports from patients surveyed.

Blood Workup

WHAT IS IT?

Blood is taken from a vein in the crook of the arm to be analyzed for levels of various hormones or other agents. Both the man and the woman usually will have a blood workup performed.

WHAT DOES IT REVEAL?

In women, lab analysis is commonly done for levels of estradiol (blood estrogen), prolactin, LH, FSH, and/or progesterone, and sometimes for antisperm antibodies or indicators of a thyroid disorder. In men, lab analysis is most often for levels of testosterone, LH, and FSH.

HOW IS IT DONE?

Your arm is tied with a rubber band above your elbow, a needle is inserted in the vein, and a tube—or more likely three or four tubes— of blood will be drawn out.

WHO DOES IT?

A nurse or lab technician.

WHERE IS IT PERFORMED?

Blood can be drawn almost anywhere. Most clinics will have a special blood-drawing room. In hospital-affiliated fertility programs you will most likely be sent down to the hospital's general blood-drawing center to sit in a huge waiting area along with patients who have come from all other departments of the hospital. You take a number and wait your turn.

When in Cycle?

That depends on which specific hormones are to be analyzed. If for estradiol, blood may be drawn at various times within the first two weeks after the period; if for progesterone, at various times within the two weeks before the next menstrual period is expected. For other blood agents, timing of the blood test may not be important.

Is it Necessary?

Yes.

Will it Need to be Repeated?

Very likely. For some hormones, such as progesterone, blood levels can vary widely from one day to the next, so that several days' tests will be necessary to establish a true picture of the level being produced.

Will it Hurt?

You've had blood drawn before, so you know how you react when it happens. Most patients find the needle-stick a minor, transitory pain, while those with thin, hard-to-find veins may find the procedure more traumatic, as the technician has to make several jabs before finding the right spot. Then there is the small percentage of patients who respond to blood-drawing with what is known as a *vaso-vagal* reaction: They become light-headed, nauseated, or may even pass out.

Could There Be Complications?

Virtually never.

Will it Be Necessary to Take Time Off From Work?

Most of the larger, more efficiently run clinics will make blood-drawing available either before or after normal working hours. At hospital clinics where you wait with perhaps dozens of other patients to have blood drawn you will need to budget some extra time for delays to avoid an occasional late arrival. This is important for those who wish to keep

> ## TIP!
>
> *I*f you really hate having blood drawn, distract yourself while it's being done and it will go by much faster. Bring along a Walkman and listen to music, or bring along a particularly engrossing book and read. But whatever happens, don't watch the needle go in!
>
> *A*nne from Washington, D.C.

their infertility care a secret from coworkers but still must account for tardiness to their employer.

ANY SPECIAL PREPARATIONS?

Wear clothing with short sleeves or sleeves that are easy to roll up. If you have ever had a vaso-vagal reaction (described above), request to have the blood drawn while you are lying down with your feet elevated. The blood-drawing room should have a special reclining chair available for patients who need it. If you find that your arm bruises easily or you have any local irritation at the site of the needle-stick, try requesting a "butterfly"—an ultrafine needle used chiefly in pediatrics.

HOW WILL I FEEL AFTERWARD?

You should have no aftereffects.

Pelvic Ultrasound (Sonogram)

WHAT IS IT?

It's an image projected on a TV-like monitor showing certain views of your ovaries and uterus.

WHAT DOES IT REVEAL?

Shape, size, and position of the uterus. Shape, size, and position of the ovaries and presence or absence, size, and number of any follicles found within each ovary. May also reveal presence of fibroid tumors, ovarian cysts, or overgrowths of endometriosis.

How is it done?

Ultrasound can be performed by either of two methods: abdominally or transvaginally (the more common way). In the abdominal ultrasound, a disk-like object (called a transducer) is lubricated with a blue gel and then moved around your bare skin over the part of your abdomen containing your ovaries and uterus, until the technician finds the best spot to get a view of the organ being scanned (the view will generally be improved if you have a full bladder, so you may be instructed not to urinate for a certain period of time before the test is performed). The transducer sends out inaudible sound waves that bounce off the organ being scanned. The reflected sound waves are translated into a visual image on a monitor screen. The image will appear very dark and grainy to your untrained eye, though not to the skilled sonographer. In transvaginal ultrasound the transducer is a probe, shaped very much like an erect penis. It is covered with a condom to which lubricating gel is applied and then is inserted into the vagina. Once inside the vagina the transducer will be tilted toward the right or left, to send sound waves in the direction of the right or left ovary being scanned.

Who does it?

A specially trained ultrasound technician, nurse, or doctor.

Where is it done?

In a sonogram room. Independent fertility clinics will have their own sonogram machines. Small group practices or solo practitioners may need to refer patients to a medical facility that has the equipment for an ultrasound scan. In a hospital-affiliated program, you may be sent to the radiology department, where you will sit alongside patients waiting to have their kidneys, prostate glands, or other organs scanned.

When in my cycle?

Your first pelvic ultrasound will usually be scheduled during or just after your menstrual period. This test, called the *baseline ultrasound,* will show your doctor what your ovaries look like when they are at rest. Subsequent ultrasounds may be ordered around the expected time of your ovulation, showing changes inside the ovaries after they have produced, or are about to produce, a mature egg follicle (or follicles). In the **luteal phase** following ovulation, your doctor may schedule yet another ultrasound to observe what has happened to the follicle after it has released its egg. The uterus may be scanned at any point in the cycle.

IS IT NECESSARY?

There are other tests (e.g., laparoscopy and hysteroscopy) that can provide the same information, but as they are generally more invasive, expensive, and painful, most women would willingly choose a sonogram instead. However, if it has already been determined that these other tests will be performed, the pelvic sonogram could be a redundant expense.

WILL IT NEED TO BE REPEATED?

Very likely, especially if you end up taking certain powerful fertility drugs (for example, Pergonal). Then you will be required to have sonograms each morning for several days in a row (see section on **monitoring** on page 232 for more information on how repeat sonograms are used).

WILL IT HURT?

It shouldn't. Women on occasion do report that the technician inserts the probe too abruptly or moves it around inside the vagina too roughly, but the first complaint can be avoided by asking the technician to let you insert the probe yourself. In fact, many clinics let the patient do the insertion as a matter of course.

COULD THERE BE COMPLICATIONS?

Ultrasound machines have been in widespread use for a variety of diagnostic needs for many years, and no harm has been shown to result. But because they have not yet been in use over the average lifespan, it is impossible to say conclusively that there is no long-term effect; however, given all the study data compiled so far, ultrasound appears to be very safe.

Will it be necessary to take time off from work?

At the bigger clinics and at hospital-affiliated centers, the sonogram room usually will be open before normal working hours. Most smaller group practices that have a sonogram machine will be open only during office hours. Solo practitioners and group practices that do not own their own sonogram machine will refer you to a larger medical facility that may well have extended hours.

Any special preparations?

Your doctor will tell you if it is necessary for you to come in with a full bladder. It's best to wear separates, so that you can remove your clothing from the waist down without having to get totally undressed. Wearing socks or kneehighs rather than pantyhose will also speed up the process of getting dressed to get back to work. For transvaginal ultrasound, take along a pantyliner to wear afterward to catch any dripping gel.

How will i feel afterward?

The ultrasound scan itself will leave no physical aftereffects. There could be emotional aftereffects, however, if there is bad news in what the sonographer sees on the screen, and she is insensitive enough to just blurt it out without regard to your feelings. I talked to one woman who thought she had a confirmed pregnancy, only to have a thoughtless sonographer point to the fetal sac and announce, "No heartbeat. It's dead." (An incident such as this should certainly be reported to your doctor, and you would probably be better off switching to another program that employs more considerate staff.)

Hysterosalpingogram (HSG)

What is it?

An X ray of your uterus and fallopian tubes after a special X-ray dye has been injected into your reproductive system.

What does it reveal?

If the dye travels through your uterus and flows out the ends of both fallopian tubes, then the test reveals that you have normal, open (patent) tubes. Any obstruction will show up at the point at which the dye flow stops. The dye also allows the shape of the inside of the uterus to be seen more clearly on the X ray.

How is it done?

You lie on a table with your feet up in stirrups. First the doctor inserts a small thin tube through the opening of your cervix (which has been dilated), and the dye is shot in through the tube. Then the X-ray machine takes pictures of the dye as it travels through your system. The whole procedure takes no more than five minutes.

Who does it?

Your doctor or a trained radiologist.

Where is it done?

Most likely in the radiology department of a hospital. You might also be referred to a separate radiology office in a medical facility. Some of the larger fertility clinics or group practices will have their own X-ray equipment.

When in my cycle?

The HSG is generally done prior to ovulation, often a day or two after the end of your last menstrual period.

Is it necessary?

Yes, in most cases. Tubal obstruction is one of the most common causes of infertility, and even if other causes have already been identified, the HSG should be performed to verify that no additional tubal problem exists. I can think of only one situation in which a woman would not have an HSG: if she and her doctor have already determined that she will undergo IVF, a procedure that completely bypasses the fallopian tubes. In such a case the doctor knows from the woman's medical history that she has an irreparable tubal problem (for example, past ectopic pregnancies necessitated the surgical removal of both tubes) and that IVF is her only chance at pregnancy.

Will it need to be repeated?

No, with one exception: if you have had a normal HSG and then an event has occurred which could have caused damage to your tubes (for example, a severe pelvic infection), a second HSG may be called for to assess the damage.

Will it hurt?

Yes, but how much is difficult to say. Some women report that the HSG is one of the most painful experiences they have ever undergone, while others (I was one of them) say it really wasn't bad at all. Interestingly enough, women tend to find either the HSG or the **endometrial biopsy** to be awful, but few women say that *both* were bad. The injection of the HSG dye can cause cramping as it rushes through the uterus, and the crampy, painful feeling may last for a few hours.

Could there be complications?

Very rarely. An HSG performed by an experienced radiologist using the proper equipment should be brief and safe. Of course, any exposure to X rays carries with it a slight increment in the long-term risk of cancer, but today's X-ray machines are tuned to give the smallest dose possible to accomplish the job. The benefits far outweigh any potential long-term risk.

Will it be necessary to take time off from work?

Yes, a minimum of an hour of time off. Though the test itself should only take a few minutes, you'll need to take into account your travel time to and from the hospital, the time spent undressing and dressing, and then the time spent just waiting around to talk to the doctor afterward. Those who find the HSG painful will also want to go home afterward and lie down for the rest of the day.

ANY SPECIAL PREPARATIONS?

Ask your doctor what painkiller he recommends you take beforehand. If the answer is aspirin, ibuprofen (Advil), or acetaminophen (Tylenol), wait until about a half hour before the procedure is to be done, then take the maximum dose of the extra-strength version of the product. If you are worried that you will experience severe cramping afterward, you might also want to ask your doctor to give you a prescription for a drug to take at home.

HOW WILL I FEEL AFTERWARD?

You may feel perfectly normal (I did) or you may feel perfectly rotten, or most likely you will feel somewhere in between. Be sure to call your doctor if you still feel crampy and miserable more than twenty-four hours after the test. Some spotting or thick discharge may appear later on the same day of the test. Call your doctor if it continues.

Endometrial Biopsy (EMB)

WHAT IS IT?

A scraping of tissue from the lining of the uterus (**endometrium**).

WHAT DOES IT REVEAL?

Whether the lining of the uterus is "in phase"—referring to whether the lining has been thickened by the action of the hormone progesterone to the level expected on a specific day of your cycle. If the uterine lining is not sufficiently thickened on the day of the test, you will be told how many days "out of phase" you are.

HOW IS IT DONE?

You will lie on a table with your feet up in stirrups, while the doctor dilates your cervix enough to allow him to insert a thin, sterile implement with a pointed tip. He will make one quick jab, just deep enough to scrape a bit of tissue from the wall of your uterus. This should take less than a minute. You go home, wearing a sanitary napkin to catch any posttest bleeding, and then call your doctor on the day your period begins, to enable him to interpret your test results based on the number of days in that month's cycle.

WHO DOES IT?

Your doctor.

WHERE IS IT DONE?

In an examining room in your doctor's office.

WHEN IN MY CYCLE?

You will try to schedule your EMB for two or three days before your next expected period. This can be difficult to judge if you are irregular, and it's easy to lose a month or two because you guessed your period would come later than it did, or because the best testing time before your period that month fell during a three-day weekend when the doctor's office was closed.

IS IT NECESSARY?

Most doctors say the EMB gives a more reliable picture of the luteal phase of the cycle than does repeated blood testing for progesterone levels. However, if you have been charting your BBT for several months and consistently show less than ten days of elevated temperature following ovulation, and several blood tests have shown your progesterone levels to be low, your doctor should be able to conclude you have a luteal-phase defect without subjecting you to the discomfort of the EMB.

TIP!

If the doctor has already told you he will do a **hysteroscopy**, ask whether the EMB could be performed at the time of the hysteroscopy, to get two painful tests over at the same time.

WILL IT NEED TO BE REPEATED?

Hopefully not. But this is one test some doctors like to do two or three times. Progesterone levels tend to fluctuate a lot, and it's hard to know for sure whether an "out of phase" reading results from a luteal-phase defect or is just part of this normal variation. Also, test results may be ambiguous or difficult to interpret (because, for example, the woman experiences a lot of posttest spotting and thus is unable to be sure when her period actually begins). A doctor may wish to repeat a test to confirm or clarify the previous month's finding. If a luteal-phase defect is diagnosed, the doctor may also wish to do an EMB after a cycle or two of treatment (usually progesterone suppositories) to gauge the effectiveness of the medication.

Should you consent to having a second or third EMB done? If the doctor is persuasive as to the *necessity* (not mere utility) of new test results in determining your treatment, and if you did not find your first EMB to be too painful, then you might want to consider it. But keep in mind that repeat EMBs could be an indicator that your doctor is prone to order excessive tests, and may spend too many months collecting data on you when he could be treating your problem. Since treatment for luteal-phase defect is usually with progesterone suppositories, a natural chemical with few side effects, some doctors will prescribe the treatment for patients who had an ambiguous EMB result, rather than put the patient through a second test.

WILL IT HURT?

Yes, but how much is difficult to say. Several patients reported to me that the EMB was the worst single experience of their treatment. Others found it not too bad at all. For some, the initial pain of the tissue-sticking tool was the bad part; for others the slight jab was hardly felt, but much later, they were doubled over with cramps and backache. Is there a way to predict how you are likely to react to this test? Since women tend to find either the HSG painful or the EMB painful, but not both, schedule your HSG first. If you find it excruciating, take heart: you probably won't mind the EMB all that much. If you think the HSG wasn't so bad, then fortify yourself with a lot of painkiller a half hour before you go in for your EMB.

Could there be complications?

Rarely. If cramping doesn't abate within a day or two, or if bleeding afterward continues to be heavy (and if it doesn't have the color, consistency, or odor of your normal menstrual period), call your doctor. Also watch for any fever, chills, or nausea that could indicate a possible infection (though with the use of a sterile sticking-implement, an infection would be unlikely).

Will it be necessary to take time off from work?

Yes, enough to allow for travel time to and from the clinic, time for undressing and dressing, and the usual waiting around for the doctor to be ready for you. You won't have to wait around afterward for the results, since no conclusion can be reached until after you have reported getting your period, and the test findings can be analyzed in the context of your cycle's length. After the test is over, you may also want to give yourself a few more hours, or even the rest of the day off, to go home and lie down until you feel recovered from the cramping you may experience.

Any special preparations?

Yes! To be absolutely sure that your uterus does not contain an embryo that the EMB could cause to be aborted, you *must* go in for a pregnancy test the morning of the day before the EMB is scheduled. The test must be for hCG levels in the blood, not in the urine (a less sensitive test), and the results must be back the same day if the information is to be of use. If your doctor does not suggest that you go in for the pregnancy test the day before your EMB, insist on it. A negative hCG level is the only way to get peace of mind that you are not having the test while pregnant.

Also beforehand, ask your doctor whether you should take aspirin, acetaminophen (Tylenol), or ibuprofen (Advil) or any other drug to ease the pain. Take the maximum dose of the extra-strength formula of whichever remedy he suggests. If you suspect that you are particularly susceptible to pain and cramping, you might even ask for a stronger prescription drug that you can take after you get home.

How will I feel afterward?

Within a day you should be feeling all right again. Those who found the experience not so bad reported feeling pretty normal within a few hours. If you still feel as bad twenty-four hours after the test as you did the day it was done, report your symptoms to your doctor.

I was told by my doctor to expect menstrual-like cramps. I thought that the test shouldn't be too bad, so I told my husband it wasn't necessary to go with me. The test, for me, turned out to be excruciating. I almost passed out from the pain and was extremely shaky and dizzy for about fifteen minutes afterward. My doctor said that most people don't have the pain I did. How could she know? She didn't go through it.

*M*arie from Illinois

Author's comment: Her doctor *was* right, in a sense: the EMB was not that bad for most of the patients I interviewed. It's hard to know how you'll react if you've never had one. My advice: Go in expecting to feel pain, and if it turns out that you don't, you'll be pleasantly surprised. And if it's bad, well, at least you'll be prepared for it!

Postcoital Test (PCT, or Sims-Huhner Test)

What is it?

Well, yes . . . it *is* what it sounds like—but don't panic: you won't have to "do it" in the doctor's office. The sexual intercourse part (*coitus,* as your doctor may call it) you will have at home in your own bed (or on the floor or hanging from the chandelier, if that's your thing). Two to twelve hours afterward, the woman goes to her doctor's office to have a small amount of her cervical mucus examined to see if it provides a hospitable environment for sperm.

What does it reveal?

Normal cervical mucus will appear clear, copious, and "stretchy" (with the quality of **spinnbarkeit**, described on page 46), and will contain a high percentage of live sperm (assuming that the husband has been tested and found to be fertile). A high percentage of dead sperm would lead to further testing to see if the mucus contains **antisperm antibodies** (also called an immunological response, or "allergy" to sperm), and if it has the correct pH (level of acidity or alkalinity).

How is it done?

The woman lies on the examining table with her feet in stirrups, and the doctor inserts a speculum, just as for an ordinary pelvic exam, and then swabs off a sample of mucus and puts it on a glass slide. The removal of the sample should only take a few seconds.

Who does it?

Either a doctor or a nurse.

Where is it done?

In an examining room in your doctor's office.

When in my cycle?

Timing is crucial for this test. You must test your urine with an ovulation test kit every morning starting a few days before your expected ovulation. The day you get a positive result (meaning that your LH surge has begun and your mucus should be optimal for sperm), you will call the doctor's office and schedule your PCT for sometime the next day. If the time of the test is the next morning, you and your husband should have intercourse late on the night before. If your test is not until the afternoon, then wake up early and have intercourse before you go to work. Although a PCT may be done up to twelve hours after intercourse, doing the test only three or four hours after intercourse may yield more useful data about the percentage of sperm that can swim in the cervical mucus medium.

WEEKEND ALERT!

*W*omen sometimes miss out on the month's only opportunity to have the PCT performed because they happen to ovulate over the weekend when the clinic is closed. Tip for avoiding this problem: If you get your positive LH urine test result on a Friday morning, call the doctor's office immediately and see if you and your husband should have intercourse right away, to have the PCT performed two hours later. If your positive LH result occurs on a Saturday, then test your urine again on Sunday. If the test stick is still blue (or pink, depending on the brand you use) and you can insert your finger and feel clear, stretchy cervical mucus in your vagina, then leave a message with your doctor's answering service asking whether it is advisable for you to have a PCT on Monday. Make love very late Sunday night or very early Monday morning before you go in for the PCT.

IS IT NECESSARY?

In most cases, yes. If the doctor has already determined that donor sperm will be used because the husband is infertile (and current medical technology can't be used to fix his problem), then the PCT is superfluous. Similarly, if the couple has already decided to try **intra-uterine insemination (IUI)**, or IVF or GIFT, then the cervical mucus will be bypassed, and so does not need to be investigated for its quality as a medium for sperm.

WILL IT NEED TO BE REPEATED?

In certain circumstances, yes. If the couple has been found to have a problem (for example, the mucus contains antisperm antibodies), and the problem is treated for a period of time, the doctor will suggest another PCT to see whether the treatment has succeeded in eliminating or reducing the problem. Women taking the fertility drug Clomid are also advised to have a second PCT to see whether the Clomid has adversely affected the quality of the cervical mucus (as Clomid has frequently been reported to do). But if the doctor wants to repeat the test and you are not aware of any change in your life-style or medication that could affect the results, closely question the doctor as to why he believes a repeat test is necessary.

Will it hurt?

Removal of the cervical mucus is painless. As for what you do beforehand to bring the sperm into contact with the cervical mucus, that's up to you, but for most people it's a pleasurable experience.

Could there be complications?

I have not read about or heard of any complications during my research for this book.

Will it be necessary to take time off from work?

Yes. Though the exam itself is very brief, you will still have to schedule it during regular office hours and allow the usual travel and waiting time. If your positive LH urine test happens on a Friday and you wish to be tested that same day (to avoid delaying the test by another month), then you and your partner will both have to take enough time off from work to make love that morning.

Any special preparations?

You and your spouse grow anxious with each new day's ovulation test. Another negative result. Should we make love tonight, or hold off, to be sure we're not too tired if we "have to do it" the next day? Many doctors instruct couples to abstain from sex for a few days until the positive LH test occurs. Then the day comes that you're finally allowed to do it, but by then the man feels pressured and finds it hard to get aroused. The woman is tense and just lying there waiting for her partner to finish. This happens to a great many couples before the scheduled PCT, so don't feel bad if it happens to you. If you are the type to get easily embarrassed and don't want to tell your doctor you did not have intercourse the night you were supposed to, then go ahead and invent an excuse (a relative got sick and needed you, or you had to go out of town). Or just call the doctor's appointment secretary and say you can't make it in that day—no reason needed. Then don't think about it anymore and just try again next month. But maybe this time try early in the morning, when you're not so tired, instead of the night before. Or first have some champagne in bed, with soft sensual music playing in the background. Only you and your partner can come up with the ideas that will work best to put you in the mood.

How will i feel afterward?

Fine, unless your coworkers somehow discover what you are going in for. Even the most unsecretive, "let-it-all-hang-out" types will want to protect their privacy surrounding the PCT. It's fine if you decide to tell friends that you're trying to get pregnant with medical help, but they don't need to know what exact dates you're trying to get pregnant on. Still, when it comes to decisions about childbearing, people can be nosier than you'd ever imagined possible, so prepare yourself to answer questions like "Why did you go to the doctor?" with a polite but firm defense of your privacy.

Hysteroscopy

What is it?

A view of the inside of your uterus through a tiny fiber-optic tube.

What does it reveal?

Any abnormalities of the shape of the uterus, such as a dividing piece of tissue (**septum**), or presence of any growths such as **fibroid tumors** or polyps, or any adhesions that may have resulted from infections.

How is it done?

The patient lies on an examining table with her feet in the stirrups. (She has been prepared by being given either a local anesthetic and sedative, or else general anesthesia.) The doctor dilates the cervix, allowing him to insert a thin fiber-optic tube with a light at the end that will allow him to see inside the uterus. Usually the uterus is expanded for better viewing by injection of carbon dioxide gas or a clear liquid solution. In some cases if the doctor finds small abnormalities, he will be able to insert an instrument right then to correct the problem on the spot.

Who does it?

An OB-GYN or fertility specialist with experience in the procedure.

Where is it done?

If performed under local anesthesia, it may be done in the doctor's examining room. If done under general anesthesia, it must be done in a hospital, in case the patient has an allergic reaction to the anesthetic used.

When in my cycle?

That depends on what the doctor is planning to do during the hysteroscopy. If he is just going to have a look around, then the beginning of the cycle is best, when the uterine lining is relatively thin and the opening to the fallopian tubes may be seen. If he is also intending to do an EMB at the same time (a common practice, and one that saves women from the discomfort of two separate procedures), then the hysteroscopy must be scheduled two or three days before the next expected menstrual period.

Is it necessary?

Not always. If your doctor is intending to do a **laparoscopy** (see next section for description), a hysteroscopy may be superfluous. If you have already had a sonogram and an HSG and your uterus appears normal, and you have no symptoms or family history (such as a mother who took DES while pregnant with you) to indicate uterine trouble, many doctors say a hysteroscopy is not needed.

Will it need to be repeated?

If years have passed since you had the first one done and there is reason to suspect that fibroid tumors, polyps, or adhesions have developed in the intervening time, then yes. For all other women, no.

Will it hurt?

Yes. Even doctors interviewed who are used to talking of "discomfort," not pain, admit that hysteroscopy will hurt. The question is, Are you willing to pay a lot more money, spend a lot more time, and take a small amount of increased risk in order to reduce the pain of the procedure? If the answer is yes, then have your hysteroscopy done in a hospital under general anesthesia. If you have a fairly high tolerance for pain (you can have teeth drilled, for example, without novocaine, but just on "laughing gas"), then let the doctor do the procedure in his office more quickly and easily while you are under local anesthetic and a sedative. Whichever way you have it done, make sure you have something to take to ease pain afterward. If carbon dioxide gas is injected to expand your uterus, some time later you will feel pain in one shoulder (why this is so, I don't know, but all the hysteroscopy patients I interviewed reported it).

COULD THERE BE COMPLICATIONS?

Hysteroscopy carries a slight risk of infection or excessive bleeding afterward. If you have a fever, nausea, or are bleeding heavily (and are not having a menstrual period) call your doctor at once.

WILL IT BE NECESSARY TO TAKE TIME OFF FROM WORK?

Yes. Take the whole day off (you'll be glad you did). If possible, schedule your hysteroscopy on a Friday, so that you don't have to return to work the next day.

ANY SPECIAL PREPARATIONS?

If your hysteroscopy is scheduled for the postovulatory phase of your cycle, you should have a blood pregnancy test first, to make sure that there is no embryo present that could be dislodged by the procedure. You should have the blood test the morning before the hysteroscopy, and get the results back the same day. If your doctor does not suggest this, insist on it. You will need it for your peace of mind as you go in for the hysteroscopy.

It's a good idea to take your husband or a close friend along to drive you home afterward (especially if you've been given a strong sedative). Bring along a thick sanitary napkin, because there will be moderate bleeding for the rest of the day, and spotting for a few days after that. Avoid wearing any tight-fitting skirts or pants: you will not feel like having anything pressing against your uterus when you are ready to get dressed again.

How will i feel afterward?

Not like going dancing till dawn. But you should feel much better within twenty-four hours, especially if you pamper yourself, have dinner in bed, and get plenty of sleep.

Laparoscopy

What is it?

A surgical procedure in which the doctor inserts a fiber-optic viewing scope into the woman's abdominal cavity through a small incision made usually inside her navel, which allows him to see the outside of her uterus, her fallopian tubes, and her ovaries.

What does it reveal?

Evidence of **endometriosis** (overgrowths of tissue from the lining of the uterus found on the fallopian tubes, ovaries, or elsewhere in the abdominal cavity). The doctor may also observe adhesions (scar tissue) or malformations of any of the reproductive organs.

How is it done?

The woman, having received general anesthesia, lies on a table in an operating room. The doctor first injects carbon dioxide gas into her abdominal cavity, inflating it to give him more room to see the organs. After making a small incision inside or just at the lower edge of her navel, he inserts a thin fiber-optic tube with a light at the end. Usually, but not always, there will be a second incision just below the pubic hairline through which an instrument is inserted that allows the doctor to gently manipulate the pelvic organs to view them better from various angles. If the doctor discovers endometriosis or adhesions that can be treated then and there, he will also insert the proper instrument needed to repair the damage found. After the operation is over (usually about a half hour to forty-five minutes), the doctor closes each incision with one stitch, and covers the wound with a small piece of gauze held in place by a small adhesive bandage (leading to the term "Band-Aid surgery" to describe laparoscopy and other small-incision procedures). The patient is wheeled into a recovery room and given an hour or two to lie down (or sit in a reclining chair) until she is able to walk steadily enough to get to the bathroom on her own and urinate.

WHO DOES IT?

An OB-GYN or fertility specialist with experience at performing this surgery.

WHERE IS IT DONE?

In the operating room of a hospital—usually in the one-day surgery department, for patients who will be going home the same day as the operation.

WHEN IN MY CYCLE?

May be performed at various times in the cycle, depending on what the doctor is looking for, and whether the procedure is to be combined with any other tests (such as an HSG or a hysteroscopy). It is frequently performed at just about the time of or just after ovulation, so that the doctor can see whether the ovaries have produced a normal follicle and egg.

If you are set to have a laparoscopy around the time of expected ovulation, ask your doctor about the merits of performing PORDL at the same time. *PORDL* stands for "programmed oocyte recovery during laparoscopy," and is a technique that allows the patient to have a chance at conception even though having surgery during the ovulation phase of her cycle (otherwise, she would have to go home, unable to have intercourse, and that month's egg—oocyte—would be wasted). PORDL adds to the cost of laparoscopy, but since the diagnostic part of the procedure is considered medically necessary, insurance companies usually will pick up most of the costs without question, leaving the patient with no bills to pay, or only the bills for the lab work involved in preparing the embryo for reinsertion in the woman's uterus. PORDL, as you can see, is a kind of IVF, but without the use of powerful and expensive fertility drugs to cause the ovaries to produce multiple eggs. Ordinarily, an IVF cycle would cost between $6,000 and $10,000 dollars, but with PORDL the cost to the patient may be kept below $3,000.

Is it necessary?

Not in all cases. A few of the people I interviewed, looking back on their testing histories, felt that the laparoscopies they had undergone proved to be of little use in arriving at a diagnosis and treatment plan—either because previous tests had already pinpointed the most likely cause of infertility, or because previous tests had indicated that all appeared normal, and the laparoscopy findings did not turn up any new evidence to the contrary. Laparoscopy is most useful in finding endometriosis that does not show up on other tests, but if the woman has no symptoms leading the doctor to suspect the condition, then laparoscopy may well turn out to be an unrevealing procedure. Doctors can and do treat patients for **unexplained infertility** without a laparoscopy; if after several months of treatment (usually fertility drugs) the patient still does not conceive, then a laparoscopy to continue to search for a cause of the infertility might make more sense.

Why then do some doctors routinely order laparoscopies in the absence of symptoms suggesting the procedure? The following are some possible explanations: (1) the procedure pays well; (2) the procedure can confirm the results of other tests; (3) the doctors were trained to regard the operation as a routine part of the infertility workup; (4) the doctors benefit from the experience of performing many laparoscopies; (5) the doctors think if they *don't* do the procedure, and then it turns out that you have a disorder that could have been detected and treated by laparoscopy, that the patient will sue them for malpractice for failure to have performed one.

Will it need to be repeated?

Occasionally, yes. If the doctor made repairs to damaged organs during the first laparoscopy, he may schedule a second several weeks later to assess whether the first operation worked. If your laparoscopy was performed to diagnose endometriosis, and it turns out that you have a moderate or severe form of the disease, you are very likely to need to repeat the procedure to treat regrowths of adhesions several months, or years, later. Laparoscopy also plays a role in the reinsertion of sperm and eggs, or embryos, during a GIFT or ZIFT cycle (some clinics also retrieve eggs for IVF via laparoscopy, although at the more advanced clinics a nonsurgical procedure, needle-guided ultrasound, is used).

Thus, the number of laparoscopies you undergo may depend on the number of GIFT or ZIFT cycles that you go through.

WILL IT HURT?

Of course—surgery always does. Upon awakening you will feel groggy and possibly nauseated. Some women feel pain at the incision site right away, while others will only feel some soreness an hour or so later. Within the next several hours most women report experiencing an odd, sometimes sharp, pain in one shoulder. This is a consequence of the injection of carbon dioxide gas into your abdomen to expand your insides—though why it should end up affecting your shoulder I have not been able to discover. If it doesn't go away in a day, call your doctor.

Your doctor may have prescribed a painkiller for you to take after you get home (if he doesn't bring it up before surgery, be sure to ask). How much pain relief women will require is a highly individual matter. I have heard from women who said that they got up an hour after the operation and went back to work with only minor discomfort. And I have spoken to a lot more women who said they were in bed for three days after the operation, and had intermittent pain for more than a week. To help you predict how you are likely to react, think back to any previous minor surgery you have had. Have you had your wisdom teeth out? Or your tonsils? If you tolerated that sort of procedure well, then you should bounce right back from a laparoscopy, which is quicker and involves less cutting.

COULD THERE BE COMPLICATIONS?

Any surgery brings with it the risk of infection, bleeding, swelling, and formation of permanent raised scar tissue (keloid scarring). Anytime general anesthesia is used, there is risk of an allergic reaction that could have serious consequences. That is why it is important to be sure that your doctor is experienced and skilled at the procedure, and that there is an anesthesiologist present who is familiar with your medical history, especially any allergies or breathing problems in the past. Your doctor will inform you of certain symptoms (such as heavy bleeding or a high fever) that could indicate a postoperative problem requiring immediate attention. Statistics show that when performed by a careful doctor at a clean, competently run hospital, laparoscopy is one of the safest operations you could have.

Will it be necessary to take time off from work?

Yes. You should take off at least one full day, and possibly two or three. You may find it helpful to schedule your laparoscopy on a Friday, so that you can have the full weekend to recover.

Any special preparations?

Yes. The hospital will instruct you as to what you are allowed to eat or drink before surgery. Read and follow all instructions exactly. When I had my laparoscopy I was required to go in several days ahead of time to be interviewed by the anesthesiologist about anything in my background that could point to an allergy to the anesthetic to be used; you most likely will, too, or at least you will be asked to fill out a questionnaire that the anesthesiologist will read. Be sure to bring up anything you believe could be of relevance, even if you don't see a question specifically on that topic on the questionnaire.

Other preparation advice: Wear a loose shift or housedress if you have one. You won't feel like having anything pressing on the incision site after the operation is over. Avoid wearing high heels, because you may walk a bit unsteadily at first. And be sure you have someone to drive you home when the hospital says you can leave.

How will I feel afterward?

Anywhere from "pretty rotten" to "not so bad after all." If you are not feeling substantially better within two or three days, call your doctor. Weeks after surgery, some women discover that the incision inside the navel has left a thick, raised scar, ruining the way they look in a bikini. This can be depressing if it happens to you, but there is one consolation: if you do conceive (something the laparoscopy ultimately is supposed to help bring about), pregnancy will ruin your figure far worse than the laparoscopy did—and that's what you *want,* isn't it?

Semen Analysis

What is it?

The man produces a semen specimen, normally through masturbation, that is taken to a laboratory where it is analyzed for a variety of factors.

*M*y doctor didn't think a laparoscopy was necessary, but he performed one after I insisted that something was wrong [because of the terrible menstrual cramps this patient had been having]. During the procedure he discovered that I had mild endometriosis and a grape-sized cyst on one of my fallopian tubes, and adhesions and scar tissue covering my other tube and ovary. He used a laser to remove the patches of endometriosis, the scar tissue, and the cyst. If I hadn't insisted on the procedure, I would probably still be wasting a lot of time and money on fertility drugs!

*N*icole from Texas

WHAT DOES IT REVEAL?

Whether the man is producing sperm in sufficient quantity ("sperm count") to make conception possible; whether sperm are normally shaped ("morphology"), whether they have good swimming ability ("motility"); whether the fluid of the ejaculate is of normal volume and chemical composition; whether the fluid contains antisperm antibodies; and other factors, such as presence of certain harmful bacteria. Your medical history will tell your doctor if there are specific problems he should be looking for.

Some doctors also order a "hamster penetration assay," or simply "hamster test," in which the sperm are put in proximity to a hamster's egg to see if the sperm are able to penetrate the outer layer. No, this doesn't mean that your sperm will actually fertilize the hamster's egg—so don't start having any science fiction nightmares about some half-human, half-rodent conception that carries around your genetic message. But the hamster's egg is similar enough to a woman's egg to allow the doctor to get a sense of the sperm's ability to cause a baby to be conceived.

HOW IS IT DONE?

The man is handed a "collection cup," is instructed to masturbate and catch the ejaculate in the cup, and bring it immediately to the lab for analysis. (Men whose religion forbids them to masturbate to collect the sperm can turn to Chapter Ten for alternatives.)

Who does it?

After the man does his part, a lab technician performs the various tests on the semen specimen. The man's doctor then analyzes and interprets the findings.

Where is it done?

Where the man "does his thing" depends on the rules of the clinic or doctor he goes to. Many clinics have a room set aside for this purpose, stocked with erotic magazines or equipped with a VCR and erotic movies. In smaller, less fancy practices, the man may simply be sent off to the bathroom or to an unused utility closet where he has to hope no one will barge in. There are some doctors who allow the man to collect his semen in the privacy of his home. If he lives within a short drive of the lab to which the specimen must be delivered, he may be told that all he has to do is to keep the cup warmed to body temperature by putting it inside his shirt and holding it under his armpit.

When in my wife's cycle?

It's best to avoid giving the sample during her fertile time of the month. Doctors usually advise that a man abstain from intercourse for two to three days before producing the semen for analysis, and you don't want to be barred from sex just at the time that her ovulation is expected.

Is it necessary?

Absolutely. Even if a problem with the female reproductive system has already been identified, the man should still have himself checked out. Up to 20 percent of all infertility cases involve problems in both partners of the couple. Another 20 to 40 percent of cases (experts disagree on the figures) are the result of infertility in the male partner alone.

Will it need to be repeated?

Yes, quite likely. Sperm production can vary significantly from day to day, and it is quite possible that the man with a low sperm count on his first sample will test normal on his second and third. If the man's test is normal on his first, however, then he is probably fertile, and does not need to be retested.

WILL IT HURT?

Not if you're doing it right.

COULD THERE BE COMPLICATIONS?

Despite what your gym teacher told you, there are no harmful side effects.

WILL IT BE NECESSARY TO TAKE TIME OFF FROM WORK?

Big clinics will often have lab hours early in the morning or after normal working hours, so you can produce the semen in a room somewhere, before the regular patients start to arrive or after they have all left. In smaller group practices you will probably have to come in during part of your normal workday. If allowed to produce the sample at home and deliver it, you may only need to be absent from work for a short time.

ANY SPECIAL PREPARATIONS?

Bring along whatever material (pictures, magazines, etc.) you find most stimulating. And leave your watch at home (you don't want to feel any pressure that you must produce by a certain time).

HOW WILL I FEEL AFTERWARD?

You should have the findings fairly soon, so how you feel will probably depend on whether you are given good news or bad. If a problem is discovered, it's important to remember that there is no connection whatsoever between sexual performance and fertility. You are not less virile because your sperm are not functioning as they should—just as your wife cannot be considered less feminine if her ovaries are not producing eggs. Sexuality is a component of our personalities, and it remains a part of us regardless of the physical state of our reproductive organs and tubes.

Male Chlamydia Test

WHAT IS IT?

A test for the presence of the sexually transmitted chlamydia infection.

The Sperm and the Jar
Men Tell What It's Like to "Deliver the Goods"

*I*t's different for men. You're brought up to think of yourselves as strong, capable, in charge of things. It's okay for women to have problems, and to turn to doctors for help with an intimate matter. Female plumbing is kind of complicated, and it always needs tinkering with . . . right? But then one day someone suggests that the reason for your childlessness might be that *your* system isn't up to the job. It's hard not to take this notion as an assault on your manhood. Then, to make matters worse, they hand you a little cup, tell you to go off to the bathroom, and "produce." At seven in the morning. With a waiting room full of pregnant women outside the door.

Your wife doesn't give you much sympathy, either. She tells you about the four painful tests she's already been through. And yours doesn't even *hurt.* So you don't say any more about it—you just go in, try to shut out the rest of the world, and do what you're there for. Maybe months, or even years from now, you'll be able to talk about it without that awful, guilty feeling that you have right now.

I talked to one man, Frank from Washington, D.C., who had a particularly refreshing and straightforward attitude toward semen collection: "It doesn't embarrass me. I don't feel I'm doing anything furtive. I'm irritated at a society that tries to make you feel you have to skulk around and feel weird about being a man who produces sperm."

What troubled Robert, also of Washington, more than the test itself, was the uncertainty about the meaning of the results. Like many women patients, he felt that no doctor had treated him as an equal, or had ever taken the time to explain the findings to him in intelligible terms. (I believe his experience is fairly common.) "I've had four different sperm analyses by three different doctors," he told me. "One was very normal in all categories, but that one was a long time ago, before I was even thinking about having children. The next two were after we started seeing a fertility doctor. My wife's gynecologist recommended a urologist. These tests were somewhat low. A sonogram showed a varicocele. The fourth test, with a different doctor, the numbers were much, much higher. None of the doctors ever made it clear to me what these numbers meant, or really answered my questions satisfactorily. My wife and I did a lot of research on our

(continued)

own, and it seems that there is a lot of disagreement among doctors on the meaning of these numbers."

And then there's another thing about that semen sample—getting it to the lab. This can involve logistical difficulties you never imagined you'd be faced with. But it does help to keep a sense of humor about the thing—as did Mike and Diane from Indiana, who told this story: "Mike wasn't able to take as much time off from work as I was. He had to use his lunch hour to come home and collect the semen. Then I had to place the glass jar, with its precious cargo, between my breasts inside my bra to keep it warm. I had to drive one hundred miles with the jar in my bra. I had to drive fast to get to the lab before the two-hour time limit was up. The whole way I prayed that I wouldn't have an accident where someone would have to explain why I had broken glass and semen between my breasts!"

Bob Bookman wrote about two such incidents from his fertility treatment days in "Coping with Male Infertility," which appeared in the *Washington Post* on March 27, 1990. On one occasion, he relates, he decided to make use of his boss's office, since it was located only five blocks from the hospital lab where the sperm sample would be analyzed. Of course he never expected that his boss would come to work at seven in the morning . . . but he was less surprised to see her than she was to see him! And then there was the time that he had to stop by the Pentagon on some business directly after leaving his semen sample at the lab. The security guards there were highly amused by the nature of the magazines they found when they searched through his briefcase!

Though his newspaper piece was filled with humorous stories, he ends with this reflection: "I wish I could tell my male friends who are a little hesitant to see a doctor about a possible fertility problem that going through the infertility experience has been worth it to me from the standpoint of enriching my relationships with my wife, my friends. . . . This would be hogwash, even though I have learned a lot from the experience. While it hasn't been pleasant, I know it is worth it when I stroke my child's head as he's falling asleep on my chest."

WHAT DOES IT REVEAL?

The presence of chlamydia bacteria.

HOW IS IT DONE?

The man is given a sterile cotton swab to insert into the opening at the tip of his penis. The swab is then sent to the lab to be cultured and analyzed.

WHO DOES IT?

A lab technician does the culturing and the doctor reads the results.

WHERE IS IT DONE?

At the doctor's office, usually in an examining room or in the bathroom, sometimes at the same time the man is asked to produce his semen specimen.

WHEN IN MY WIFE'S CYCLE?

It doesn't matter.

IS IT NECESSARY?

Yes. Chlamydia is a tremendously widespread infection and it's easy to have it without knowing it. If the man is infected he will most likely infect his partner, whose reproductive system could become permanently damaged before she realizes it and has the chance to seek treatment. The chlamydia bacteria can remain in the system for a long period of time, and there are strains that are resistant to antibiotics, so that even if you were treated for it a long time ago, it's quite possible that you are still infected, and so should be tested.

WILL IT NEED TO BE REPEATED?

Not unless you or your spouse has been engaging in sexual activity that could introduce outside bacteria into your reproductive tract.

WILL IT HURT?

Getting the swab into the urethral opening is somewhat irritating, but the irritation quickly passes.

Could there be complications?

As long as you have kept the swab sterile (you haven't touched it to any surfaces or to any other part of your body), the test has no risk of complications.

Will it be necessary to take time off from work?

It takes only a second to do the test, so you shouldn't have to be gone too long. You may be asked to do the chlamydia test at the same time you come in to produce your semen specimen, in which case you lose no extra time from work. However, you will be required to do the chlamydia test first, and then your penis will feel slightly irritated, not making it any easier to produce the semen under already trying conditions.

Any special preparations?

None needed.

How will I feel afterward?

You should feel perfectly normal.

Testicular Biopsy

What is it?

A surgical procedure in which the doctor, after first anesthetizing the patient, removes a small sample of tissue from the inside of the testicle.

What does it reveal?

Whether the man has normal hormone-producing cells and sperm-producing structures, whether there is a malignant growth, or whether there are any other abnormalities that could interfere with the production of sperm.

How is it done?

The man can have general anesthesia, or local anesthesia and a sedative beforehand. The doctor makes a small incision, inserts an instrument to take the tissue sample, then closes the incision with a few stitches. The whole procedure usually takes less than half an hour.

Who does it?

A urologist or male fertility specialist with surgical experience.

Where is it done?

If performed under general anesthesia, in the operating room of a hospital. If performed under local anesthesia with a sedative, the procedure can take place in the examining room at a properly equipped clinic or doctor's office.

When in my wife's cycle?

If the reason for the biopsy is **azoospermia** (no sperm) or **oligospermia** (very low sperm count), then it probably doesn't matter when you have it done. But if there is reason to believe that you are producing at least some sperm with the ability to fertilize an egg, then you should probably set the date for the test after your wife has already ovulated for the month. That way, by the time she ovulates again you will have fully recovered from the test.

Is it necessary?

In most cases, no. Testicular biopsy should only be performed if your semen analysis or your blood hormone levels lead your doctor to suspect that there is a structural or chemical problem in your testicles. It should certainly not be routine for a man with normal or near-normal sperm. The decision to perform the biopsy should be based on at least three separate sperm samples taken several weeks apart, to rule out the possibility of the abnormal sample being a chance event.

Will it need to be repeated?

No.

Will it hurt?

Yes, as with any procedure requiring an incision there will be pain, but probably a lot less than you'd expect. The site of the incision will be sore after the anesthetic wears off, and most men will feel a general ache in the testicle for a day or so afterward, but a good painkiller should keep it within bearable limits. Ask your doctor to write you a prescription ahead of time, so that you can have it on hand to take the minute the anesthetic begins to wear off.

COULD THERE BE COMPLICATIONS?

Yes, surgery always entails some risk of infection, swelling, and scarring, but if your biopsy is performed by an experienced doctor, your chances for complications should be minimal.

WILL IT BE NECESSARY TO TAKE TIME OFF FROM WORK?

Yes, at least one full day, and preferably two. It makes sense to schedule your biopsy on a Thursday, take Friday off as well, and then have a full weekend to rest before going back to work.

ANY SPECIAL PREPARATIONS?

Yes. If your biopsy is to be performed under general anesthesia, you should first be interviewed by the anesthesiologist for any information about past allergic reactions or other points in your medical history that could affect the choice of the anesthetic drug to be administered. Go wearing the loosest, most comfortable underwear you own. You will probably want your wife or a close friend to go with you, to drive you home afterward, especially if you have had general anesthesia, or were given a sedative before administration of local anesthesia.

HOW WILL I FEEL AFTERWARD?

Well, you won't feel like doing any bareback horseriding for a while, but you should feel a great deal better within a day or two. If you don't, call your doctor. Some men report that wearing an athletic supporter for the next few days is helpful.

Vasography

WHAT IS IT?

An X ray of the vas deferens after the injection of a radio-opaque dye.

OVERTESTING VERSUS UNDERTESTING

Which to watch out for?

Both!

After analyzing over a hundred surveys and interview notes I found that the majority of patients had cause for complaint, either about overtesting or undertesting. Some patients said that they languished far too many months in the testing phase, with time running short for treatment. Other patients were not tested enough, leading their doctors to miss the true cause of their infertility and put them through months of useless and expensive drug therapies.

Which problem is the more prevalent? The answer was surprising to me (since my own experience of too many tests had led me to assume that this would be the case with others), but more of my respondents reported lack of adequate testing than those who reported too much. As a result I heard many stories such as this one:

After being unsuccessful with IUI [intra-uterine insemination] for five cycles, more testing was recommended. I later discovered that these tests should have been done *before* IUI.

Rhonda from Connecticut

. . . and this one:

My OB-GYN assured me that hormones could not possibly be my problem, as he had done a single blood test during my first appointment. This was a serious mistake. My past medical history indicated problems in the area of hormones. Low levels of progesterone were later discovered through proper testing by a specialist. I remain angry at the enormous amount of time lost in my pursuit of having a child—not to mention the financial implications.

Meg from California

. . . and this one:

My first doctor put me on Pergonal without doing a laparoscopy, though I did have some symptoms of endometriosis. Not abdominal

(continued)

cramping, but cramping in other parts of the body, but no other symptoms, so the doctor said a laparoscopy wasn't necessary. When I went to another clinic to pursue more advanced treatment, they did a laparoscopy and found endometriosis, and cleaned it out.

*E*llen from New Jersey

*F*rom talks with patients from both sides of the testing dilemma, a few commonsense rules emerge:

On undertesting: If you have been in treatment for your infertility more than six cycles without success, and you have *not* had all the tests described in this book, you could be missing some valuable information about your condition that you could get from further testing. Ask your doctor about the advisability of any test you have still not had. If the doctor cannot give you a very persuasive reason why the test is not worthwhile, seek a second opinion on it.

On overtesting: If you have been more than six months in the testing phase and have had all the tests listed in this book once (and perhaps some more than once, or you have had some other tests not listed here), then you are probably being overtested. It's time to take the plunge and try a treatment. If your doctor does not agree, then it's time to find a new doctor.

WHAT DOES IT REVEAL?

A blockage at the point in the man's tubes where the dye stops.

HOW IS IT DONE?

First the doctor injects the dye through a small incision in one of the sperm ducts. As the patient is X-rayed, the doctor watches to see how the dye flows through his system. Sometimes this procedure is done at the same time as the testicular biopsy, either with the patient under general anesthesia (as described in that section) or under a local anesthetic with a sedative—though the combining of the two tests is controversial. Since the vas duct is such a tiny, delicate thing, it is quite susceptible to damage as the dye-laden needle is introduced; therefore some doctors argue that a vasogram should always been done separately, and only when the urologist is equipped to perform microsurgery on the spot to repair any damage that may occur. If your doctor suggests scheduling your vasogram at the time of your testicular biopsy, you might consider seeking a second opinion.

Who does it?

A urologist, or male fertility specialist, or radiologist experienced at the procedure.

Where is it done?

In the radiology department of a hospital, or if done at the same time as the testicular biopsy, in the hospital's day surgery department (for patients who will go home the same day). Some large fertility clinics or urologists' offices may have their own X-ray equipment.

When in my wife's cycle?

Since the reason most men have the test is that their semen contains no sperm, then it doesn't matter when.

Is it necessary?

For most men, no. Vasography is indicated only when there is some cause to suspect an obstruction. If the scrotum on careful examination appears normal, without any swelling or indication of infection, and the man has a normal or near-normal sperm count, and no past history suggesting that a blockage could be the problem, then this test is one to be avoided.

Will it need to be repeated?

No. Subsequent semen analyses should be sufficient to tell whether treatment has repaired the problem.

Will it hurt?

Yes, it's uncomfortable. If done under a local anesthetic and sedative, you can expect some soreness afterward at the point of the insertion of the dye, but within a day or two you can expect to start feeling back to normal.

COULD THERE BE COMPLICATIONS?

Yes, the vas duct may be damaged when the dye needle is introduced, as described above. This needs to be repaired microsurgically soon after it happens.

WILL IT BE NECESSARY TO TAKE TIME OFF FROM WORK?

Yes, at least a half day off, and quite possibly a full day, to recover completely. It may be a good idea to schedule the test on a Friday, so that you will have the weekend to relax.

ANY SPECIAL PREPARATIONS?

Wear your loosest, most comfortable underwear.

HOW WILL I FEEL AFTERWARD?

Sore for a day or two, but after that, back to normal. Call your doctor if any discomfort persists.

CHAPTER FOUR

DIAGNOSIS AND PROGNOSIS

(Meaning, What's Wrong and
Your Chances of Fixing It)

All right, now we're getting somewhere. You have had all your tests and your doctor has told you what's wrong. You've got *googliopigosis*. What does *that* mean? you ask your doctor. She responds: Googliopigosis is an insufficiency of the hormone googliop created by dysfunction of the Pagoogli gland located behind the wazoo.

Okay, you say, not wanting to look stupid . . . but you really have no clue as to what your doctor has said. Maybe you thought of some questions to ask at the time but didn't get the opportunity to ask them, or maybe you did ask them, but found that the doctor's explanation needed further explanation. Don't call and ask again. Just find your diagnosis in this chapter to read answers to the following four questions:

What is it?

What are my options for treatment?

Are there any controversies surrounding this diagnosis?

How does my patient profile—*that is, my age, medical and family history, degree of severity of the condition, and attitude toward medical intervention—affect my prognosis?*

This chapter cannot possibly cover every identified cause of infertility, but it will cover the most commonly diagnosed problems, including female hormonal and ovulatory disorders; endometriosis; blocked fallopian tube(s); uterine abnormalities; recurrent miscarriage; polycystic ovarian disease; premature menopause; pituitary tumor(s); thyroid gland problems; immune system response problems; sperm problems, varicocele; epididymitis and other male infections; excessive testicular heat; retrograde ejaculation; unexplained infertility; and combinations of causes.

154

After you have read about your condition in this chapter, consult the chart in Chapter Five to see what the options are for conservative, moderate, or aggressive forms of treatment. To help you discover which form of treatment you would find most suitable to your personality and physical condition, complete the questionnaire that begins on page 187.

Chapters Six and Seven will contain more detailed discussion of what's involved in each of the different treatment options.

Female Hormonal and Ovulatory Disorders

WHAT IS IT?

You are told you do not ovulate, or that your ovulation is abnormal, because you are producing too many androgens (male hormones), or too much prolactin (a milk-producing hormone that tends to suppress ovulation), or too little estradiol (estrogen in the blood), or too little progesterone for too short a time following ovulation (**luteal-phase defect**).

OPTIONS FOR TREATMENT

There are drugs specifically tailored to certain problems, such as bromocriptine (Parlodel) to suppress prolactin levels or progesterone suppositories to increase the level of that hormone. Also commonly used, either alone or in a wide variety of combinations, are ovulation-inducing drugs, such as Clomid (clomiphene citrate, a relatively mild drug), Pergonal (an extremely potent drug) and Metrodin (also extremely potent). If pregnancy does not result after a certain time period on the drugs prescribed, the doctor will usually increase the dosage or change the type or combination of medication used, or recommend moving on to one of the **assisted reproductive technologies** (**ARTs**), such as **GIFT, ZIFT,** or **IVF.**

CONTROVERSIES

Hormonal disorders tend to be fairly straightforward problems, not difficult to pin down. Research has established what the normal levels of each of the necessary hormones should be. But that does not mean that doctors will generally agree on the best drug to be tried to correct the problem found. More about the controversies surrounding certain drugs in the specific section dealing with each drug (in Chapter Six).

One of the most common problems that different doctors tend to approach differently is luteal-phase defect (insufficient progesterone production in the time between ovulation and the next menstrual period). Some doctors say that this condition (generally identified after an **endometrial biopsy**) is greatly overdiagnosed, and that a one-time abnormal test result is not enough evidence to prove that the problem exists. These doctors will urge that a second or even third EMB be done before prescribing treatment. Other doctors will go ahead and treat the patient with progesterone suppositories based on the results of a single EMB, reasoning that the treatment is low-tech, is relatively inexpensive, and has few side effects, so even if it doesn't help, there is no harm in trying it.

PATIENT PROFILE

Overall, doctors tend to be very successful in inducing ovulation in women with hormonal disorders. Studies have shown that up to 70 percent of nonovulating women can be caused to ovulate on Clomid, and up to 90 percent will ovulate on Pergonal. Of course the odds of conceiving each time you ovulate are much lower—between 6 and 25 percent per cycle, the large variation depending on your age (the older you are, the lower your chances), the influence of outside factors (such as quality of sperm, your cervical mucus, etc.), and a host of other influences, including many that are not yet understood—as well as pure luck.

Patients who are within the normal, medically accepted weight range for their height, whose overall health is good, and who are under thirty-five, have a better response rate to treatment than do those who are either underweight or overweight, those who must contend with other health problems (such as diabetes), or those over thirty-five. After age forty the woman's response to fertility drugs begins to drop off dramatically, and it can be difficult to impossible in many cases for her to get pregnant using her own eggs. A donor egg program may be the ultimate best hope for a woman who seems to be getting nowhere after months on strong fertility drugs.

Endometriosis

WHAT IS IT?

This condition is the overgrowth of tissue from the lining of the uterus (called the **endometrium**) in places outside the uterus. Endometriosis may be found on the **fallopian tubes,** on the outside of the uterus, on the ovaries, or in other parts of the abdominal cavity. The cause is not well understood, although the most prevalent theory is that some of the woman's menstrual flow is going out through her fallopian tubes during her monthly period, instead of flowing down her vagina. Endometriosis can cause painful periods and occasionally pain during intercourse, although it is also possible to have the condition in a mild form without having any symptoms at all.

OPTIONS FOR TREATMENT

Endometriosis can be treated by drugs; three commonly prescribed ones are danazol (brand name: Danocrine), Lupron, and GnRH (sometimes dispensed in the form of a nasal spray under the brand name Synerel). Endometrial adhesions can also be removed either by conventional surgery through an incision in the abdomen (**laparotomy**) or by surgery performed through a tiny incision in the navel (**laparoscopy**), through which a laser is inserted to burn off endometrial adhesions. Moderate to severe endometriosis may involve both drug therapy and surgery. In extreme cases, where endometriosis rapidly grows back despite treatment and causes severe pain, a hysterectomy may ultimately be recommended. (If this should unfortunately turn out to be the result in your case, make sure that your surgeon preserves your ovaries. That way you will still have the option open to you of using a **host uterus** to have a genetically related child.)

Doctors who believe that there is little direct relationship between endometriosis and infertility (see section immediately below for controversy) will urge patients not to bother with the usual six-month drug regimen, but move right to high-tech methods, such as IVF, to attempt to have a baby.

CONTROVERSIES

Endometriosis is one of the most hotly debated topics in the entire infertility field. Some doctors believe the condition is responsible for up to 40 percent of all cases of female infertility. Other doctors argue that endometriosis can be found to one degree or another in the majority of women who are perfectly fertile, and that it is only rarely the real reason behind a woman's failure to conceive. To see how widely divergent the views of different, respected, mainstream doctors are, let's look at what three different doctors have to say about endometriosis.

First, let's hear from Dr. Robert R. Franklin, writing (with Dorothy Kay Brockman) in *In Pursuit of Fertility: A Consultation with a Specialist:* "A 'benign' invasive disease that affects between four and ten million women in the United States alone, endometriosis is one of the major causes of infertility" (p. 26). "Adhesions—the enemy of fertility—are one of the most common complications associated with endometriosis. . . . Adhesions can be filmy and cobweblike or dense and fibrous. . . . Even the delicate weblike adhesions can cause infertility if they keep the fallopian tubes (oviducts) from picking up the egg. . . . The weblike adhesions can be removed during a minor surgical procedure, but major surgery is necessary to eliminate dense scar tissue" (p. 27).

Now read what Dr. Sherman J. Silber has to say in his book *How to Get Pregnant with the New Technology:* "Among some doctors 'endometriosis' is considered the major cause of infertility. . . . In truth, endometriosis is a more controversial condition than some would give it credit for, and although it is an extremely frequent diagnosis associated with hospital and surgery bills for infertility-related procedures, its relationship to infertility is highly mysterious and the treatment of it is questionable" (p. 202). "Controlled studies have demonstrated that women who have 'moderate' or 'minimal' lesion endometriosis that is treated have no greater pregnancy rate than women who go with no treatment at all. So the question comes up whether endometriosis actually causes infertility or is in some way caused by some other factors that are associated with infertility. If that were the case, then removing the endometriosis would do nothing to improve the woman's fertility" (p. 203).

And now for the views of Dr. Derek Llewellyn-Jones in *Getting Pregnant: A Guide for the Infertile Couple:* "One rather picturesque theory [for how endometriosis causes infertility] is that the endometrial tissue produces substances that seduce the ovum away from the entrance to the fallopian tube. . . . Another theory is that the endometriosis provokes the body to release immunologically competent microphage cells into the fallopian tube, where they 'eat' the egg or the sperms" (p. 135). "These results [of a survey discussed in a preceding paragraph] indicate that moderate to severe endometriosis found unexpectedly during infertility investigations, and all cases of endometriosis that produce menstrual pain or pain on intercourse, require treatment. . . . The more extensive the disease, the greater is the need for surgery, and the lower the subsequent pregnancy rate. Less extensive endometriosis responds to the use of hormonal drugs, especially danazol" (p. 136).

Well, with that degree of disagreement, what's the poor patient to think? Sensible advice and support from others who have been there before you can best be found through membership in the Endometriosis Association, a patients' self-help organization (address listed in the Resource Guide at the back of this book) or through RESOLVE.

Nearly all doctors (even those who argue that endometriosis is not a significant causative factor in infertility) agree that the more extensive and long-term your endometriosis is, the more difficulty you will have in getting pregnant. Much depends on what other factors, if any, are found along with endometriosis. The woman with the condition who gets pregnant but then experiences an early miscarriage each time at least will be reassured that she is fertile, and her prognosis for treatment to allow her to carry a fetus to term is generally optimistic. The woman whose endometriosis is linked to ovulation problems, on the other hand, may find herself facing a dilemma: the fertility drugs normally given to boost the production of eggs commonly will increase the growth of endometriosis, too. She may find herself leaning toward surgery as the preferred means to eliminate the growths, to allow her to use ovulation-inducing drugs with less worry about side effects. Of course, much depends on the patient's depth of desire to have a child and her willingness to subject herself to surgery rather than first try other, slower, drug-therapy approaches.

The truly aggressive patient, especially if she is over thirty-five, may find her most favorable course of action is to go straight to one of the high-tech (and enormously high-cost) ARTs, such as IVF (if the endometriosis has affected her fallopian tubes) or GIFT or ZIFT (if her tubes are completely normal).

Blocked Fallopian Tube(s)

WHAT IS IT?

The egg is not able to travel from the ovary to the uterus, or sperm are not able to swim up from the uterus to reach the egg, because of an obstruction, or **occlusion**, somewhere along the fallopian tube. If both tubes are blocked, the woman has no chance of conceiving normally without treatment. If only one tube is blocked, then she still may be able to conceive—but seen over the long term, her odds of doing so are only half as good as a woman with both tubes open (or **patent**, as your doctor might put it). Tubes may be blocked, either partially or

GETTING A DIAGNOSIS OF ENDOMETRIOSIS

Three Washington, D.C., Patients Talk About Their Experiences

I had pain for ten years. I saw eight doctors. Endometriosis is a mysterious disease. I didn't fit the pattern, so it was hard to diagnose. I only had pain after my period had stopped. I had pain with bowel movements. We ended up doing a lot of research on our own in a medical library. I had to bring information on my condition to the doctor, to help him arrive at the diagnosis.

Cheryl

*E*ndometriosis is a "disease of decisions." There is no one right answer for it. The patient has to keep doing a cost-benefit analysis, to weigh how much you can take physically and mentally. You need a doctor who will give you information. If you don't have that, you have the wrong doctor.

Helen, who serves as a patient-contact for the Endometriosis Association (a volunteer self-help network)

I ended up researching my own problem. My endometriosis symptoms did not match up with the doctors' textbook understanding of the disease. My husband went to a medical library and read the latest journals (books are not as good, since they become outdated quickly). One book said that bowel pain was a symptom, which was what I had. I told my doctor what I'd learned, but he pooh-poohed it. He still didn't think I needed a laparoscopy. He said I still had "unexplained infertility." After switching doctors I found one who agreed to do a laparoscopy. I wasn't looking forward to it—it was *not* fun—but it was worthwhile. Now I advise other patients to find a doctor who is knowledgeable about endometriosis and is willing to *listen* to you.

Sharon

completely, by scar tissue left over from past **pelvic inflammatory disease** (**PID**), from endometriosis, or from scar tissue caused by past abdominal surgery, or the blockage could even be congenital (present since birth). A related problem to blocked tubes is lack of *cilia,* the tiny hair-like structures that line the inside of the fallopian tube and help to push the egg along its path to the uterus.

OPTIONS FOR TREATMENT

The blockage may be removed surgically, either by burning it away with a laser or by cutting it out with a scalpel. A relatively new method is the balloon tuboplasty, a procedure in which a tiny uninflated balloon is threaded inside the tube and then inflated, causing the tube to open up. If only one tube is damaged, some doctors, rather than subject the patient to surgical attempts at repair, will simply try to boost the woman's chance to conceive each month by making the ovary on the "good side" work harder, by giving her ovulation-inducing drugs to produce multiple eggs each cycle. If both tubes are so badly damaged that surgery is unlikely to restore normal tubal functioning, then the woman's remaining option is IVF, a procedure which bypasses the tubes entirely—although the overall success rates for IVF at most clinics are only 10 to 16 percent.

CONTROVERSIES

A blockage is a mechanical defect that is either there or not. Everyone agrees that blockages prevent conception, and everyone agrees that removing the blockage is a logical approach to take to facilitate conception. But many women still do not conceive within the first six months after the blockage has been repaired. The question is, How long is it reasonable for the couple to keep on trying in the normal (medically unassisted) way before moving on to fertility drugs or IVF? If your doctor has scheduled an operation to open your tubes, you will be wise to find out beforehand what his views are on this point. That way, if your view and his view turn out to be very different (say, he wants you to wait at least a year before trying fertility drugs, while you are intent on boosting your odds to conceive as soon as possible), you will be able to look around for another doctor to operate on you who is in sync with your personal timetable.

The major factor with blocked tubes is whether one or both are impaired. Obviously the patient with one working tube has a much more optimistic prognosis than the one with none. Also affecting outcome of surgery is the patient's tendency (predictable by her reaction to any past surgeries) to form thick scar tissue afterward around the site of any cutting. If new scar tissue forms, the operation could result in additional blockages and actually make things worse. Her age and overall health, as always, play a role in determining her likelihood of conceiving after treatment.

Uterine Abnormality

What is it?

In the case of a uterine abnormality, the woman's uterus cannot sustain an embryo because it is too small, or because it is poorly positioned (it may be prolapsed, or sinking down into her vaginal canal), or because it contains abnormal growths such as polyps or **fibroid tumors,** or because it is divided into two chambers (**bicornuate**), or because it consists only of one side (**unicornuate**), or because there is a partial dividing wall of tissue (a **septum**) in the middle. Many of these conditions are found in women whose mothers took the antimiscarriage drug DES when they were pregnant with their daughters.

Options for treatment

A dividing wall or septum needs to be surgically removed. Fibroids and polyps are also excised on the operating table, and the prolapsed uterus will be surgically "pinned" in place. The woman whose uterus is too small may conceive but will often miscarry early or midway through her pregnancy (see the section on **recurrent miscarriage** for more detail); many doctors say that the uterus may be stretched by pregnancy and so be left in a better condition afterward to carry a subsequent pregnancy to term—although most women will be left unhappy by the thrust of this advice. It's disconcerting to be told your best chance to have a baby is to suffer a late miscarriage and hope that next time your uterus will be more hospitable. In cases that cannot be surgically improved, the couple's best hope of having a genetically related child is to find a woman willing to serve as a host uterus and carry the couple's fertilized egg (implanted through a ZIFT or IVF cycle) to term for them.

Doctors disagree most often about when to consider a patient's uterine problems too severe for her to have a reasonable chance of ever carrying a baby to term. Conservative doctors will advise their patients not to subject themselves to operations, or not to go on conceiving and miscarrying in the hope of delivering safely, when they could be using their time productively in pursuing adoption or some other alternative. More aggressive-minded doctors will encourage their patients to continue trying to have a baby, with or without surgical intervention, until there is finally not even a very slight degree of reproductive capability left.

PATIENT PROFILE

The degree of the problem is what determines how good the chances are that you can be helped by surgery (or that you could conceive and carry a baby to term without surgery). Past reproductive history provides important clues, too: for example, if you have been able to conceive before, even if you miscarried, then your prognosis is better than if you haven't. In assessing yourself, think long and hard about the kind of hardships you are willing to undergo (operations or miscarriages) for perhaps only slightly improved odds of carrying a pregnancy to term. Make sure your doctor is providing you with a bluntly realistic picture of the efficacy in your case of any operation he recommends.

Recurrent Miscarriage

WHAT IS IT?

Recurrent miscarriage—your doctor will probably prefer the term *habitual abortion*—is possibly the saddest of all diagnoses. The woman is able to conceive and the embryo will implant itself in the uterine wall but then will abort (the medical term), or miscarry (the colloquial term), typically before twelve weeks' gestation. Causes may be poor hormonal production or uterine abnormality (discussed in previous sections), or production of antibodies that attack the embryo (discussed under Immune System Response Problems, page 172). A frequent cause of miscarriage in the population at large is known as *blighted ovum,* which occurs when the genetic material inside the fertilized egg is faulty, and the embryo does not receive the instructions it needs to develop normally. However, this type of genetic error is thought to occur randomly and thus a miscarriage due to blighted ovum is believed to be unlikely to happen to the same woman twice.

OPTIONS FOR TREATMENT

Progesterone by suppository or injection is generally given when poor hormonal production is suspected, usually through the first eight, twelve, or sixteen weeks of the pregnancy. After the first trimester (as the first twelve weeks are called) bed rest (complete or partial) may be ordered. If the woman is prone to contractions of the cervix (called "premature labor," and sometimes attributed to a condition known as **incompetent cervix**), the doctor may perform a **cervical cerclage** (also called a Shirodkar stitch), in which, under local anesthesia, the doctor sews up the opening of the cervix to prevent the cervix from dilating and releasing the fetus too soon. The stitch is removed around the thirty-sixth or thirty-seventh week of gestation (assuming that premature labor can be held off that long). Drugs (a commonly used one is called Terbutaline) may also be given to halt or limit the contractions of premature labor. Terbutaline has been in use for many years and has generally been shown to have no harmful impact on the developing fetus.

If the woman has been tested and has been found to have an immunological response problem (her system is producing antibodies that attack the embryo or fetus), she may be put on any of a number of drugs designed to reduce or alter the production of harmful chemicals—though the efficacy of any of such drug therapies has not been conclusively demonstrated in large-scale studies.

Another possible cause of recurrent miscarriage is attack on the embryo by infectious agents in the womb. Analysis of the aborted tissue is most helpful in determining the type of antibiotic needed to eradicate the particular bacterium that is found.

CONTROVERSIES

The usefulness of progesterone in preventing early miscarriage has been called into question. Many doctors strongly believe in it, as do many of the mothers I have interviewed who had healthy, full-term babies after taking the drug, but who had experienced miscarriages without it. However, you should be aware that the FDA has classified all progestins (the class of drugs that includes progesterone) as involving risk of birth defects to the fetus, including heart, limb, and genital malformations. When I was pregnant with my daughter and taking the drug, I consulted RESOLVE to see if that organization could shed any light on the controversy. A registered nurse answered my query with a reassuring letter to the effect that only synthetic versions of the drug have been linked to fetal defects. Controlled studies of natural progesterone (which was the form of the drug that I was taking, and the *only* type that should be supplied to a pregnant woman) show no greater incidence of birth defects than that found in the population at large.

Another subject of dispute: How many miscarriages do you need to suffer to be classified as at risk for recurrent miscarriage? Two? Three? More? Can you be classified as a recurrent miscarriage risk if no underlying cause is found, or must your experience be chalked up as just bad luck? Some doctors will start treating women aggressively, after the second or even the first miscarriage, prescribing progesterone or bed rest right away. Others will tell you, even after three miscarriages, if no underlying cause is found, that you should just take it easy and have faith this time that things will go well. You will want to find a physician whose willingness to treat your condition (or leave it alone) matches your own level of desire to try drugs or other medical measures, or let nature take its course.

PATIENT PROFILE

The number of past miscarriages and the cause(s), if any are known, are key to assessing the patient's chances of carrying a baby to term. Age is also important, as the risk of miscarriage rises sharply through the late thirties, and may be as high as 40 percent when the patient is in her forties. Balanced against that statistic is the more encouraging news that some 70 to 90 percent of women who miscarry eventually will carry a baby to term. The woman's chances go up if her overall health is good (e.g., she is not diabetic or extremely overweight or underweight, does not have high blood pressure, and does not smoke, abuse drugs, drink alcohol, or work with toxic chemicals while pregnant), if she takes the prescribed dose of prenatal vitamins each day, avoids strenuous physical activity, and keeps stress to a minimum.

Horrible as this will sound, the woman who has experienced a miscarriage will improve her doctor's chance of discovering the source of her problem if she gathers up any fetal tissue she is able to recover from the miscarriage and bring it in for examination. The miscarried remains are the clearest source of information about what has gone wrong. You will feel more positive afterward if you take this step, because you will know that something beneficial has been learned that may lead you to prevent a reoccurrence and deliver a healthy child.

*M*y problem wasn't getting pregnant but staying pregnant. I went through three miscarriages before I had my son. I felt my case was mishandled by the fertility doctors I saw. They tended to think their job was over as soon as my pregnancy test came back positive. I didn't really get the attention I felt I needed until I saw an OB-GYN who specialized in high-risk pregnancy. He did tests that none of my other doctors had done. He put me on double the dosage of progesterone that I had taken with the previous pregnancies. I also think it helped that I stayed in bed most of the first three months of my pregnancy with my son [although this was not something her doctor said was necessary].

*S*hirley from New York

Polycystic Ovarian Disease (PCO)

What is it?

Polycystic ovarian disease, also called Stein-Leventhal Syndrome, is a set of symptoms indicating that the ovaries are producing too many male hormones, resulting in follicles within the ovaries that fail to release their eggs and remain as water-filled cysts. Typical symptoms include excessive facial and body hair, irregular periods, enlarged ovaries, obesity, acne, and oily skin, although many patients with PCO exhibit no outward signs of the disease.

Options for treatment

Doctors usually prescribe fertility drugs (Clomid or Pergonal) to induce ovulation. Sometimes steroidal drugs, such as prednisone or dexamethasone, will be used to suppress production of androgens (male hormones). In moderate to severe cases, surgery may be performed: either an "ovarian wedge resection" in which part of the ovary is removed to reduce the ovary's androgen-producing capabilities, or a newer operation (that now has all but replaced the ovarian wedge resection), involving "laser drilling" into the ovary to achieve the same result with less risk of scar formation. For mild cases of PCO, all that may be needed is some life-style modification. The obese patient is put on a diet of five or six very small low-fat and low-sugar meals a day; she is also urged to stick to a regular routine of low-impact aerobic exercises and to avoid overwork and stress. All of these changes are believed to bring about a change in the woman's brain chemistry, leading to improved use of estrogen in the reproductive system.

Fertility drugs may also be used in conjunction with the life-style modification program, and if after a period of time there is still no conception, GIFT or ZIFT, with or without the use of donor eggs, may be considered.

CONTROVERSIES

Older doctors will sometimes stick to the ovarian wedge resection procedure that they learned during their training, which more up-to-date doctors believe should be completely abandoned in favor of the less invasive laser-drilling procedure. But there is also a school of thought that contends that surgery is *not* the way to deal with PCO, that life-style changes—with or without the use of fertility drugs—should always be tried first. The patient diagnosed with PCO will want to find out what school her doctor follows and why. If surgery is recommended, a second opinion is a good idea. You still may end up choosing surgery, but only after you have tried the diet and exercise program for a time and have still not conceived.

PATIENT PROFILE

The earlier PCO is caught, the better the prospects for a nonsurgical cure. Severe, long-term PCO generally responds poorly to drug therapy, and even after surgery may reappear. The best the long-term PCO sufferer may be able to do is to halt the disease for a few months to a year, try by the most aggressive means possible to conceive within that time window (such as with Pergonal, GIFT, or ZIFT), and hope to succeed before the ovaries again fill up with cysts.

Premature Menopause

What is it?

The woman's ovaries start to fail years before the usual age for menopause, and she no longer produces sufficient hormones to sustain the normal cycle of ovulation and menstruation.

Options for treatment

If signs of ovarian dysfunction have just begun, it may be possible to stimulate ovarian activity and hormone production needed for conception with high doses of powerful fertility drugs. However, success rates with this treatment are usually low. ARTs such as GIFT and ZIFT may also be recommended, but with odds for success far less than those for women whose infertility has other causes. One study I saw concerned women who sought treatment just as the first signs of menopause appeared. The pregnancy rate as a result of GIFT and ZIFT on these patients (called *premenopausal,* rather than prematurely menopausal) was no better than 5 percent. However, in those premenopausal patients who attempted GIFT and ZIFT using donor eggs, pregnancy rates very closely approximated those of nonmenopausal women in the study group.

Controversies

Many clinics will limit the number of treatment options for prematurely menopausal women, barring them from entering programs of IVF, ZIFT, or GIFT on the grounds that the chances for success are too low (and also, that these hard-to-treat patients will lower the clinic's overall success statistics). Other clinics will take all comers, but may not fully inform their prematurely menopausal patients of the high odds against them, letting them spend tens of thousands of dollars on failed cycle after failed cycle.

When a woman is experiencing menopause early, but not so early as to be classified as premature (let's say she is forty-three or forty-four), debate has sometimes centered on whether she is too old to try for first-time motherhood. Articles in medical journals have questioned the ethics of devoting so much of our limited medical resources toward achieving pregnancy in women at the end of their childbearing years, who may lack the stamina and longevity needed to take on the twenty-year commitment to child rearing. Responses to these articles, on the other hand, have pointed to studies showing that first-time mothers over forty these days have a life-expectancy in the mid to upper eighties and generally show an extraordinary degree of love and commitment to their late-born children.

Another, far more inflammatory ethical issue surrounds the use of donor eggs. For a discussion of a few of the pros and cons on that subject, see page 281.

PATIENT PROFILE

Age and point at which the condition is diagnosed are most strongly correlated with patient's chance of success. The earlier in the patient's life that the menopausal symptoms set in, the worse her prognosis for reversal. But if treatment can be initiated soon after the first signs of ovarian failure appear, then she may have a reasonably good chance at conceiving a child before full menopause sets in. For women who choose to use donor eggs, age is far less significant a factor.

Pituitary Tumor(s)

WHAT IS IT?

Pituitary tumors (also called "prolactinomas") are benign, very tiny (even microscopic) growths on the pituitary gland in the brain. The tumors can affect the production of the hormone that in men stimulates the testicles to produce sperm and in women stimulates the ovary to ripen the egg.

OPTIONS FOR TREATMENT

Pituitary tumors may be treated with drugs, such as bromocriptine (Parlodel) to reduce excessive prolactin levels associated with the condition, though some doctors still advise removing the tumors surgically, despite both risk and expense to the patient.

CONTROVERSIES

The question of surgery for prolactinoma excites passions in the infertility field. Opponents say that the brain operation is dangerous and not necessarily more effective than drug therapy, while proponents say that in many cases without surgery the patient's condition will worsen to the point where it can no longer be fixed by any means. To illustrate the debate, let's take a look at what two eminent fertility specialists have written.

In his book *In Pursuit of Fertility: A Consultation with a Specialist*, Dr. Robert R. Franklin states his opinion that a tumor should be excised before it becomes too big to treat successfully with drug therapy. "Once a tumor reaches an advanced stage, pregnancy is less likely." The operation he favors is the "formidably named 'transnasal trans-sphenoidal resection,' [which] has a low mortality rate (between 0 and 2 percent) in highly skilled hands. The prognosis generally is excellent, especially if the tumor is small and the prolactin level has not skyrocketed. The tumor is eradicated, or at least significantly reduced in size. Since the patient's prolactin level often normalizes, pregnancy may follow, or at least the patient is rendered more susceptible to the medications that induce ovulation. The initial cure rate after surgery for small prolactinomas is high, and many patients remain symptomless for years" (p. 148).

Now hear what Drs. Gary S. Berger and Marc Goldstein have to say about surgery as a treatment option in their book (also coauthored by Mark Fuerst) *The Couple's Guide to Fertility:* "The best treatment is therapy with the drug bromocriptine (Parlodel) to lower prolactin levels and reduce the size of a tumor, if present, that's producing the excess prolactin. About half the impotent men taking bromocriptine become potent again. Surgery to remove tumors within the man's brain has been tried, but can be dangerous, and generally is no longer recommended" (p. 213).

The upshot of the doctors' disagreement is, as usual, that the couple must make a tough decision though not themselves expert at evaluating the pros and cons—either that, or place blind faith in their doctor's judgment.

PATIENT PROFILE

How you respond to a recommendation for brain surgery depends a great deal on your attitude toward surgery in general. Some people seek to avoid being cut into at all costs, and will certainly be more at ease seeking out a doctor who will try to reduce the prolactinoma with drug therapy alone. Others, whose primary goal is to get rid of whatever stands in the way of pregnancy by the quickest, surest means possible, will not blanch at the prospect of an operation, but will be relieved that something real has been discovered that can be excised. Those who opt for surgery should still seek a second opinion, however—just as a safety precaution (also because most health insurance policies will require it). It's also wise to seek out the best neurosurgeon available, even if it means exceeding your insurance company's reimbursement limits to pay the surgeon's fee. You can then proceed to the operating room with peace of mind that you are in the most skilled hands you could find.

Thyroid Gland Problem

WHAT IS IT?

The thyroid is a gland in the throat that affects the body's metabolism. An underactive gland produces a condition called hypothyroidism, which is sometimes the underlying cause of fertility problems in both women and men. In women hypothyroidism is most often indicated by excessive levels of the hormone prolactin.

OPTIONS FOR TREATMENT

Most common and effective is use of synthetic thyroid hormones. The length and dosage will vary according to the severity of the case being treated.

CONTROVERSIES

Many doctors who find excessive prolactin levels in their patients do not think it necessary to seek out the underlying cause. They simply put the patient on bromocriptine (Parlodel) to bring the prolactin level down to normal. Other doctors follow the rule that any time you find an excessive prolactin level you do a follow-up blood test for thyroid stimulating hormone (TSH), to see if a malfunctioning thyroid gland could be the cause. If it is, then you correct that problem, not its symptom.

PATIENT PROFILE

Thyroid problems are associated with a variety of bodily ills, not just infertility. Patients often must struggle with eye problems, sudden weight loss or gain, or overall feeling of fatigue or depression. The fertility problem may need to take a backseat to care for the patient's general health. It may be a good idea to get your TSH level normalized first, then continue the investigation into your reproductive functioning to see if any other impediments to conception exist, or if measures to boost ovulation are warranted.

Immune System Response Problems

What is it?

Either the man or woman may produce antibodies (substances manufactured by the body's immune system to fight disease) that attack the sperm as if they were invading germs. In the man's case the antibodies kill his own sperm; in the woman's case the antibodies create a hostile environment for the sperm in her cervical mucus, and they die, or become unable to navigate through the mucus to find the egg, or else become too weakened to fertilize the egg when they find it. Cervical mucus may also become an inhospitable medium for sperm if it becomes too acidic or too thick. When a woman produces "hostile cervical mucus," she is sometimes referred to as having an "allergic reaction" to sperm. Antibodies may also be produced in response to the presence of an embryo in a pregnant woman, in which case she will suffer recurrent miscarriage (discussed on page 163).

Options for treatment

Either husband or wife, or both, may be prescribed steroids such as cortisone, prednisone, or dexamethasone to reduce the body's immune system response. However, serious side effects can result, including high blood pressure, complications to pre-existing ulcers, hip-joint problems, and increased risk of pneumonia.

If the immune system response is believed to be a temporary sensitization, then "condom therapy" may be recommended for a period of time (six months on average). The couple use condoms each time they have intercourse, limiting the woman's exposure to the man's sperm to allow her body's immune system to stop producing the antibodies. After the couple is allowed to resume intercourse without condoms, the woman has a **postcoital test** (see page 129 for description) to determine whether her cervical mucus has returned to normal.

When the woman's cervical mucus response is in the form of incorrect acidity, she may simply be instructed to douche regularly with a specific solution to bring the pH of her vagina to the proper level.

Another simple—though somewhat expensive—option is to bypass the cervical mucus altogether, putting the sperm directly into the woman's uterus through the artificial insemination procedure known as **IUI** (intra-uterine insemination). A newer procedure may also be available, ITI, or intratubal insemination, in which the husband's sperm is loaded into an ultrafine catheter, which is guided up through the uterus and into the opening of the fallopian tube, where the sperm are then deposited.

For the couple seeking a more aggressive treatment course, the woman's egg production may be increased through use of strong fertility drugs, and then her eggs may be retrieved and mixed with sperm in her fallopian tubes through the GIFT procedure, or fertilized in a lab dish and reinserted in her uterus in the IVF procedure.

CONTROVERSIES

Yet another hotly debated subject in the fertility field. This is because the body's immune system functioning is not one of the better understood processes in our bodies (if it were, we would have a cure for AIDS by now). We still don't really understand why some people's bodies will manufacture antibodies to attack natural substances like sperm, or like a developing embryo, that the normal body not only tolerates but actually nurtures. Different researchers offer different speculations, leading clinical physicians to lean toward different approaches in treatment.

Then there is a school of thought that suggests that a poor immune system response is not a cause of infertility at all. In his book *How to Get Pregnant with the New Technology,* Dr. Sherman J. Silber says that the diagnosis may sometimes be the result of testing the woman at the wrong time in her cycle, when her mucus is naturally hostile to sperm; poor mucus may also be due to hormonal deficiencies, not antibodies. In any case, he concludes that six months of condom therapy is nearly always a waste of the couple's precious time, and that prednisone's side effects can be so severe that the drug should be avoided if at all possible (pp. 163–164).

Furthermore, a problem exists with the present methods used to diagnose a problematic immune system response. Tests, whether of blood, semen, or cervical mucus, can give ambiguous results, leaving the doctor unable to tell whether the antibodies found are a response to sperm or to some bacteria in the man's or woman's system. Dr. Attila Toth, in his highly controversial book *The Fertility Solution: A Revolutionary Approach to Reversing Infertility,* argues that bacteriological infection is the single most underdiagnosed cause of infertility, and that couples with high levels of antibodies in their systems would be best advised to try some intensive antibiotic therapy to rid themselves of suspect bacteria, before trying six months of condom therapy.

PATIENT PROFILE

The couple whose infertility is attributed to an immune system response problem should first consider their own medical histories to see if either could have picked up a perhaps symptomless infection that could be producing the immune response. Past infections that were treated but not eradicated could also be culprits. Since a course of antibiotics is less onerous to the couple than six months of condom therapy, they may wish to explore that treatment path first.

The couple who are most anxious to achieve pregnancy in the quickest way should probably go right to a program of fertility drugs combined with IUI.

The doctor checked my husband's sperm for antibodies. The results weren't very good. The doctor told me, "If you ever needed proof you were not going to get pregnant, this is it—your husband has shitty sperm." Not only was I outraged that he would talk to me that way, but I knew it wasn't true. [This couple had already had one child without medical intervention and were trying to have a second.] I knew you couldn't reach that conclusion on the basis of a single sample. My husband had another sperm sample analyzed somewhere else and the results were excellent. I called the doctor three months later to let him know I was pregnant.

Emily from New York

Sperm Problems

WHAT IS IT?

Sperm may be infertile or less fertile for a variety of reasons. Semen may have too few sperm present (oligospermia), or no sperm present (azoospermia), too many sperm badly shaped (have two tails, or no tail, or the wrong-size head, or two heads, or other malformations) or too many sperm that can't swim well (poor motility). Underlying causes for the sperm problem may be hormonal (e.g., poor production of FSH or LH) or structural (e.g., a blockage in the sperm ducts or absence of the sperm-producing cells in the testicle) or part of a complex syndrome linked to a disease or condition (such as diabetes, which is sometimes associated with **retrograde ejaculation**—discussed separately on page 181).

OPTIONS FOR TREATMENT

There are basically five ways to approach a sperm problem:

1. try to fix the sperm through drug therapy
2. surgically correct a defect found in the testicles or elsewhere in his reproductive system that is preventing the production or ejaculation of fertile sperm
3. try to make the wife/partner superfertile so that the few sperm that are present and capable of fertilizing an egg will encounter many eggs in the fallopian tubes
4. attempt to control fertilization in the laboratory through micro-manipulation of sperm and egg (for example, by drilling a micro-scopic hole in the egg and injecting a single sperm into it)
5. use donor sperm to artificially inseminate the woman (though tech-nically this is not really a "treatment" for faulty sperm)

Any of the first four options may be tried in various combinations.

CONTROVERSIES

Improving sperm count and sperm quality is a tricky business. Drugs commonly have a variety of unpleasant side effects and are not highly effective. In cases of severe oligospermia or with azoospermia, many urologists find drug treatment to be pointless. How soon and under what conditions the doctor will recommend use of donor sperm varies greatly from doctor to doctor.

Whether the doctor advocates trying to make the woman superfertile at the same time as the male is undergoing treatment depends to some extent on what specialty the doctor practices: a fertility specialist who treats both sexes is more likely to advocate measures for both partners, while a male-only specialist will concentrate entirely on his male patient's problem. If the couple wish to be very aggressive in their attempt at conception, and the male-specialist doctor does *not* refer the woman to a doctor who can boost her fertility, the couple should raise the question with the doctor themselves, or perhaps seek treatment at a facility equipped to work with both husband and wife.

PATIENT PROFILE

The degree of the sperm problem is closely correlated to the chance of rectifying it. That is to say, the lower your sperm count, the less likely it is that drugs will make a difference.

When both the man and woman are put on powerful fertility drugs, both must be of the same mind as to what risks and sacrifices they are willing to undertake to try for pregnancy. Women treated under the superovulation approach can easily find themselves resenting having their bodies manipulated and made to endure side effects when it's not *their* problem. If this happens in your case, some joint counseling may be in order to help both partners come to a decision about how much they as a couple are willing to go through to have a child that is biologically related to both.

Much also depends on the patients' financial resources. The newest approach, micromanipulation of sperm and egg, is still considered "experimental" (meaning uninsurable) by virtually all health insurance companies, and only the couple who are well off (or really desperate to have a biologically related child) will be able to give this option serious consideration. The couple should also be aware that there are still very few clinics sophisticated enough to perform the micromanipulation techniques, and that so far results are not especially encouraging.

The couple who are not anxious to try everything to have the husband's genetic child may not wish to subject themselves to the expense and discomforts of any type of treatment, but will be happiest going right to donor sperm.

Varicocele

WHAT IS IT?

A varicose vein in the testicle. How and why an enlarged vein (which is what *varicose* means) should cause infertility is still unknown, but the predominant theory is that the blood which collects in the vein raises testicular temperature above normal, overheating and killing or weakening the sperm.

OPTIONS FOR TREATMENT

Surgery, choosing one of three different types: conventional surgery, done under general anesthesia, requiring an incision of several inches; microsurgery, done under spinal anesthetic, using an operating microscope to work with the man's ultrafine tubes and ducts through a less-than-one-inch incision; or "balloon" surgery, involving insertion of an extremely thin catheter containing an uninflated balloon into the testicular vein, guided in place through X ray, and inflating it to block off the varicose segment.

CONTROVERSIES

First, there is controversy about which method of surgery is the most effective with the least risk. Microsurgery and the balloon technique both require a high degree of skill to perform; conventional surgery, less so. But conventional surgery creates a larger incision and requires the man to spend more time in the hospital. The balloon procedure is done with the smallest incision used in any of the three procedures, but it carries with it the grave (though numerically slight) risk that the balloon could lodge in one of the other vital organs, resulting in, for example, the loss of a kidney. When selecting a procedure, make sure you have heard all the pros and cons for *each* of the choices, not just the reasons in favor of the particular operation your doctor has recommended.

A second, perhaps more crucial controversy concerns whether varicoceles really need to be repaired at all. The majority of infertility specialists say yes, but there is a vocal minority who question the relationship between male infertility and varicocele. Dr. Sherman J. Silber is one of the sharpest critics of the conventional view. In a section called "The Varicocele Scandal" in his book *How to Get Pregnant with the New Technology,* he decries the practice of "some urologists who find a varicocele in almost every 'infertile male' they see" (p. 131). Up to 40 percent of all male infertility patients, he notes, may be told they have a varicocele, yet "nobody could explain why 15% of the world's fertile men have a large varicocele and yet suffer no apparent harm" (p. 132). Silber goes on to tell how studies that attempt to prove that varicoceles cause infertility have been faultily conducted, while others that reach the opposite conclusion are methodologically correct. "The fact is, [Silber charges,] many urologists who treat male infertility depend heavily on varicocelectomy for their income" (p. 132). His final verdict (p. 135): "Drugs and hormones administered in the usual way do not increase sperm count, and neither does varicocele surgery."

Patient profile

Not surprisingly, perhaps, in light of the controversy discussed above, is the fact that those doctors who believe in varicocele surgery will describe the varicocelectomy patient's prognosis as good, while those doctors who don't believe in the procedure will generally offer a more mixed prognosis: good for men with borderline sperm counts and poor for men with poor counts or no sperm at all.

Whether a man is willing to undergo surgery to try to improve his fertility depends on several factors, including his attitude toward surgery in general, his confidence in his doctor's analysis of the merit (or lack of merit) of the varicocele removal procedure, and the severity of his fertility problem (even the most enthusiastic advocates of the varicocelectomy will admit that it rarely helps a man who produces no live sperm).

Epididymitis and Urinary-Tract Infections

What is it?

Epididymitis is swelling or infection of the epididymis, the long, coiled tube that stores and conveys sperm. The functioning of the epididymis or of the urinary tract may be compromised by any of several thousand varieties of germs, the most common of which are chlamydia, mycoplasma, and anaerobic bacteria. One of the more unusual infections is called "weird tuberculosis," which can appear in the epididymis, causing swelling and extreme pain, requiring between six and eighteen months of drug treatment to eradicate completely.

Options for treatment

The drug of choice will depend entirely on the germ that has caused (or is suspected of causing) the infection. The standard treatment for the standard urinary-tract infection in men is ten days of the antibiotic doxycycline. Unfortunately, these days antibiotic-resistant strains of bacteria are on the rise, and the standard treatment may not be enough to wipe out the infection or prevent recurrence. In such cases long-term antibiotic therapy, or massive doses of a mixture of antibiotics over the short-term, and even possibly intravenous administration of antibiotics may be in order.

CONTROVERSIES

Debate is heated over just how much infertility may be traced to infectious organisms. In 1991 Dr. Attila Toth put forward in *The Fertility Solution* the astonishing figure that up to 50 percent of all infertility cases may be attributed to bacteriological infection of either the male or the female partner or (since the organisms usually can be passed back and forth during sexual intercourse) both partners. Dr. Toth's views are decried by many physicians, yet he claims a 60 percent success rate in patients treated with his (often intensive) antibiotic therapy.

If you believe your infertility could possibly be linked to any past unrecognized or untreated urinary-tract infection, but your doctor disagrees, you will probably want to read Dr. Toth's book and discuss his conclusions with your doctor, who may also direct you to read some contradictory articles by other doctors on the subject.

PATIENT PROFILE

Most important is the patient's medical, sexual, and contraceptive history. If a man has no memory of ever having had a urinary-tract infection, and has no symptoms such as swelling in the testicles, itching, or pain during urination, and has only had monogamous relationships, and is not aware of any history of infections in any of his lovers in the past, or if he has consistently used a condom in all his past relationships—then it will be highly unlikely that that man's fertility problem will be bacteriological in origin (although Dr. Toth believes that some mothers with pelvic infections will pass the organisms on to their babies, who will then be systemically infected and become infertile adults as a consequence).

However, if you have any reason at all to suspect that you could have picked up a urinary-tract infection from anywhere, then it may well be worth your while to have this possibility investigated. Cultures may be done to try to identify bacteria found in your blood or semen, or a biopsy (the taking of tissue from an organ) may be required. If your urologist is not convinced that this search will be productive, but you still want to go ahead, you should seek out an infectious-disease specialist or a urologist who specializes in urinary-tract infections. And keep in mind, a few weeks of antibiotics is a whole lot easier than several months (or even years) of Pergonal.

Excessive Testicular Heat

What is it?

The temperature inside the testicles is higher than the normal 94°F. When the testicles are warmer than they are supposed to be, sperm production is diminished, and the sperm that are produced are more likely to be malformed or unable to swim well.

Options for treatment

Until recently all the man could do was try to get some cooling air circulation around his testicles by wearing loose cotton boxer shorts and avoiding tight-fitting pants. He might also try to identify and eliminate heat sources in his daily routine (such as working at a desk too close to a heating vent), and give up bicycling or rowing or other temperature-elevating exercises. None of these measures tended to be very successful. But now there is a new treatment available called a testicular cooling device, a jockstrap-like contraption that the man wears under his clothes containing a cooling unit which is held in place against his testicles. Because the treatment has been in use only since 1985, there are few long-term studies available on its success rate, and some of those that have been done contradict each other in their findings.

Controversies

As with any new device, there are those who believe a great breakthrough has been achieved, and there are those who are skeptical. The latter say that the preliminary data tend to suggest that the treatment is effective only when the cause of elevated temperature is external to the patient—for example, a baker who stands all day near a hot oven. The former have their anecdotes of individual patients whose wives got pregnant after they had worn the device for a period of time. To make a truly informed choice, the patient may need to do a lot of research on his own in medical journals, listen to conflicting experts' opinions, and then judge in his own mind which side's evidence he finds most persuasive.

The man with the best chance of restoring sperm fertility is the one who is able to identify a cause for the elevated temperature and eliminate it. If the cause is external, such as a source of heat in the workplace (as in the baker's example, cited above), the man is probably best advised to change jobs rather than try to cool down his testicles by wearing an experimental appliance against his skin. If an internal reason can be found such as varicocele, then the man is advised to seek expert care for that problem in the hope that his temperature will return to normal when the root cause is eliminated.

Retrograde Ejaculation

WHAT IS IT?

A relatively rare condition in which the man ejaculates not out the end of his penis but into his bladder. The condition is most often seen in diabetics and men who have had prostate surgery.

OPTIONS FOR TREATMENT

Doctors usually will first try antihistamine drugs to attempt to get the valve at the opening to the man's bladder to tighten up, to keep the semen from entering during orgasm. Another approach is to attempt to retrieve live sperm from the man's urine and then use that sperm to artificially inseminate the wife—but the recovered sperm are usually of poor quality, not capable of penetrating an egg. Micromanipulation of the egg and sperm may be necessary to achieve fertilization. That means the woman must have her eggs retrieved in an IVF or ZIFT cycle and the resulting **pre-embryo** must be reinserted into her body, a procedure that even in very fertile women carries a low chance of success.

CONTROVERSIES

There are many urologists who think of all the available treatments as poor prospects, and the ones that are most expensive (sperm recovery from urine and micromanipulation) as being a waste of everyone's time and money. Some clinics claim better-than-average conception rates, so the man looking for any chance at all to have a genetically related child may still be willing to investigate some of the techniques offered by the more successful clinics.

Patient profile

Some men do respond to antihistamine therapy, especially those whose bladder valve will still function at least partially. Men who are not bothered by financial constraints may be free to pay out of pocket for the still-experimental micromanipulation techniques of sperm and egg. Men who are most intent on becoming fathers quickly (and not so stuck on the idea of being the child's genetic-material supplier) would probably be far less frustrated if instead of trying chancy treatment after treatment, they quickly moved to donor sperm.

Unexplained Infertility

What is it?

It's the diagnosis that is left over after all the other known causes have been ruled out. Unexplained infertility shows the limits of our knowledge about human reproduction.

Options for treatment

Most doctors try drugs, mainly Clomid, progesterone, Pergonal, or Metrodin. Various combinations are possible. If drugs fail to produce a pregnancy after the end of a set period of time, some doctors will urge the couple to try a few cycles of GIFT or IVF. In women over forty the use of donor eggs may be recommended to greatly improve the chance that a GIFT cycle will succeed.

Controversies

The major disagreement that doctors have is over the number of cases that will remain unexplained after thorough testing has been done. Some doctors report that up to 20 percent of their cases are labeled unexplained; other doctors pride themselves on their persistence in digging for the root cause of infertility. These doctors say that after checking and rechecking test results, only 3 percent of cases should still remain unexplained. However, before submitting themselves to repeat endometrial biopsies, repeat sperm analyses, repeat postcoitals, and other tests, the couple should be sure to ask the doctor two questions: (1) Will our treatment definitely be changed if we are reclassified from unexplained infertility to a particular problem? and (2) Would it perhaps be worthwhile to try a drug therapy—Clomid, for example— for a few months, and then if it doesn't work, continue the investigation to try to pinpoint the cause of the problem?

If the doctor responds with some assurance that repeat testing will this time succeed in discovering a problem, and that problem will be treated very differently than the treatment for unexplained infertility, then (and only then) should you consider undergoing the repeated tests.

PATIENT PROFILE

The number of months or years that the couple has been trying to conceive gives the best clue to the couple's prognosis. The couple who has been trying only six months to two years may not be infertile at all, but simply stuck with a run of bad luck. With ovulation-boosting drugs this couple's chances should be greatly improved. If the couple has been trying for more than five years with no luck—especially if they are under thirty—that suggests there is an underlying problem; it just has not been found yet. Couples under thirty will not feel as pressured by the passage of a few more months spent in the testing phase, and so may prefer to continue the investigation until a root cause can be discovered and treated.

Combinations of Causes

WHAT IS IT?

The couple's infertility is not caused by a single factor but by two or even three or more problems combined. The man may have a problem with sperm quantity or quality, while the woman ovulates infrequently; or the woman may suffer from endometriosis, which has interfered with her fertility in more than one way—for example, affecting both the functioning of her fallopian tubes and her ovaries. Almost any combination of factors is possible.

184 / How to Be a Successful Fertility Patient

SOMETIMES "UNEXPLAINED INFERTILITY" REALLY IS EXPLAINABLE

*M*y regular OB-GYN couldn't find a reason for my infertility. He looked at my temperature charts and did a few blood tests, but nothing more. He kept insulting my intelligence by saying we were "missing the fertile time," or we were "too tired," or "trying too hard," etc. . . . After one year of nothing I was finally referred to an infertility specialist, who did the right tests and found the problem [her fallopian tubes were blocked].

*M*olly from Ohio

OPTIONS FOR TREATMENT

All the treatments described for each of the conditions individually will still apply, but in cases of combined causes, clinics tend to urge couples to take a relatively aggressive course of action. For example, in a woman who had blocked tubes *and* poor ovulation, some doctors would not advise trying the usual tubal surgery and then waiting to see if the problems have cleared up. Even if such a woman takes fertility drugs to improve her ovulation, it will still be difficult to tell if her inability to conceive is due to poor response to the drugs, or some residual tubal problem not cleared up by her surgery. In such cases the doctor might advise the woman to go straight to IVF, to bypass the tubal problem and have ovulation induced, all in the same cycle. The woman with blocked tubes whose husband has very few fertile sperm may be urged to let the doctor try micromanipulation of sperm and egg in the laboratory to bring about conception, rather than put the woman through tubal surgery and put the man on sperm-enhancing drugs.

CONTROVERSIES

Debate is generally focused on how hopeless a case must be before the doctor should advise the couple to quit seeking a medical solution. Some doctors pride themselves on their willingness to help every patient who wants help; they believe that even when the odds are high against success, a few couples will have babies and the rest will at least have known that they tried. We'll call doctors who take this position "treaters."

Another school of thought says that the right thing to do is to avoid giving couples false hope, but bluntly tell them how poor their chances are, and advise them not to invest their time, emotions, and money in treatment, when other nonmedical alternatives are available. We'll call these doctors "nontreaters."

The treaters tend to imply that the nontreaters are simply not as skilled at the techniques of infertility treatment and give up much too soon on couples who could be helped. The nontreaters tend to imply that the treaters are primarily profit-driven, taking desperate couples' money and in far too many cases giving nothing in return.

If your doctor has diagnosed multiple problems in your case, you should certainly find out whether your doctor is basically a treater or a nontreater. If the doctor's philosophy is at odds with your own inclinations, you will certainly want to change to one who suits you better.

PATIENT PROFILE

Logically enough, the more problems that contribute to infertility, the worse the couple's prognosis will be, and the fewer problems, the better. With more than one problem, your chances of success can only be as good as your chances at fixing the most difficult of the problems you have. The severity of each problem is also crucial to assessing the chance of success.

CHAPTER FIVE

CHOOSING A TREATMENT

Treatment Classifications:
Conservative, Moderate, and Aggressive

Now that you have some idea of what's wrong and have learned
something about the techniques doctors use to treat the problem, it's
time to make a choice. But how do you know which treatment is best
for *you?*

The usual way most people decide is simply by following their doctor's recommendation.

That's good for those who have an excellent relationship with their
doctor, with confidence that their doctor understands not merely their
physiology but also their psychology—just how far they are willing to
go for just how slim (or how good) a chance to have a child. My interviews with couples have led me to conclude that such a thorough understanding on the part of the doctor is relatively rare, and that quite
often doctors will misread their patient's intentions and recommend a
course of action the patient finds intolerable, while not even mentioning
other options that the patient would find more acceptable. Just as often
the patient is not very good at letting the doctor know what types of
things she or he is willing to do. There can be miscommunication all
around.

The table on pages 188–191 and the two questionnaires following
are designed to help patients discover what they really want. The table
lists the major infertility problems and classifies the most common treatment options as conservative, moderate, or aggressive. The questionnaires, one for women and one for men, are designed to help couples
understand better their own goals and attitudes toward treatment, so
that they can know which form of treatment suits their own physical
and emotional needs best.

Questionnaires for Self-analysis Regarding Treatment Goals

Should I . . .

. . . seek the most aggressive treatment for my infertility?

. . . take a moderate course of action?

. . . first try a cautious, conservative approach?

. . . stop and reflect more on my needs and emotions before seeking treatment?

The multiple choice questions and statements that follow have been designed to help you reflect on your own emotional and physical readiness for treatment and guide you toward the type of treatment most suited to your level of determination to have a child. You do not need to know what type of infertility problem you have in order to complete this questionnaire.

Of the two questionnaires, one is for women and one is for men. Answer the one appropriate to your sex. Read each question or statement and choose the answer or completion of the sentence that comes closest to describing your feelings or your physical state. Record your answers in the margin, on a separate sheet of paper, or however you feel comfortable. After you are done, have your spouse or partner complete the other questionnaire—preferably without reading the responses you have chosen or being influenced by you during the selection of choices. Scoring information is provided at the end of this section to tell you how to interpret your responses.

When you have each figured out your scores, you should sit down together and compare the results. A wide divergence in your answers indicates a major difference in approach to your infertility problem, a difference that the two of you will need to work out before pursuing any of your available treatment options.

Whatever treatment category you end up in, you should keep in mind that this questionnaire is just a tool, a way to set you thinking about yourself and how the treatment you choose might affect your life. You must not feel bound to take the approach suggested by your score if it conflicts with the best advice of a doctor you trust, or if it differs from your own deeper reflections on the problem. If, on the other hand, your doctor wants to put you on a highly aggressive course of medical

TREATMENT OPTIONS*

	Conservative	Moderate	Aggressive
Female hormonal disorders	Drug therapy to correct deficiency or excess of specific hormone Progesterone for luteal-phase defect. Parlodel for excess prolactin	In addition to drug therapy to treat specific hormonal problem, use Clomid to increase monthly odds of conception. May also try • Clomid with hCG • Clomid with hCG, IUI	In addition to drug therapy to treat specific hormonal problem, use Pergonal to increase monthly odds of conception. Or • Pergonal with IUI • GIFT • ZIFT
Endometriosis	Danazol Lupron GnRH	Laser surgery to remove adhesions. May be followed or preceded by drug therapy. Ovulation-boosting drugs (Clomid, Pergonal) may be used to increase monthly odds of conception for limited time before endometriosis symptoms return.	If endometriosis has damaged fallopian tubes, IVF

(continued)

	Conservative	Moderate	Aggressive
Blocked fallopian tubes	If only one tube is blocked, use Clomid or Pergonal to boost chances that conception will occur in open tube	If both tubes blocked, attempt to clear blockages through balloon tuboplasty or microsurgery	IVF
Polycystic ovarian disease	Life-style modification Prednisone, dexamethasone, possibly with Clomid	In addition to one or more of the conservative measures listed, use Pergonal or Metrodin, possibly with IUI	Laser or conventional surgery to reduce androgen-producing elements in ovaries
Premature menopause	—	—	Donor egg Embryo transplant Surrogate mother
Uterine septum, other abnormalities	Hysteroscopic or laparoscopic repair of abnormality	Surgical repair, followed by use of fertility drugs to increase monthly chance of conception	If uterus appears unable to sustain pregnancy to term, try host uterus

(continued)

	Conservative	Moderate	Aggressive
Pituitary tumor	Parlodel	Parlodel and Clomid Parlodel and Pergonal Parlodel, fertility drugs, plus IUI	Brain surgery to remove tumors Surgery, followed by fertility drugs, possibly with IUI
Thyroid problems	Synthetic thyroid hormone Parlodel	Parlodel and Clomid Parlodel and Pergonal Parlodel, fertility drugs, IUI	GIFT
Immune system problems	Condom therapy Steroid treatment Natural-cycle IUI	Clomid, IUI Pergonal, IUI	GIFT
Sperm problems	Various male drug therapies	Use fertility drugs to boost wife's ovulation along with drugs to attempt to improve sperm production IUI Donor sperm	IVF, ZIFT Micromanipulation of sperm and egg

(continued)

	Conservative	Moderate	Aggressive
Varicocele	No treatment/let nature take its course Search for other factors affecting couple's fertility	Microsurgical repair Balloon procedure	After surgical repair, use fertility drugs to increase wife's fertility IUI GIFT
Various male urinary-tract infections	Standard doses of antibiotics	Antibiotics, followed by fertility drugs to increase wife's ovulation IUI	Massive doses of antibiotics IV antibiotics
Retrograde ejaculation	Antihistamine therapy	Attempt to retrieve sperm from urine and use for IUI	GIFT IVF or ZIFT with micro-manipulation of egg and sperm
Unexplained infertility	No treatment— "keep trying" Continue testing to attempt to find cause	Clomid Clomid with hCG Clomid, hCG, IUI	Pergonal Pergonal with IUI GIFT ZIFT

*Note: Three of the conditions described in Chapter Four are not included in this table. They are recurrent miscarriage, excessive testicular heat, and combinations of causes. It is not possible to classify treatment options as conservative, moderate, or aggressive in these cases without having some information about the underlying cause for the condition. Recurrent miscarriage, for example, might be the result of immune system problems or hormonal disorders (both listed on this table). Excessive testicular heat could be caused by a varicocele or by working too close to an external source of heat. Treatment of the couple diagnosed with a combination of causes depends very much on which causes are found in the couple.

intervention but your score indicates that you would be more comfortable starting out with a conservative approach, by all means discuss your misgivings with your doctor and ask him to explain what other options might exist and why (or why not, in his opinion) they might better suit your particular case.

> We learned the hard way about the importance of selecting a compatible doctor. It seems obvious now, but when we started two and a half years ago we just focused on finding someone who was qualified and knowledgeable. But our first doctor's philosophy was, "Find the problem, fix it, then let nature take its course." That led us down a lengthy path that we didn't have the stamina for. During years of unsuccessful treatment, I was never told about the advantages or disadvantages of trying more advanced or intensive treatments. Switching to a doctor who could do IVF was a huge relief for us. Yes, it's more effort, but we feel we have a much better chance this way.
>
> Janet from Massachusetts

QUESTIONNAIRE FOR WOMEN

1a. I am . . .

    (a)   under 30
    (b)   30–35
    (c)   35–40
    (d)   over 40

1b. My husband/partner is . . .

    (a)   under 40
    (b)   40–50
    (c)   50–55
    (d)   over 55

2. We have been actively trying to have a baby . . .

    (a)   for less than a year
    (b)   1–3 years
    (c)   4–7 years
    (d)   over 7 years

3. I have . . .

    (a) one biological child or more.
    (b) an adopted child, foster child, or stepchild I regard as my child; or godchildren, nieces, or nephews, or foster children, or a protégé(e) with whom I have a close, quasi-parental relationship.
    (c) no close relationships in which I play a maternal role.
    (d) no one in my life that I feel needs me very deeply/no one to love me unconditionally.

4. My marriage/relationship has been stable for . . .

    (a) less than 18 months
    (b) 18 months to 5 years
    (c) 5–10 years
    (d) over 10 years

5. I have had . . .

    (a) no miscarriages
    (b) one miscarriage
    (c) two miscarriages
    (d) three or more miscarriages

For numbers 6 through 15, pick the one statement from the choices given that most closely describes your feelings.

6. (a) I have ambivalent feelings about having children—sometimes I deeply long for them, but other times I am not certain.
    (b) I am sure I want children, and if I can't have a biological child, I will probably find some other way to add to my family.
    (c) My strongest desire now is to have a biological child; at this point I don't want to think about adoption, or living a child-free life, or any other alternatives to having a child except through pregnancy and birth.
    (d) I feel an overwhelming need to have children; if I don't, I fear my marriage might be in trouble, or I could become deeply depressed.

7. I believe . . .

    (a) my husband/partner would not be unhappy if we continued as we are now.

    (b) my husband/partner wants children but more important wants me to be satisfied with whatever course we pursue.

    (c) my husband/partner shares equally my intense desire to have children.

    (d) my husband/partner wants to have children far more than I do/my partner believes the success of our marriage depends largely on our having a baby.

8. If I hear about any activities, habits, or substances that may possibly be linked to infertility (such as caffeine consumption or excessive amounts of exercise), I . . .

    (a) wait to see how mainstream scientists evaluate the data before I let it affect my own behavior or consumption of the substance.

    (b) try to cut down on the substance/activity—but not if it means a major disruption in my life-style.

    (c) immediately cease the activity/give up the substance—even if it means doing without something that has till now been an important part of my life.

    (d) feel confused, upset, or depressed—it seems that every day scientists find some new cause of infertility and I feel helpless and don't know what to think or how to react.

9.   (a) I consider myself extremely sensitive to pain and/or fearful of surgical procedures or the use of highly potent drugs.

    (b) While I'm nervous about the pain or side effects of surgery or certain types of drug therapy, if I have confidence that the treatment is the right one for my condition, then I have no hesitance in going ahead with it.

    (c) My attitude is, give me the treatment that will get results the fastest. I am not especially anxious about or frightened of pain or side effects. I want to do whatever is necessary to get pregnant in the least amount of time.

    (d) Sometimes I feel ready to undergo any procedure to get pregnant; other times I think, why should people subject themselves to surgery or system-disturbing drugs for an outcome that can't be guaranteed?

10. (a)   In the past I have generally avoided seeing doctors for medical problems/gone to the doctor only when I had to (because the problem wouldn't go away by itself or I couldn't treat it with home remedies any longer).

   (b)   I look on doctors as professionals that I hire to help me or work with me on whatever health problems that I may develop. I want to understand the doctor's diagnosis and treatment advice so that I can participate fully in my own recovery.

   (c)   I want a doctor I can trust to keep up with the latest medical advances, find out what my problem is, and fix it. If I hear of some new treatment that another doctor is using with success on patients like me, I will either ask my doctor about trying it, or switch to a doctor who is doing this effective new technology.

   (d)   I'm uneasy in my relationships with doctors. I get intimidated by their medical jargon, or I find it embarrassing to be examined by them or to talk to them about sensitive matters, especially sexual ones.

11. If my treatment regimen required that I cancel an important business trip, or miss a family wedding, or be absent from work often enough to injure my career, I most probably would . . .

   (a)   want to abandon or change the treatment. I still want to live a normal life, and not have to explain to outsiders about my medical and personal choices, or have to invent frequent excuses for my absence. I can always go back to the treatment at a more convenient time.

   (b)   try to reach an accommodation between the demands of treatment and the demands of my work and family. Sometimes my infertility problem would be subordinated to my other goals; sometimes it would take priority. It all depends on the nature of the event I planned to attend, and whether or not my problem required immediate attention.

   (c)   cancel my plans so that I can receive the treatment I need. Having a baby is top priority, and if I must, I will put competing activities on hold until I achieve my goal.

   (d)   wait until the situation arises before I decide what I would do. Thinking about questions like this is very stressful for me. I would really just hope I don't end up having to make this type of choice.

12. In general I would say I . . .

    (a) don't like taking risks/hate to lose.
    (b) try to analyze the odds objectively/feel neither luckier nor unluckier than anyone else.
    (c) feel pretty lucky/am happy to take a chance if it gives me a fair shot at something I want.
    (d) don't really believe in chance or randomness; but those who win are somehow favored by God or have some inner power that accounts for their success, while losers are somehow being punished or are lacking in some indefinable quality that is necessary for success.

13. The following best describes my sex life:

    (a) Since we started trying to have a baby it's become a little stressful. Sometimes I don't enjoy it or am unable to have orgasm; there's been a problem with spontaneity and passion on occasion during the fertile time of the month, when I feel we "have to do it."
    (b) Our sex life hasn't changed in any major way since we began trying to have a baby. We still make love regularly, two or more times a week, even when it's not the fertile time of the month.
    (c) Trying to get pregnant seems to have motivated us to make love more frequently, or at least to be sure to do so when it's the fertile time of the month. I have no problem getting aroused, even though we are sometimes planning our lovemaking according to the calendar rather than our own spontaneous desires.
    (d) We've been having some real problems: we seldom make love anymore/make love only when we think it might be the fertile time of the month/don't enjoy sex anymore/there is a possibility that one of us has fallen out of love or may be having an extramarital affair.

14. If the type of treatment we chose caused me to have mood swings, gain ten pounds, have hot flashes, and/or require two weeks of bed rest, I most probably would . . .

    (a) look for a different form of treatment, or cease treatment altogether.
    (b) stick with the treatment for a certain number of months. If after that period of time I didn't get pregnant, I would make

an appointment to sit down with the doctor and ask for an evaluation of how the program was affecting my health and an assessment of its chances for success in the future.

(c)   keep reminding myself that these side effects happen to many women who go on to have a baby. I would get off the program only if my doctor thought my health was seriously threatened or that the odds for success were very low.

(d)   go on with the treatment but try to keep my husband/partner from finding out about my side effects, or at least minimize the discomfort I was feeling. How the treatment affects me really is something I'm going to have to deal with on my own/I'd just be afraid that he would worry needlessly over me.

15.   If we had a baby through medical intervention I would . . .

(a)   prefer that my friends and family believe it occurred naturally.

(b)   want my good friends and close family members to know how the pregnancy came about/not feel strongly about other people's knowing how it happened.

(c)   not mind if everyone learns what steps we took to start a family.

(d)   be extremely upset if it got out that we were having some kind of a problem and turned to outside help.

In this next section, choose the statements that you feel approximately describe your feelings or your condition. Don't worry if you agree with one statement that seems to contradict another statement you have chosen. If you only partly agree with the sentiment expressed, go with your initial "gut" reaction to the statement.

16.   I have always found it very uncomfortable to get shots or have blood drawn. (A)

17.   When I'm faced with something unpleasant but medically necessary, I just grit my teeth and get on with it. (B)

18.   Whenever the doctor is performing some procedure on me—even an unpleasant one—I'm very interested in what's going on/I always ask a lot of questions about what the doctor is doing/I like to see my X rays, sonograms, or other test results. (C)

19. When faced with unfamiliar tests or painful medical procedures I sometimes will cancel or postpone appointments until I feel able to face them, or I might go in for the appointment only after having taken painkillers in advance. (D)

20. When I hear news reports of some new super-high-tech method of creating life in a test tube, I can't help but wonder if all this experimentation on human life is really ethical. (A)

21. When I hear news reports of new fertility treatment techniques— no matter if they're applicable to couples in our situation or not— I feel like cheering, because more people who want children will be able to have them. (B)

22. Every time I hear of some new advance, I want to learn more about it; I can't help thinking that maybe this is the breakthrough that will work for me/my partner. (C)

23. Most health problems will resolve themselves on their own in time if the person can just maintain a positive attitude. (A)

24. Life is really a great mystery. Despite all the advances in knowledge, we will never truly understand how conception works and why some couples just can't seem to have babies. All we can do is apply the techniques we have now and hope for the best. (B)

25. I believe that medical knowledge is advancing all the time and that sooner or later doctors will be able to fix just about any infertility problem, no matter how severe. (C)

26. A great many infertile people, if they could just face the truth, would have to admit it's their own fault they can't have children, either because they were promiscuous in the past and caught a disease that injured their reproductive systems, or because they used an unsafe method of birth control like the Dalkon Shield, or they had abortions that caused uterine scarring, or otherwise abused their own bodies. (D)

27. If I had to live my whole life without children, I'd still have a rich, full life. (A)

28. If I never have children, I know I will regret it when I'm old, especially if I become widowed and alone. (B)

29. I already feel regret for the years I've let go by without having children. (C)

30. The main thing for me is, how disappointed my parents (or my husband's parents) will be if they never become grandparents. (D)

31. I really only want a boy (girl). (D)

32. Everyone on my block has children; I feel we'd fit in much better if we had children too. (D)

33. If I miscarried a pregnancy after a successful round of infertility treatment, I think I would need some time off to consider my options before making another try. (A)

34. A miscarriage after infertility treatment would be devastating, but it's not an uncommon outcome for any pregnant woman. Unless the doctor told me that my treatment somehow had contributed to the problem, I would most likely go right back on the same program and try again. (B)

35. Sad though the event would be, I would still feel in a way encouraged by a miscarriage, because I'd at least know that I *can* get pregnant. I'd keep telling myself the great majority of women who miscarry do go on to have another pregnancy with a healthy delivery. (C)

36. If I believed that in order to have a healthy baby I was going to have to suffer through several operations, and possibly miscarry more than once, I would still do it anyway. (C)

37. If I had a miscarriage, I'm afraid I couldn't help feeling guilty— maybe something I did could have caused it. (D)

38. I consider myself a fairly private person. I don't like to involve others in my personal problems. (A)

39. When it comes to solving difficult problems (personal or medical), I try to find the best-qualified professionals to advise me. (B)

40. I'm very open to advice from any quarter, even about personal matters. You never know where you might hear of an idea that will work for you, so you should be willing to be frank with anyone who might be able to be of help. (C)

41. One of the negatives of infertility treatment in my mind is the increased risk of having twins or triplets. (A)

42. I'm not really worried about whether I have a multiple pregnancy or a single one; with careful monitoring and good prenatal care I know I'm still very likely to end up with a healthy child (or children), and that's all I really care about. (B)

43. Having twins (or even triplets) would be great! I wouldn't have to try to get pregnant again, because I'd already have all the children I want. (C)

44. My inability to have a baby often makes me feel inadequate as a woman. (D)

45. I try not to focus on my/my partner's infertility; it just causes stress, and I think that stress just adds to the problem. (A)

46. I can't help but think about my/my partner's infertility a lot—but at least I know I'm educating myself about it and doing all I can to solve the problem. (B)

47. I think about my/my partner's infertility constantly, because the goal of having a baby is really the number one thing in my life right now. (C)

48. With each month's period I get terrifically depressed/cry/feel ill. (D)

49. I take each month's cycle as it comes, and what happens, happens. (A)

50. I look to each new monthly cycle as a new chance to get pregnant. (B)

51. If I don't get pregnant this month, or next month, or next year, I'll just keep on trying until I hit menopause. (C)

52. If I knew that there was an infertility center in another state that had far superior live birth rates for those with my/my partner's particular problem than any center close by, I'd be willing to travel, or even relocate for part of the year, to take advantage of the program. (C)

53. If I thought that my/my partner's infertility treatment regimen was causing problems in my relationship with my partner, I'd give up the treatment/seek a different type of program—even if all doctors told me that only with this treatment would I have a decent chance at pregnancy. (A)

54. Whatever problems arose in my relationship because of the requirements of the treatment program, I would try to work them out with my husband/partner, with professional help if necessary—but I would still stick with the program. (B)

55. If told there was no way I could ever have a biological child, I would still want my husband to avail himself of whatever methods were available to have one. (C)

56. If I learned that it would be impossible for my husband ever to have a biological child, I would still want to do everything possible to try to have one myself. (C)

57. If a couple cannot have a biological child, I think the honorable thing is for the infertile partner to offer the fertile one the option of divorce, so that he/she can have children with someone who's normal. (D)

58. I have strong religious beliefs that I'm afraid might be compromised by certain forms of infertility treatment. (A)

59. Your religious values, your family, and doctors all have a role to play in helping you decide what's the right way for you to handle your infertility, but ultimately it will be up to you and your partner together to choose the way you will deal with your own bodies. (B)

60. I haven't answered/don't even want to think about many of the questions on this questionnaire because many of these issues are very painful/too confusing for me right now. (D)

Questionnaire for Men

1a.　I am . . .

    (a)　under 40
    (b)　40–50
    (c)　50–55
    (d)　over 50

1b.　My wife/partner is . . .

    (a)　under 30
    (b)　30–35
    (c)　35–40
    (d)　over 40

2.　We have been actively trying to have a baby . . .

    (a)　for less than a year
    (b)　1–3 years
    (c)　4–7 years
    (d)　over 7 years

3.　I have . . .

    (a)　one biological child or more.
    (b)　an adopted child, foster child, or stepchild I regard as my child; or godchildren, nieces, or nephews, or foster children, or a protégé(e) with whom I have a close, quasi-parental relationship.
    (c)　no close relationships in which I play a paternal role.
    (d)　no one in my life that I feel needs me very deeply/no one to love me unconditionally.

4.　My marriage/relationship has been stable for . . .

    (a)　less than 18 months
    (b)　18 months to 5 years
    (c)　5–10 years
    (d)　over 10 years

5.   My wife/partner has had . . .

   (a)   no miscarriages
   (b)   one miscarriage
   (c)   two or three miscarriages
   (d)   more than three miscarriages

For numbers 6 through 15, pick the one statement from the choices given that most closely describes your feelings.

6.   (a)   I have ambivalent feelings about having children—sometimes I deeply long for them, but other times I am not certain.
   (b)   I am sure I want children, and if we can't have a biological child, I will probably find some other way to add to my family.
   (c)   My strongest desire now is to have a biological child; at this point I don't want to think about adoption, or living a child-free life, or any other alternatives to having a child except through my wife's pregnancy and birth.
   (d)   I feel an overwhelming need to have children; if I don't, I fear my marriage might be in trouble, or I could become deeply depressed.

7.   I believe . . .

   (a)   my wife/partner would not be unhappy if we continued as we are now.
   (b)   my wife/partner wants children but more important wants me to be satisfied with whatever course we pursue.
   (c)   my wife/partner shares equally my intense desire to have children.
   (d)   my wife/partner wants to have children far more than I do/ my wife believes the success of our marriage depends largely on our having a baby.

8.   If I hear about any activities, habits, or substances that may possibly be linked to infertility (such as caffeine consumption or excessive amounts of exercise), I . . .

   (a)   wait to see how mainstream scientists evaluate the data before I let it affect my own behavior or consumption of the substance.

(b) try to cut down on the substance/activity—but not if it means a major disruption in my life-style.

(c) immediately cease the activity/give up the substance—even if it means doing without something that has till now been an important part of my life.

(d) feel confused, depressed, or angry—it seems that every day scientists find some new cause of infertility, and I feel helpless and don't know what to think or how to react.

9. (a) I consider myself extremely sensitive to pain and/or fearful of surgical procedures or use of highly potent drugs.

(b) While I'm nervous about the pain or side effects of surgery or some types of drug therapy, if I knew that in order for my wife to get pregnant I must have the treatment, then I would have no hesitance in going ahead with it.

(c) My attitude is, give me the treatment that will get us results the fastest. If I need treatment, I am not especially anxious about pain or potential side effects. I want to do whatever is necessary to enable my wife/partner to get pregnant in the least amount of time.

(d) Sometimes I feel ready to undergo any procedure so that we can have a baby; other times I think, why should people subject themselves to surgery or to system-disturbing drugs for an outcome that can't be guaranteed?

10. (a) In the past I have generally avoided seeing doctors for medical problems/gone to the doctor only when I had to (because the problem wouldn't go away by itself or I couldn't treat it with home remedies any longer).

(b) I look on doctors as professionals that I hire to help me or work with me on whatever health problems that I may develop. I want to understand the doctor's diagnosis and treatment advice so that I can participate fully in my own recovery.

(c) I want a doctor I can trust to keep up with the latest medical advances, find out what my problem is, and fix it. If I hear of some new treatment that another doctor is using with success on patients like me, I will either ask my doctor about trying it, or switch to a doctor who is doing this effective new technology.

(d) I'm uneasy in my relationships with doctors. I get intimidated by their medical jargon, or I find it embarrassing to be examined by them or to talk to them about sensitive matters, especially sexual ones.

11. If our schedule of treatment required that I cancel an important business trip, or miss a family wedding, or be absent from work more often than would be compatible with my career goals, I most probably would . . .

   (a) want to abandon or change the treatment. I still want to be able to live a normal life, and not have to explain to outsiders about our medical and personal choices, or not have to invent excuses for my absence. We can always go back to the treatment at a more convenient time.

   (b) try to reach an accommodation between the demands of treatment and the demands of my work and family. Sometimes our infertility problem would be subordinated to my other goals; sometimes it would take priority. It all depends on the nature of the event I planned to attend, and whether or not the problem required immediate attention.

   (c) cancel my plans so that we can receive the treatment we need. Having a baby is top priority and if I must, I will put competing activities on hold until we achieve that goal.

   (d) wait until the situation arises before I decide what I would do. Thinking about questions like this is very stressful for me. I would really just hope I don't end up having to make this type of choice.

12. In general I would say I . . .

   (a) don't like taking risks/hate to lose.

   (b) try to analyze the odds objectively/feel neither luckier nor unluckier than anyone else.

   (c) feel pretty lucky/am happy to take a chance if it gives me a fair shot at something I want.

   (d) don't really believe in chance or randomness; but those who win are somehow favored by God or have some inner power that accounts for their success, while losers are somehow being punished or are lacking in some indefinable quality that is necessary for success.

13. The following best describes my sex life:

   (a) Since we started trying to have a baby it's become a little stressful. Sometimes I have trouble getting aroused or finishing; there's been a problem with spontaneity and passion on occasion during the fertile time of the month, when I feel we "have to do it."

   (b) Our sex life hasn't changed in any major way since we began trying to have a baby. We still make love regularly, two or more times a week, even when it's not the fertile time of the month.

   (c) Trying to have a baby seems to have motivated us to make love more frequently, or at least to be sure to do so when it's the fertile time of the month. I have no problem getting aroused, even though we are sometimes planning our lovemaking according to the calendar rather than our own spontaneous desires.

   (d) We've been having some real problems: We seldom make love anymore/make love only when we think it might be the fertile time of the month/don't enjoy sex anymore/there is a possibility that one of us has fallen out of love or may be having an extramarital affair.

14. If we chose a treatment that caused my wife/partner to have mood swings, gain ten pounds, have hot flashes, and/or need two weeks of bed rest, I most probably would . . .

   (a) want to look for a different form of treatment, or urge her to cease treatment altogether.

   (b) want to see her stick with the treatment for a certain number of months. If after that period of time she didn't get pregnant, I would want both of us to sit down with the doctor and ask for an evaluation of how the program was affecting her health and get an assessment of its chances for success in the future.

   (c) keep in mind that these side effects happen to many women who go on to have a baby. As long as she was willing, and her doctor did not think her health was in serious jeopardy, then I would like to see her stick with the program for as long as her chances to succeed with the treatment appeared good.

(d)   not get involved in the decision to quit or continue. Since I really can't know what she's feeling, how can I advise her what to do?

15.   If we had a baby through medical intervention I would . . .

(a)   prefer that my friends and family believe it occurred naturally.
(b)   want my good friends and close family members to know how the pregnancy came about/not feel strongly about other people's knowing how it happened.
(c)   not mind if everyone learns what steps we took to start a family
(d)   be extremely upset if it got out that we were having some kind of a problem and turned to outside help.

In this next section, choose the statements that you feel approximately describe your feelings or your condition. Don't worry if you agree with one statement that seems to contradict another statement you have chosen. If you only partly agree with the sentiment expressed, go with your initial "gut" reaction to the statement.

16.   I have always found it very uncomfortable to have blood drawn or deal with shots. I'm afraid I'm incapable of learning to give someone else a shot. (A)

17.   When I'm faced with something unpleasant but medically necessary, I just grit my teeth and get on with it. (B)

18.   Whenever the doctor is performing some procedure on me—even an unpleasant one—I'm very interested in what's going on/I always ask lots of questions about what the doctor is doing/I like to see my X rays, sonograms, or other test results. (C)

19.   When faced with unfamiliar tests or painful medical procedures, I sometimes will cancel or postpone appointments until I feel able to face them, or I might go in for the appointment only after having taken painkillers in advance. (D)

20.   When I hear news reports of some new super-high-tech method of creating life in a test tube, I can't help but wonder if all this experimentation on human life is really ethical. (A)

21. When I hear news reports of new fertility treatment techniques—no matter if they're applicable to couples in our situation or not—I feel like cheering, because more people who want children will be able to have them. (B)

22. Every time I hear of some new advance, I want to learn more about it; I can't help thinking that maybe this is the breakthrough that will work for me/my partner. (C)

23. Most health problems will resolve themselves on their own in time if the person can just maintain a positive attitude. (A)

24. Life is really a great mystery. Despite all the advances in knowledge, we will never truly understand how conception works and why some couples just can't seem to have babies. All we can do is apply the techniques we have now and hope for the best. (B)

25. I believe that medical knowledge is advancing all the time and that sooner or later doctors will be able to fix just about any infertility problem, no matter how severe. (C)

26. A great many infertile people, if they could just face the truth, would have to admit it's their own fault they can't have children, either because they were promiscuous in the past and caught a disease that injured their reproductive systems, or because they stupidly went ahead with a sterilization without thinking enough about the future, or they used drugs or in some other way abused their bodies. (D)

27. If I had to live my whole life without children, I'd still have a rich, full life. (A)

28. If I never have children, I know I will regret it when I'm old, especially if I become a widower and end up living alone. (B)

29. I already feel regret for the years I've let go by without having children. (C)

30. The main thing for me is, how disappointed my parents (or my wife's parents) will be if they never become grandparents. (D)

31. I really only want a boy (girl). (D)

32. Everyone on my block has children; I feel we'd fit in much better if we had children too. (D)

33. If my wife/partner miscarried a pregnancy after a successful round of infertility treatment, I think we would need some time off to consider our options before making another try. (A)

34. A miscarriage after infertility treatment would be devastating, but it's not an uncommon outcome for any pregnant woman. Unless the doctor told us that our treatment somehow had contributed to the problem, I would most likely want us to go right back on the same program and try again. (B)

35. Sad though the event would be, I would still feel in a way encouraged by the miscarriage, because we'd at least know that she *can* get pregnant. I'd keep telling myself that the great majority of women who miscarry do go on to have another pregnancy with a healthy delivery. (C)

36. If I believed that in order to have a healthy baby either my wife or I would have to suffer through several operations, and possibly she would end up miscarrying more than once, I would still want us to go ahead with the program anyway. (C)

37. If my wife/partner had a miscarriage, I'm afraid I couldn't help but wonder if anything she did could have caused it. (D)

38. I consider myself a fairly private person. I don't like to involve others in my personal problems. (A)

39. When it comes to solving difficult problems (personal or medical), I try to find the best-qualified professionals to advise me. (B)

40. I'm very open to advice from any quarter, even about personal matters. You never know where you might hear of an idea that will work for you, so you should be willing to be frank with anyone who might be able to be of help. (C)

41. One of the negatives of infertility treatment in my mind is the increased risk of having twins or triplets. (A)

42. I'm not really worried about whether we end up with a single baby or more than one; with careful monitoring and good prenatal care I know the baby (or babies) most likely will be born healthy and that's the important thing, after all. (B)

43. Having twins (or even triplets) would be great! We wouldn't have to bother with infertility treatment again because we'd have all the children we want. (C)

44. My inability to father a child often makes me feel inadequate as a man. (D)

45. I try not to focus on my/my partner's infertility; it just causes stress, and I think that stress just adds to the problem. (A)

46. I can't help but think about my/my partner's infertility a lot—but at least I know I'm educating myself about it and doing all I can to solve the problem. (B)

47. I think about my/my partner's infertility constantly, because the goal of having a baby is really the number one thing in my life right now. (C)

48. Each month that my wife/partner gets her period I feel is a month of our lives down the drain. (D)

49. I take my wife's/partner's monthly cycles one at a time, and feel, if it happens this month, great, and if not, no big deal, we'll just try again next month. (A)

50. As my wife's/partner's fertile time approaches in each cycle, I get hopeful that maybe this month will be the one. (B)

51. If we aren't able to conceive this month, or next month, or the one after that, we'll just keep trying until there are no more cycles left to try. (C)

52. If I knew that there was an infertility center in another state that had far superior live birth rates for those with my/my partner's particular problem than any center close by, I'd be willing to travel, or even relocate for part of the year, to take advantage of the program. (C)

53. If I thought that my/my partner's infertility treatment regimen was causing problems in my relationship with my partner, I'd want us to give up the treatment/seek a different type of program— even if all doctors said that only with this treatment would we have a decent chance at having a baby. (A)

54. Whatever problems arose in my relationship because of the requirements of the treatment program, I would try to work them out with my wife/partner, with professional help if necessary— but I would still stick with the program. (B)

55. If told there was no way I could ever have a biological child, I would still want my wife to avail herself of whatever methods were available to have one. (C)

56. If I learned that it would be impossible for my wife ever to have a biological child, I would still want to do everything possible to see that a child was born with half my genes. (C)

57. If a couple cannot have a biological child, I think the honorable thing is for the infertile partner to offer the fertile one the option of divorce, so that he/she can have children with someone who's normal. (D)

58. I have strong religious beliefs that I'm afraid might be compromised by certain forms of infertility treatment. (A)

59. Your religious values, your family, and doctors all have a role to play in helping you decide what's the right way for you to handle your infertility, but ultimately it will be up to you and your partner together to choose the way you will deal with your own bodies. (B)

60. I haven't answered/don't even want to think about many of the questions on this questionnaire because many of these issues are very painful/too confusing for me right now. (D)

Scoring and Interpretation of Results

Count up the number of responses under each letter, A, B, C, and D. If the majority of your answers fall under one letter, then read the interpretation section for that category. If you do not find a majority of responses under one letter, then find the letter category with the greatest number of responses and read the interpretation for that category.

But what if your answers are about evenly divided, let's say, between the Bs and the Cs? You could handle it this way: Ask yourself which of the statements touch on issues that are most important for you. If items dealing with the timing of treatment are most important and your responses to those statements fall into the C category, then you should consider yourself a C. But if you feel most concerned about the items dealing with the nature of your relationship with doctors, and your responses to those items are mostly Bs, then consider yourself a B.

What if your answers are fairly evenly distributed among all the categories? In that case you probably have conflicting goals and expectations from treatment. For example, you may want as little medical intervention in your life as possible, or you may be reluctant to make significant changes in your life-style, while you still want to achieve a pregnancy as soon as possible. You may need to take some time first to sort out in advance what's most important to you. Before entering any kind of treatment program, you would probably also benefit from sitting down with an infertility counselor, or attending a support group such as RESOLVE, so that you can ask specific questions of knowledgeable sources about what to expect of different types of treatments. Once you're clear in your own mind as to what is required of patients in different situations and you have had some time to consider how you might respond to the demands of the different types of programs, then take the questionnaire again—and don't be surprised if this time you come up with a more consistent profile.

Majority or Greatest Number of Responses Under Letter A: Conservative Response

You are generally predisposed to seek the least amount of medical intervention that will help you achieve pregnancy. If you are not yet aware of any specific problem needing correction, or if you've had tests but no particular cause of infertility has been identified, then you might be happiest continuing to try to become pregnant naturally for some set period of time.

However, if you have been told of a specific problem and then offered a choice between, for example, a high-potency drug that requires daily monitoring and carries a high risk of side effects, and one that is rated somewhat less effective but also entails less risk and less supervision, you will most likely be more comfortable with the latter choice.

You are not overanxious about your infertility; you feel you have some time to work on the problem, or you have some hope that it may just clear up on its own. You also seek to balance your desire to have children against your need to keep control over your own body and avoid disruption of your private life or your career.

When seeking medical advice you should do the following:

- Try to find a doctor with a low-key personality, one who will take the time to explain all the ramifications of different treatments to you, and won't push you to enter any program until you're sure you're ready.
- Question the purpose of all tests and the course of action most often followed if a problem is uncovered. Should you decide that normal treatment regimen is not one you would undergo, then you probably don't want to undergo the test, either.
- Look for ways to minimize the impact of those tests and treatment methods that you have decided to undergo. If, for example, you are especially fearful about the pain of a procedure, you may be able to get a local anesthetic before the procedure begins. In most cases, all you have to do is ask.
- Go for a second opinion before agreeing to undertake any sort of treatment plan that promises to be highly disruptive of your life-style. It may be that the treatment is indeed the one you need if you are to have a shot at having a baby, but you'll feel more at ease about going through with it if you've heard that judgment from more than one expert in the field.

MAJORITY OR GREATEST NUMBER OF RESPONSES UNDER LETTER B:
MODERATE APPROACH

You want to do what is reasonable and prudent to overcome your infertility, even if it means having major surgery, staying for months on

Since I have no structural problems and am relatively young, we plan to try conservative treatments first (fertility drugs and IUI).

Carolyn from
Delaware

an intensive drug regimen, or submitting yourself to procedures that are still in the experimental stage. But that doesn't mean you'll do *anything* to have a baby. You will still look for less invasive procedures if they are available and effective in your case, though you are not afraid of taking on a higher level of medical involvement in your life, if that's what the objective evidence tells you.

You don't feel you have a vast amount of time; you are willing (or able) to invest only so many months or years to dealing with this problem, or endure only so much hardship (you tell yourself, for example, two miscarriages are my limit, or I'll only try this surgical operation once), before you are ready to quit and move on.

While you are willing to inconvenience yourself to a large extent, give up old habits, and rearrange your personal life to suit a treatment schedule, you would not go so far as to displace yourself permanently in your quest for a baby. You are not about to move to Australia, even if the IVF program there has had a breakthrough that might just solve your problem!

You will feel most comfortable in a program that

- will work within a set timetable arrived at after careful evaluation of your age, physical problems, and emotional needs
- will "step you up" to a more aggressive level of treatment if you haven't achieved a viable pregnancy by the end of your personal timetable
- is staffed by doctors and nurses who will treat you as a full partner in the quest to overcome infertility, who will keep you apprised of any new developments that could aid in your case, and who will listen carefully to your reactions to their advice, to be sure you are thoroughly informed and are proceeding based on a good understanding of the prognosis

I left my first clinic because they seemed too aggressive. I felt I wasn't ready for the kind of treatment schedule they advised. I went to another clinic, but after a few months I felt my case wasn't getting enough attention. I went back to the first clinic. Now I feel ready to try a somewhat more intensive approach.

*N*ancy from Washington, D.C.

𝒱 researched clinics and chose the one with the best rating for IVF. I decided to go to ———— Clinic in Virginia. I spent two weeks of each cycle there. My husband stayed with me for one cycle, using his vacation time from work. The other cycle, he just came down when he was needed. [This patient became pregnant on the second IVF attempt.]

*𝐄*llen from New Jersey

MAJORITY OR GREATEST NUMBER OF RESPONSES UNDER LETTER C: AGGRESSIVE APPROACH

No doubt about it: having a child is the number one need in your life right now. You want to bypass conservative treatments and go right for whatever gives you your best shot at conception. You don't feel you have any time to waste, either. If, for example, surgery offers you a way to get rid of your endometriosis now, you're not about to try a few months of danazol to see if you can clear the problem up that way. You want that operation scheduled, and the sooner the better. Or if the recommendation is for you to take Pergonal instead of Clomid, you're not going to hesitate, even though the recommended drug requires you to come in daily for blood drawing and sonograms; what matters most to you is the higher ovulation induction rate of Pergonal.

Though it's good that you know what you want and have the motivation to stick with the rigors of a fertility program, you would also be wise to temper your determination with a dose of cautious restraint. You may be a bit too prone to follow blindly your doctor's suggestions, and his interest could also include studying the effect of certain new procedures or drugs on you as well as helping you to achieve pregnancy. Your interest, of course, is only in the latter, but it's up to you to ask the tough questions and find out realistically what the chances are that the recommended course of action will give you the result you desire. Once you know what the probabilities are, you may need to keep reminding yourself of them. Otherwise you could be prone to work yourself into an overoptimistic "high" after each cycle of treatment, only to fall into a bitterly disappointed "low" when your period comes and it's clear the treatment has failed.

Chief among the qualities you'll want in your treatment program are

- best live-birth rate in the region (or if you're willing to move, best anywhere)
- availability and experience in the very latest of the high-tech procedures and therapies, including cryopreservation of embryos, microinjection of sperm, and whatever else is on the cutting edge of the field at the time
- willingness of staff to persist with treatment regimen for as long as you are physically and emotionally willing to keep trying
- frankness of staff, so that after every available treatment option has been tried more than enough times and has failed, you will be advised that in their best medical judgment it is time for you to quit

MORE THAN SIX RESPONSES UNDER LETTER D

Even if a majority of responses fall into another letter category, if you had more than six responses under letter D, you are not ready for treatment yet. You have some serious misgivings, inner conflicts, or problems in your relationship with your partner that you need to resolve before you can discover what course of action will be right for you:

- You may not be sure that you truly want a child now but may feel pressured by others to "produce."
- You could be pinning too great a hope on conception, believing that it will heal a damaged relationship or boost a sagging sense of self-esteem—when in fact it will probably just add more stress to your life.
- You may be in a relationship that seems to be stable now but you're worried that introducing a baby into it will change things in ways you don't want.
- You may want children very deeply but feel intimidated by medical technology or frightened by the prospect of pain or unknown side effects from treatment.

If any of these statements comes close to describing what you feel (unless you only have these sentiments fleetingly, or on rare occasions), the first thing you'll need to do is to share them with your spouse/ partner. It's no good going in for treatment if one of you is secretly reluctant.

Of course, discussing some of these issues openly may be difficult and painful. In that case you might want to look for an infertility program that offers not just medical advice but psychological counseling for couples. The larger, more complete urban fertility centers, especially those affiliated with a university or teaching hospital, would be more likely to include such a service than would a small private infertility practice.

Another, perhaps more easily accessible source of counseling or emotional support is through your local chapter of RESOLVE. RESOLVE may refer you to a therapist or counselor specially trained to help couples work through some of the emotional conflicts they're experiencing with the decisions they must jointly make about their infertility. It may well be that RESOLVE has a discussion group going in your area (either peer-group counseling, or with a trained group leader) designed to help couples like you find the solutions most appropriate for their own lives.

CHAPTER SIX

ABOUT CONVENTIONAL TREATMENTS

Drug Therapies and Surgeries

Now we come to the heart of your experience as an infertility patient: treatment, at last!

You've been through months of testing, your problem has been identified, and now your doctor has recommended a first course of action. He names the form of treatment he wants to commence, and then he briefs you about what is involved. His talk is full of terms like "contra-indication" and "GnRH agonist" and "chorionic gonadotropin," and your eyes are starting to glaze over. You'd like to ask him lots of questions, but you wonder: Will his answers really be all that helpful? After all, it's a good bet that he's never been on the receiving end of treatment. Can he really describe what it *feels* like?

You know you would learn more by talking to other couples who have already been through it. You would ask about each of the various drugs you have just been prescribed:

What is it?

How is it taken?

What are the common variations and combinations for this drug regimen?

What does it feel like?

What side effects should I watch out for?

How will it affect my life-style?

What questions or issues should I discuss with my doctor?

Based on the answers provided by my interviewees and survey respondents, I will address each one of these questions for each of the drug therapies in widespread use today. In this section following the descriptions of the drugs Pergonal and Metrodin, I will also provide answers to questions about **monitoring,** the term used by most clinics for the series of daily tests required of women who take either of these powerful ovulation-inducing medications.

Men who have received a prescription for the *testicular cooling device* will also find answers to questions about this mechanical apparatus on page 247 of this chapter.

Also in this chapter, in the section following the Drug Therapies section, I will provide information on the types of surgeries commonly performed and include a list of questions for patients to discuss with their doctor before undergoing any operation.

DRUG THERAPIES

Clomid (Clomiphene Citrate)

WHAT IS IT?

A pill you swallow on several consecutive days, starting during or just after the end of your menstrual period. The same drug is also sold under another brand name, Serophene.

HOW IS IT TAKEN?

Dosage will vary depending on the degree of your ovulatory problem. A typical dose might be two pills of fifty milligrams each taken once a day, starting on Day Five of your menstrual cycle, and continuing through Day Nine. Ovulation should occur around Day Fifteen. The woman is usually asked to keep track of her **LH** surge with an ovulation test kit, and after a positive test result, have intercourse with her partner within thirty-six hours—then wait fourteen or fifteen days to take a pregnancy test.

VARIATIONS AND COMBINATIONS?

Clomid can be started on Day Three or Four; it can be taken for longer than five days; it can be taken in combination with Pergonal, Metrodin, and/or hCG; the couple may be advised not to rely on intercourse but to schedule an **intra-uterine insemination** (**IUI**) with the husband's sperm, or if the husband is infertile, with donor sperm.

What does it feel like?

No special description needed about taking a pill—unless you get side effects, described below.

Side effects?

Most women I talked to found Clomid quite tolerable (especially if they'd ever taken any stronger drugs, like Pergonal). However, some did experience one or two of the following problems: headaches, occasional nausea, occasional light-headedness, weight gain, and hot flashes. The patient consent form given to me when I took Clomid also warned of some other possibilities (occurring in less than 2 percent of patients): breast tenderness, nervousness, insomnia, frequent urination, temporary hair loss, and visual symptoms such as blurriness, spots before the eyes or flashing lights. If you experience any of these more serious side effects you should certainly inform your doctor.

Clomid can also cause what's known as "ovarian overstimulation," meaning that your ovaries produce too many eggs, become enlarged or cystic, and possibly cause abdominal discomfort. If this happens to you (as it does to about 15 percent of all patients on Clomid), you will most likely have to stop taking the drug for a month or two to let your ovaries return to their normal state.

Effect on my life-style?

Taken by itself, not in combination with any other drug, a Clomid regimen should not require you to make any changes in your normal routine.

Questions and issues to discuss with my doctor?

Since multiple births (usually twins, but occasionally triplets or more) will occur in about 6 percent of all pregnancies resulting from Clomid, you should let your doctor know whether you view this possibility as one of the drug's risks, or one of its serendipitous effects.

You should also ask what your doctor intends to do about **monitoring** you for signs of ovarian overstimulation (described above). Some doctors routinely perform mid-cycle ovarian **sonograms** for all patients on Clomid; others simply warn patients of symptoms to watch out for and wait for the patient to call if any develop. If your doctor takes the latter approach, and you are nervous about the drug's side effects, you might want to request an ovarian sonogram during your first cycle on the drug.

If you do not have an LH surge (as detected by your use of an ovulation test kit) by Day Nineteen of your cycle, you should call and ask your doctor if a sonogram might be in order to see how the Clomid is working.

I was informed about the side effects of Clomid beforehand, but they were still horrible. Hot flashes, nausea, mood swings, fatigue, loss of appetite, depression. But there is no way around them if Clomid is your only choice.

Jennifer from Texas

Progesterone

WHAT IS IT?

A drug taken to cause the uterine lining to thicken to be better able to nourish a fertilized egg in the second half of the cycle (**luteal phase**) and through the early part of the pregnancy.

HOW IS IT TAKEN?

Usually beginning three or four days after a positive LH (ovulation kit) test, the woman begins inserting suppositories twice a day in her vagina. Once in the morning and once before bedtime is the pattern most women follow, continuing medication until a menstrual period occurs, or, if pregnancy is confirmed, until the end of the first eight, twelve, or sixteen weeks of gestation.

VARIATIONS AND COMBINATIONS?

The drug may also be administered by injection, especially if the use of vaginal suppositories has caused vaginal irritation or spotting. I interviewed one patient who was taking a new form of the drug, by lozenges slowly dissolved under the tongue for twenty minutes (she said the lozenges were bitter, despite some added peppermint flavoring). Progesterone is frequently used as a part of the drug regimen of **IVF, GIFT, ZIFT,** or other **ARTs.** It may also be used in the second half of an ovulation cycle stimulated by Clomid, Pergonal, or Metrodin.

What does it feel like?

It's messy! The inactive ingredients in the suppository melt in the heat of your vagina and then drip out all day long. It's necessary to wear a sanitary napkin both day and night for the whole of the time that you are taking the drug. Tampons are banned because they interfere with the drug's absorption into your bloodstream. Some doctors recommend that you lie down for a half hour after insertion, to try to prevent some drug loss from dripping.

If you take the drug by injection, you avoid the mess, but then you will need to prepare and receive a shot—given with a rather long, thick needle—every night or every other night, and by the end of your time on the drug, your buttocks will feel like an overused pincushion.

Side effects?

If you are not pregnant, you will experience a longer than normal wait till your menstrual period arrives, and during the extra days you will almost certainly start imagining that you are pregnant. This is because progesterone mimics many of the same sensations you would feel if you had actually conceived: bloating, breast tenderness, occasional light-headedness, nausea, and elevated **BBT.** A few women also reported experiencing diarrhea, depression, and irritability while on the drug.

If you are the type to research the effects produced by any drug you are taking, and you look up progesterone in a medical reference book, you may be alarmed to see that it carries an FDA warning about potential birth defects if taken during pregnancy. This is misleading because the studies showing a higher incidence of birth defects all were done on women taking the *synthetic* form of the drug only; no study has ever shown an increased birth defect rate in the babies of mothers who took natural progesterone. But when you pick up your prescription it's a good idea to check with your pharmacist to be sure that you are getting only the natural form. Even if your insurance company will only reimburse you for using the cheaper synthetic form, *you must use the natural form to be safe.*

Effect on my life-style?

Progesterone will affect any travel arrangements you may make. It must be kept cool, so you will need to have a refrigerator available in your hotel room or wherever you stay. If you will be taking a long car trip you will need to pack the progesterone in a small cooler with ice or with those special frozen gel packs. You must also have on hand sufficient sanitary napkins wherever you are, both for day and night.

Questions and issues to discuss with my doctor?

Ask your doctor about the pros and cons of using suppositories or injections (especially if you have any vaginal irritation or spotting after a month or two of suppository use). Also, since progesterone will lengthen your cycle by anywhere from a few days to over a week, ask about coming in for a blood pregnancy test between fifteen and seventeen days after ovulation. If the test is negative, you can then discontinue the drug, get your period soon thereafter, and start getting yourself ready for another cycle.

Pergonal

What is it?

Pergonal is the brand name for a powerful fertility drug produced only by Serono Laboratories. It consists of "**human menopausal gonadotropins**" (**hMGs**), and it is extracted from the urine of postmenopausal

I asked one doctor I had seen about progesterone and he said, "It's a placebo." Then I saw a specialist in Boston who has a theory about recurrent miscarriage. He says it's caused by a feto-toxic antibody. It's subclinical [without symptoms]. Progesterone is a mild immuno-suppressant. This doctor advocates 200-milligram progesterone injections, morning and night. I heard of a patient who had had nine miscarriages before she went to see this doctor.

Emily from New York

> ## TIP
> ### Learning to Give Shots
>
> Serono Labs (the manufacturer of Pergonal and other injectable fertility drugs) has an excellent videotape on the preparation and administration of shots. Narrated by a registered nurse, the tape shows a real couple going through all the steps to give a shot. The viewer can follow along, stopping the tape as needed, before going on to the next step. Your doctor's office may own and lend out a copy of this tape. If not, try calling Serono's toll-free number (listed in the Resource Guide in the back of this book) to find out about viewing the tape.

women. When it enters the system, it fools your body into thinking that you are not producing enough hormones to ovulate, and so your body compensates by producing an overabundance. The high hormone levels in turn cause the ovaries to work overtime, turning out multiple eggs per cycle.

HOW IS IT TAKEN?

By injection in the woman's buttocks or upper thigh. Usually the woman's partner learns to give the shot, but the woman may also learn to give herself a shot. Most clinics offer classes to give couples careful instruction in preparing the Pergonal solution and administering the mixture by injection, including letting couples practice injections on an orange during the teaching session until they feel confident about doing it correctly at home.

The timing, number, and dosage of the injections will vary depending on the woman's ovulatory needs. Starting about Day Three or Four of her menstrual cycle, she will start receiving the injections as instructed by her doctor. Starting usually on Day Eight, she will come in to the clinic every morning for two tests (an ovarian sonogram and a blood test) to see how her ovaries are responding to the drug, and to enable her doctor to set the correct dosage for that evening's shot. This testing routine is called **monitoring,** and it is an essential part of a drug regimen involving either Pergonal or Metrodin, to protect the woman against some of the riskier side effects the drug occasionally will produce. Because of the importance of monitoring all patients who are on Pergonal or Metrodin (this includes all patients undergoing ovarian stimulation in preparation for an IVF, GIFT, or ZIFT cycle, too), the whole monitoring routine will be described in more detail in its own separate section, beginning on page 232.

When the results of the daily monitoring tests show that the woman's ovaries have produced enough egg **follicles,** and they are of sufficient size and maturity, and when her blood hormone levels are high enough (but not so high as to be a warning sign of ovarian hyperstimulation), the doctor will inform the woman that she is ready for an injection of **hCG,** which causes the follicles to release their eggs approximately thirty-six hours after the shot. The couple will be instructed to have intercourse two or three times within that "window of opportunity" for maximal chance at fertilization. Alternatively, the couple would not rely on intercourse to achieve fertilization, but the man would produce a semen specimen, which, after laboratory processing, would be inserted into the woman's uterus in the procedure known as IUI (described in a separate section beginning on page 259).

VARIATIONS AND COMBINATIONS?

Pergonal may be taken in combination with either Clomid or Metrodin. When the follicles are large enough, hCG is nearly always given to trigger the eggs' release. Progesterone is sometimes prescribed to boost hormone production after ovulation has taken place.

More and more doctors are also prescribing the drug Lupron for patients to take in the week or two prior to beginning Pergonal. Lupron has the opposite effect of a fertility drug: it causes the ovaries to shut down production of hormones so that they will be in a state of rest when the Pergonal stimulation begins. When Lupron, Pergonal, hCG, and progesterone are all used in sequence, your doctor will be in control of your body's hormone production from the beginning to the end of your cycle. You may end up feeling as if you are caught in an episode of that old science fiction TV show *The Outer Limits,* in which the unseen announcer's booming voice warns, "*We* are in control of your television set. *We* control the horizontal, *we* control the vertical. Do not attempt to adjust your set"—only it's not your TV that is put beyond your control: it's the inner workings of several major organs of your own body!

What does it feel like?

The injections are done with a fairly slim needle and so are not as painful as most people expect. After a week or so of shots on alternating buttocks, however, your whole backside will feel pretty sore.

Side effects?

Both plentiful and powerful. Most women report bloating, weight gain, and a feeling of fatigue. Hot flashes, depression, and mood swings are also common. Blurring of vision or headaches should be reported to your doctor, as should any sudden or constant abdominal pain. You will probably be instructed to weigh yourself daily while you are on the drug, and to report any sudden weight gain (more than two pounds in one day) to your doctor.

Pergonal also carries with it the risk of certain possibly severe side effects. "Ovarian overstimulation," meaning that the ovaries have become enlarged and are producing too many follicles, is a condition that happens to about one in five women being treated with Pergonal. To reverse the condition the woman must go off Pergonal for the next cycle or even the next two cycles, and get as much rest as possible, allowing the ovaries to return to normal.

"Ovarian **hyperstimulation**" is an even more dangerous side effect. This side effect occurs in 1 to 2 percent of women, generally in the two-week time period after they have stopped taking the drug. The ovaries suddenly become enlarged, blood hormone levels skyrocket, and excess fluid may collect in the abdominal cavity or in the lungs. Cysts that have formed within the ovaries may rupture, causing internal bleeding. Rarely, blood clots will develop, which can be fatal. Because of all these dangers it is *extremely* important that you inform your doctor at once of any unusual symptoms or pain you may develop. Before going on Pergonal make sure your doctor has provided you with a telephone number to be used during the off-hours to get hold of medical help in an emergency.

Other problems associated with Pergonal therapy include risk of ectopic pregnancy (about 3 percent, as opposed to the 1 percent risk found in the general population); risk of miscarriage (about 25 percent, as opposed to 15 percent in the general population); and risk of multiple births (15 percent of the patients who conceive on Pergonal have twins; another 5 percent have triplets or more).

TRAVEL TIPS FOR PERGONAL USERS

*W*hen traveling without your partner during the period when shots are necessary, be sure you make arrangements in advance to have someone give you your injections at the proper time (unless, of course, you have learned to give yourself the injections). Most cities and towns have visiting nurse services that can send someone out to your hotel room to prepare and administer the injection according to your doctor's instructions. But these visits are usually expensive, and are seldom covered by insurance.

When traveling abroad, be sure you bring your prescription along, proving that you are authorized to possess needles and syringes for injectable medication. You don't want to have to try to explain how fertility treatment works to a foreign customs agent, and you certainly don't want the agent jumping to any other conclusions about your need for drug paraphernalia.

EFFECT ON MY LIFE-STYLE?

When you are on this drug, you had better be prepared to have your daily life turned around for a week or two. First, you will be bound to a certain schedule each evening (or perhaps twice a day) of preparing and administering injections. Let's say your injection is supposed to be given at ten P.M. and you're invited out to a dinner party that night. You can decline the invitation so that you can get your shot in the privacy of your home—or you can do as one Washington couple did and pack up the syringes, needles, and drug vials in a plastic bag, hide them in the woman's pocketbook, and at the proper time, retreat to the bathroom together, lock the door, and give the shot. Just be sure you remember to bring a jar with a screw-on lid to store the used needle in so that you can bring it back home for safe disposal. Otherwise, your hosts may find the used drug paraphernalia in the trash and conclude that one of you is a heroin addict!

Once monitoring begins, you will have to arrange your working day to allow yourself to spend one to two hours every morning at the clinic for your blood test and sonogram. By then you will be experiencing a variety of side effects from the drug, and will probably be tired, short-tempered, and depressed. By the time you are instructed to have intercourse (or come in for IUI), you may feel about as sexy as a blimp—and your husband may feel like a walking sperm bank.

During the last two weeks of the cycle, when you are waiting anxiously to see if the fantastically expensive drug has worked, you will probably feel alternately overly optimistic and overly despairing. Then the day will arrive that you go in for your blood hCG test to find out whether you are pregnant—and how you feel then will of course depend on the news you get.

QUESTIONS AND ISSUES TO DISCUSS WITH MY DOCTOR?

Do not consent to begin a Pergonal regime without having a detailed discussion with your doctor that covers each of the subjects listed below:

1. *Aggressiveness of approach.* What are the advantages of Pergonal in our case over a milder drug like Clomid?
2. *Cost.* Unless your health insurance company is picking up the tab, expect to pay anywhere from $40 to $65 for each vial of Pergonal used (some women will be required to use up to two, three, or even four or more vials per shot, and/or more than one shot a day, over a period of six to twelve days). Find out whether you are required to buy the drug through the clinic, and if so, whether you must pay in advance for the expected dosage for the entire cycle, and whether any leftover Pergonal may be returned for a refund.
3. *Possible measures to increase the chance of conception with Pergonal.* Should we consider doing IUI? Adding progesterone in the luteal phase? Taking any other drugs, or avoiding any substances?
4. *Abortion.* You should face this issue squarely before you start, because Pergonal does entail risk of four or five or even more embryos developing, and such a pregnancy would almost inevitably endanger your health. If you find abortion morally unacceptable under all circumstances, you are probably best advised not to begin a Pergonal regime. For those who *are* willing to contemplate abortion in such a situation, there are a few doctors skilled in a procedure that goes by the rather horrible euphemism "selective reduction." This means that the doctor will cause a few of the developing embryos to be aborted, while (if all goes well) twins or triplets will remain and develop normally to term. Selective reduction is highly risky, and available only in a few big-city hospitals, so you should find out ahead of time whether you would be able to avail yourself of the procedure should the need arise.

Metrodin

WHAT IS IT?

The brand name of a drug produced by Serono Laboratories that is pure **FSH (follicle-stimulating hormone)** in composition, identical to the FSH your body produces naturally. Metrodin differs from Pergonal in that Pergonal consists of both FSH and LH (luteinizing hormone). When a woman takes Pergonal and her ovaries respond by producing too much LH in relation to FSH, or if she experiences ovarian hyperstimulation, she will usually be switched from Pergonal to Metrodin for her next treatment cycle.

Because Metrodin is so similar to Pergonal, both in the way that it is taken and in its physical and emotional effects on the patient, all the answers to questions about Metrodin (*How is it taken? Variations and combinations? What does it feel like? Side effects? Effect on my life-style? Questions and issues to discuss with my doctor?*) will be similar to the answers provided for Pergonal, in the preceding section.

One Patient's Progression

I have done eight cycles of Clomid, including Clomid with hCG, three cycles of Clomid-Pergonal combination with hCG, and I am now in my third cycle of Metrodin-hCG. I intend to do only six cycles of Metrodin. . . . After that, I don't really have any choices except to go on to IVF, GIFT, ZIFT, etc.

*R*ose from Washington

Lupron

WHAT IS IT?

The brand name for the drug leuprolide acetate, produced by TAP Pharmaceuticals. Lupron chemically is a "GnRH agonist," which means that it is an agent that will cause the ovaries to shut down production of hormones and enter a state of rest, rather similar to what would happen if you were entering menopause. By causing your ovaries to stop working, your doctor is able to gain control over what day they will start working again. Your cycle can then be coordinated with that of many other women in the same clinic's fertility program, and you can all have your orientation class at the same time, begin your Pergonal or Metrodin injections at the same time, and have any other procedures that may be performed (such as egg retrieval for an IVF, GIFT, or ZIFT cycle), done at about the same time of the month.

Not all clinics use Lupron this way. Some doctors administer it only to reverse ovarian overstimulation that was caused by the woman's response to Pergonal in the previous cycle. It is also commonly used in the treatment of **endometriosis,** freeing the woman from having menstrual periods for a certain amount of time, and at the same time freeing her from producing any excess endometrial tissue.

How is it taken?

By injection, usually administered by the woman herself into her upper thigh. Dosage and number of shots per day will vary greatly, depending on the reason the drug is given and the severity of the condition being treated. When used as a treatment for endometriosis, a single monthly injection may be sufficient. You may also want to ask your doctor about the availability of a relatively new form of a Lupron-like drug for daily use, administered by nasal spray (brand name: Synarel).

Variations and combinations?

As discussed above, Lupron is commonly used along with Pergonal or Metrodin, especially if the ovarian stimulation will be followed by a procedure such as IVF, GIFT, or ZIFT.

What does it feel like?

Of all the injectable medications taken as part of a fertility program, Lupron is the most comfortable. The Lupron needle is so fine that you can't even feel it going in (and I'm fairly squeamish about needles, so I wouldn't be saying this unless it had felt okay to me). Most women who swear at the outset that they would *never* learn to give themselves an injection will find, after the first painless shot or two (given to them by their partners), that it's not difficult at all to stick the needle in by themselves.

FYI

If You Live in a Remote Small Town

It's frustrating that the pharmacies here don't carry the drugs I need. I needed to start my daily Lupron injections and my local pharmacy said they could get the medicine and have it the next day. It didn't come in, and we had to drive two hours to Austin to get it.

Carla from Texas

SIDE EFFECTS?

Since Lupron is used to simulate a menopause-like cessation of ovarian function, it is not surprising that it can also bring on many menopause-like symptoms, including hot flashes, irritability, depression, decrease in breast size, vaginal dryness, and increase in body hair growth. For my part, I also experienced a little spotting when I first began taking the drug, but my doctor said that Lupron could not have been the cause. I still think it was.

EFFECT ON MY LIFE-STYLE?

Since a woman usually will be able to administer her own Lupron medication easily, she will not be as restricted in how and when she can travel, as she is with Pergonal or Metrodin. If she needs to go on a business trip apart from her husband while taking Lupron, she won't need to find someone qualified to administer her shots while she's away. And since the Lupron needle is identical to that used by diabetics for insulin, she can more easily explain what she is doing with drug paraphernalia, if anyone happens to ask her about it.

As with any injectable medication, when traveling abroad you must always have your prescription on hand to prove to customs agents your legitimate medical purpose for possession of needles and syringes.

QUESTIONS AND ISSUES TO DISCUSS WITH MY DOCTOR?

Lupron is not strictly a necessary part of any ovary-stimulating drug regimen, but its use may make it easier for a doctor to coordinate his services to many infertility patients, by having them all ovulate around the same time of the month. If this is the main reason your doctor has put you on Lupron, and you find its side effects difficult to tolerate, then you should certainly discuss discontinuing the drug, or seek treatment at a clinic that does not routinely prescribe Lupron to its patients.

Monitoring

WHAT IS IT?

Monitoring is the way that your doctor will keep track of the effect of very powerful fertility drugs (Pergonal, Metrodin) on your reproductive organs. Monitoring is absolutely essential for providing the patient with some degree of protection against the risks of ovarian overstimulation or hyperstimulation (described in section about Pergonal). *You should never agree to take Pergonal or Metrodin without being monitored daily, beginning no more than eight or nine days after Day One of your cycle.* In the past there have been clinics that have failed to keep patients on strict monitoring programs, resulting in tragedies such as the conception of octuplets who all died at birth. There have even been a few patient deaths due to ovarian rupture, deaths that could have been prevented had proper monitoring procedures been observed. In California a former fertility patient sued and won a substantial judgment against her clinic, which had failed to monitor her properly, leading her to conceive septuplets who were born extremely prematurely and severely handicapped. Fortunately, nearly all of the clinics that failed to monitor their patients have been driven out of business, so few patients today will encounter this form of fertility malpractice.

Monitoring also allows your doctor to determine what is the appropriate dosage for you to take to cause the development of egg follicles to continue at the proper pace. Here is what takes place:

On the morning monitoring begins, the woman goes to her clinic or to a designated hospital or medical facility to have two tests performed. She will have blood drawn from her vein for same-day lab-testing to determine the level of the hormone estradiol, and she will have an ultrasound of her ovaries to see how many follicles are being produced and to measure the size of any that appear to be near maturity.

The blood test is performed just as any blood test would be (for description, see under Blood Workup in Chapter Three).

The ultrasound is performed by the transvaginal method described in Chapter Three under Pelvic Ultrasound. (Presumably you had a baseline ultrasound done during the middle of your last menstrual period;

all subsequent ultrasounds may be compared against your baseline ultrasound, which showed what your ovaries looked like prior to stimulation by fertility drugs.) When the technician has got a view of your right ovary on the monitor, she will begin to measure any follicles that are over ten millimeters in length. The follicles will appear on the screen as round, black, blobby objects, and you will soon learn to recognize what they look like when you have produced a satisfactory number that have developed to the proper size (sixteen millimeters or more is considered good). It will take the technician a minute or two to measure each follicle in the right ovary and record the results on the machine; then she will run through all the same steps to measure and record the size of any follicles found in the left ovary. Finally, she will look at your uterus and note whether any fluid is present in it or around it.

After the ultrasound is over, the woman dresses, while the ultrasound technician writes up her findings on a report like the one shown on page 234.

Most clinics try to set up their monitoring procedures to reduce as much of the inconvenience of these daily visits as possible. You may find that you are allowed to come in for your monitoring tests anytime between, for example, six-thirty and eight A.M., and that you can choose to have the blood work or the ultrasound done first, as you prefer. The blood-drawing room may be right next to the ultrasound room, to reduce the amount of time you spend running from one part of the clinic to another.

However, at some clinics far less trouble has been taken to minimize hassle for the patient. I talked to many women who were patients at a hospital-affiliated program that required them to go to one building to have blood drawn and another building two blocks away to have the ultrasound performed. At other clinics, the patient had to go to a room on the top floor for the ultrasound, then ride the elevator to the basement to have blood drawn. If convenience is of importance to you in selecting a fertility center, you would be well advised to ask where and how monitoring is performed before signing up with a program.

Another common cause of concern is the handling of monitoring on weekends. Many clinics are closed then and must send their patients elsewhere (to a hospital, usually) to have the two tests done. There are even clinics that are closed on weekends but make no alternative arrangements; monitoring just stops on Saturday and Sunday. *You should not sign up for any program involving monitoring that does not provide for full coverage on weekends.* Always check to make sure you understand what the procedures are for weekend monitoring, if they are different from the weekday routine.

ULTRASOUND FOLLICULAR MONITORING REPORT

Patient's name _Peggy Robin_   Date of birth _06_ / _19_ / _53_

Doctor _P.R.G._   Account Number _1234567890_

Program: IVF ☐ GIFT ☐ ZIFT ☐ Pergonal ☑ Lupron ☐ Clomid ☐

natural ☐ evaluation ☐ other ☐

Follicles:

	Right Ovary		Left Ovary

Right Ovary

1. _16_ x _16_ x _17_ = _16_
2. _15_ x _17_ x _17_ = _16_
3. _13_ x _12_ x _10_ = _12_
4. _10_ x _10_ x _11_ = _10_
5. ___ x ___ x ___ = ___
6. ___ x ___ x ___ = ___

Left Ovary

1. _12_ x _12_ x _12_ = _12_
2. _13_ x _10_ x _13_ = _12_
3. ___ x ___ x ___ = ___
4. ___ x ___ x ___ = ___
5. ___ x ___ x ___ = ___
6. ___ x ___ x ___ = ___

Additional follicles < 10 mm _4_   _2_

Cysts:

___ x ___ x ___ = ___   ___ x ___ x ___ = ___

Uterus: _normal_

Cul de sac fluid: none ☐ minimal ☑ moderate ☐

Remarks: _____

sonographer _L.G._

WOMEN'S COLLEGE HOSPITAL
WOMEN'S HEALTH CENTRE
THE RESOURCE CENTRE

I actually ended up enjoying the early-morning drives to the clinic. This was a quiet time for me to daydream and hope. I looked forward to the supportive atmosphere created by the staff and other patients in the waiting room. At times it felt like I was in a women's support group. We rejoiced for each other's follicles and anguished for a canceled cycle. And the event that kept us addicted, of course, was a positive pregnancy test.

*C*andy Levine
Licensed Clinical Social Worker from Washington, D.C.

Each day after you have been monitored, the test results are made available to your doctor. She will evaluate them to determine whether to increase, maintain, or decrease your next dose of Pergonal or Metrodin. She will get in contact with you at a phone number you have given her to call between certain hours (for example, between three and five in the afternoon). If you are not able to receive confidential calls at work, you may prefer to have your doctor call your home and leave the dosage information on your answering machine.

When the doctor has determined that your follicles have matured to a sufficient size and that your estradiol level is sufficiently high (but not so high as to be a sign of overstimulation), then she will tell you that it's time for your hCG shot, to trigger your follicles to release their eggs. Between twenty-four and thirty-six hours after the shot, you should have intercourse, preferably once in the morning, then again that same night, and then first thing the next morning—if you're not too exhausted by then. If IUI is planned, the man will be instructed when to come into the office to provide the semen to be processed and inserted in the woman's uterus.

In IVF, GIFT, and ZIFT cycles the woman will be told when to come in for her egg retrieval, and her husband will be instructed about providing the semen.

VARIATIONS AND COMBINATIONS?

Some clinics also monitor cervical mucus. The woman comes in for a pelvic exam at a certain time during her cycle and a bit of cervical mucus is swabbed out of her vagina and examined to see if it is clear and stretchy. It will also be put on a glass slide and looked at under a microscope.

What does monitoring feel like?

Most women find the daily blood drawing and ultrasound tolerable—but no one would call it fun. You may feel either hope or anxiety as you watch your ovaries appear on the ultrasound screen each day and see either good or bad development of follicles (good means you have several follicles that appear to be developing toward maturity; bad means that few or no follicles are developing, or else you are producing far too many follicles, or the follicles are not growing to sufficient size). When told your follicles are poor, it's easy to start feeling discouraged and upset, especially if the ultrasound technician uses words like "inadequate" or "abnormal," or tells you that your ovaries are "polycystic."

I talked to women who were so upset at bad ultrasounds that they left the ultrasound room in tears. But more often, women reported that the ultrasound technician was sensitive of their feelings, and good at gently explaining what she was seeing as she moved the probe around.

Side effects?

The main purpose of monitoring is to prevent dangerous side effects. The only complaint most women have about it (not counting the incredible inconvenience and expense!) is that after a few days of consecutive blood-drawing, the site of the needle-stick will look bruised and feel tender. It helps somewhat to have blood drawn from the opposite arm each day to give each puncture an extra day to heal.

Effect on my life-style?

Yes, yes, yes! It is impossible to lead a normal life on any drug regimen that entails monitoring. For a week or more of your life you must find the time each morning to go in to the clinic and have your tests done. If you have far to travel and have to wait a while each time for your tests, monitoring may take several hours out of your day. You cannot go away on a business trip or a vacation during this time. You will spend your afternoons most likely waiting for the phone to ring, to hear your doctor comment on your ovarian progress and issue instructions for preparing your next shot. Being on the receiving end of a daily phone call from your doctor will make it difficult for you to hide the fact of your infertility treatment from coworkers or other family members.

Do you recall hearing an announcement from newscaster Connie Chung that she was going to cut back on her work schedule for CBS so that she and her husband could "aggressively pursue" their quest for a baby? Well, making time for monitoring was undoubtedly what she was talking about.

QUESTIONS AND ISSUES TO DISCUSS WITH MY DOCTOR?

Make sure your doctor knows what phone number to use to deliver the information about the dosage for your next shot. If there are certain phone numbers that should *not* be used for the calls, make sure he knows that, too. A reliable answering machine that may be accessed remotely is essential for those who cannot sit by the phone for hours at a time. At certain points in the cycle the doctor may need to get hold of you directly, in which case a telephone pager (or beeper) or cellular phone may prove most useful. You can rent either of these devices by the month or week, if you don't want to buy one.

If you have access to a fax machine for personal use, find out whether your doctor would be interested in faxing you dosage information or receiving any information from you by fax.

Find out what arrangements are made for monitoring over weekends and on national holidays.

If you have any obligations, such as religious devotions or business travel, that cause a conflict with your monitoring schedule, make sure your doctor is informed of the problem at the outset, and find out whether rescheduling (say, from early-morning monitoring to after-work monitoring) can be arranged for a limited period of time.

Danazol

WHAT IS IT?

A drug (brand name: Danocrine) taken to reduce or eliminate **endometriosis.**

HOW IS IT TAKEN?

In pill form, with the dosage varying depending on whether the endometriosis is classified as mild, moderate, or severe. Typically, starting toward the end of the menstrual period (to ensure that the patient is not pregnant, since danazol can cause birth defects), you will take the drug three or four times a day, staying on the medication from four to six months.

Variations and combinations?

In moderate and severe cases, danazol will often be prescribed in conjunction with surgery, either beforehand, to reduce growths, or afterward, to prevent recurrence.

For patients who find danazol's side effects intolerable, alternative drug therapies are available: Provera is a synthetic progestin that works to inhibit endometriosis by simulating some of the physical conditions of pregnancy (when a woman is pregnant her symptoms of endometriosis are usually alleviated or eliminated); Lupron is a GnRH agonist (see Lupron section for further explanation) that suppresses female hormone activity, therefore preventing endometrial overgrowths, without increasing the production of male hormones.

Danazol suppresses female hormone production (it's actually an anabolic steroid), and it works to counteract endometrial overgrowths by reducing or eliminating the buildup of the uterine lining that occurs in the latter half of the menstrual cycle. As you might imagine, taking a steroid can make you feel "masculinized"—plus you will be rendered completely infertile for the duration of the treatment, so you will probably feel frustrated at knowing that, at least for the short term, you can't even *try* to have a baby. Your mood may improve if you can keep reminding yourself that the majority of patients who start danazol therapy for endometriosis do go on to have a baby.

Side effects?

The following symptoms are suffered by between 50 and 85 percent (depending on which medical text you read) of women taking the drug: weight gain, excess facial and body hair growth, acne, muscle cramps, voice deepening, decrease in breast size, hot flashes, loss of libido, increased cholesterol level. *All* of the danazol takers I interviewed had at least a few of these effects.

Effect on my life-style?

To help to counteract some of the side effects, some modification of your regular routine may be beneficial. Weight gain and increased cho-

> *I* did Danocrine after surgery [for endometriosis]. It gave me leg cramps and made me moody—but I wouldn't describe the side effects as all that bad. Then I did Lupron-Depot, one monthly injection. It cost $340 a shot, but I only had to go in once. It was fairly effective on the endometriosis. I had no cramping. It made me feel very emotional, though that could also have been from other causes.
>
> *C*arla from Texas

lesterol levels may be prevented by adhering to a low-fat, low-sugar diet of frequent but very small meals. A program of regular exercise (preferably low-impact aerobics) will help avoid water retention and muscle cramping. Generous use of lubricants should prevent discomfort during sex. While you are on danazol, your doctor will probably have you use birth control to avoid the chance of an embryo being affected by this birth-defect-causing drug. You may find it annoying and frustrating to have to mess with diaphragms and jellies, or use condoms, when all you want to do is have a baby, but you may be able to keep your aggravation to a minimum by keeping the long-term outlook in mind.

QUESTIONS AND ISSUES TO DISCUSS WITH MY DOCTOR?

First you should find out how your doctor views the question of the causal relationship between endometriosis and infertility, discussed under Endometriosis in Chaper Four. You should not undertake a long course of steriodal treatment unless your doctor is able to explain to you in very persuasive terms how he believes that danazol will work to create the conditions you need to become pregnant.

If your endometriosis has been classified as severe, and you have *not* been told you need surgery, ask your doctor whether he believes that danazol alone will be effective enough in reversing your endometriosis and restoring your fertility, or if he believes there is a good chance that surgery may still be required later on. If the latter is the case, you may not want to try out a drug with considerable side effects for six months when you possibly could "get it all over with" in a single operation.

If you are already in your mid or late thirties or older, you might not want to spend six months taking a drug that renders you completely

I researched danazol thoroughly before I went on it. I didn't think it would do anything for me, because it turned out [after a laparotomy to remove endometriosis] that I had incredibly dense adhesions. But my doctor said it would clear up what he couldn't get to in surgery. I had all the side effects: mood swings, bloating. . . . My new doctor okayed going off it, since my endometriosis was so severe. I had more surgery—six or seven times, total. I eventually became pregnant through IVF.

*H*elen from Washington, D.C.

infertile when you could be trying one of the ARTs, such as IVF or GIFT. If the doctor uses the laparoscopic method of egg retrieval as part of the program, at the same time he can insert a laser to burn off any endometrial adhesions he can see.

Also, be sure your doctor is aware of the extent of your insurance coverage. As with most fertility medications, danazol is expensive. Six months of this drug, unless covered by insurance, will be burdensome to most couples. If a less costly alternative is available that your doctor believes could be equally effective, you may want to consider it.

Parlodel

What is it?

The brand name of the drug bromocriptine, a prolactin suppressant. (Prolactin is a hormone normally produced during breastfeeding; the hormone inhibits ovulation.)

How is it taken?

In pill form, the dosage varying according to how elevated the woman's prolactin level is.

Variations and combinations?

Parlodel is sometimes prescribed in conjunction with Clomid, Pergonal, or other fertility drugs.

What does it feel like?

No special comment needed about pill-taking routine.

Side effects?

Nausea, stuffy nose, headache, dizziness, and a feeling of fatigue are all common, so the patient should check to see if she is on the lowest dosage that will still be effective.

Effect on my life-style?

Unless the side effects are so severe as to keep you from working normally, there should be no special impact on your daily routine.

Questions and issues to discuss with my doctor?

Is an elevated prolactin level the cause of my infertility, or could it be the outward symptom of some other problem, such as pituitary tumor or thyroid gland dysfunction? Are these other conditions worth investigating in your opinion, and if not, why not?

Antibiotic Therapy

What is it?

Treatment with drugs such as doxycycline, erythromycin, Flagyl, penicillin compounds or other antibiotics for fertility-impairing infections such as **chlamydia,** gonorrhea, mycoplasmas, unreaplasmas and other female **pelvic inflammatory diseases (PIDs)**, male urinary-tract infections, or **sexually transmitted diseases (STDs)**.

How is it taken?

Dosage and length of time on medication will vary greatly, depending on the infection being treated and its degree of drug resistance. A typical treatment for chlamydia, for example, might consist of ten days of doxycycline, in 100-milligram doses, taken three times a day. It is extremely important to follow the doctor's instructions about what time of day to take the medication and whether to take it with food or not. Doctors will sometimes be puzzled that an antibiotic course appears to be in-effective, when the real problem is that the patient either did not take the drug exactly as prescribed, or else was not adequately briefed about the proper way to take it.

Variations and combinations?

The list of available antibiotics is lengthy and their use in combination with one another seemingly limitless. If the infection remains after one course of treatment is finished, a different drug or drug combination will be tried. In infections caused by drug-resistant strains of bacteria, treatment with a week, or even several weeks, of intravenous antibiotics, administered during a hospital stay, may be the only effective course of action. Intravenous antibiotic administration is also possible outside of a hospital setting, through the use of a small battery-operated pump that you can wear on a belt around your waist, which will infuse the medication at set intervals through a catheter into your vein. When antibiotics are administered in the hospital, the cost will usually be picked up by the health insurance company without question; however, antibiotics received by an outpatient are frequently excluded from cov-erage, and the cost of IV medications will be high—perhaps as much as $1,500 per day! So expense may play a large role in which form of medication delivery system you choose.

What does it feel like?

Taking pills for a week or two requires no special comment. Receiving the drugs intravenously, whether you are in the hospital or not, will range from mildly uncomfortable to actually painful, depending on what type of drug is being administered, whether you have "good" veins (meaning, easy for the nurse to find for an IV start), how often you are to receive the medication, and how long it takes for each dose to drip into your system.

Side effects?

Short-term use of antibiotics seldom results in anything worse than occasional bouts of diarrhea, heartburn, or nausea. You will also become more susceptible to yeast and other fungal infections. Long-term or intensive use will occasionally cause severe side effects, such as liver or intestinal damage, or weakening of the immune system. If you find yourself suffering from indigestion and heartburn while on antibiotics, resist the urge to take antacids. Most antibiotics have the effect of reducing the normal population of protective organisms in your intestinal tract, leaving your more susceptible to food poisoning. Stomach acids can help to kill off harmful bacteria such as salmonella, but not if you have eliminated those acids by taking Tums, Rolaids, or a similar product. Salmonella, unchecked, has been known to cause perforation of the colon, a life-threatening condition, so be especially careful to avoid undercooked chicken or eggs (the most common sources of salmonella) while on your antibiotic program.

EFFECT ON MY LIFE-STYLE?

Little effect when taken in pill form for less than a month. Your doctor may warn you to eliminate or cut back on your use of alcohol, so as to avoid irritating your stomach, liver, or other organs. You may also be instructed about other foods or medications to avoid. If hospitalized for intravenous administration, then your normal life will be put on hold for the duration of your stay.

QUESTIONS AND ISSUES TO DISCUSS WITH MY DOCTOR?

If your doctor has not specifically instructed you already, be sure you understand all the details about how the drug is to be taken, including whether it must be taken with meals or not, whether alcohol is to be avoided, whether there are any other over-the-counter or prescription medications to be avoided, and whether anything in your past medical history (such as an allergy to penicillin) might pose a problem when you are on this drug.

Since many antibiotics are unsafe to take while pregnant, ask your doctor about the advisability of using some form of birth control (but not an oral contraceptive, which when combined with an antibiotic, will almost always result in a yeast infection).

Before beginning an intensive antibiotic regimen (especially if intravenous antibiotics are prescribed), you should have a thorough discussion with your doctor to find out his views on the relationship between your bacterial infection and your fertility problem. Since antibiotic therapy for infertility is in many cases controversial (see section in Chapter Four on infections for further discussion), you will want some assurance

My OB-GYN looked at my husband's sperm test, which was somewhat abnormal. He didn't think about varicocele, which was the most likely explanation. Instead of sending us to a urologist, he sent us to a specialist in bacterial infection, who recommended oral antibiotics for my husband. The next sperm test showed improvement, so he said the treatment was working. The test after that was abnormal again. The doctor was talking about putting my husband on intravenous antibiotics. We were coming to the conclusion on our own that bacteria wasn't the problem. Everybody has *some* bacteria. We stopped seeing the doctor. I did get pregnant, but miscarried. When we went back to the [bacterial] specialist, he made me feel it was my fault I had miscarried because we didn't stick with the antibiotics. He did another test that showed none of the first bacteria he had tested my husband for, but this time a different bacteria. He prescribed more antibiotics, but by then we'd had it. We saw another doctor, who specialized in high-risk pregnancy as well as fertility. I got pregnant and that pregnancy was fine.

Carol from New Jersey

that your doctor has positively identified certain harmful organisms that are disturbing your reproductive functioning, and that the antibiotic course prescribed is what is needed to restore your fertility potential.

If the infection is one that can be passed on to your partner (and most reproductive-tract infections are), be sure to ask your doctor about the advisability of treating your partner—whether or not your partner has tested positive for the same organism. Testing for some infections can be imprecise, yielding false negatives, so it is often a good idea to treat both partners, even if only one appears symptomatic.

Hormone Therapy for Men

What is it?

A fairly wide variety of drugs can be used, either alone or in combination, to try to improve sperm quantity or quality. These drugs include Clomid, hCG with Pergonal, Parlodel, FSH, GnRH, **testosterone,** and tamoxifen. However, the use of fertility drugs in men is seldom as effective in improving the production of sperm as it is when used in women to improve the production of eggs. This may be because the woman's body has been the subject of more intensive research and the relationship between each of the hormones and her fertility is better understood. Standard doses of the various hormones for women are well established, and doctors can often predict which patients will respond well. With men, on the other hand, there is a much greater range of treatments, as doctors are less certain as to which drugs will get which response from which patient.

How is it taken?

Given the number of drugs that have been used in male hormone therapy, it is not possible to describe methods of administration for each. Some may be in pill form, others (Pergonal, for example) may be by injection. Clomid is often prescribed to be taken one pill per day for several consecutive months. The hormone hCG might be given by injection three times a week for a period of six months. Your doctor will provide instructions for your particular prescription, and then retest your semen periodically to see if the drug is helping.

Variations and combinations?

Different urologists will favor different drug combinations. Often the doctor must try out several different drugs or drug combinations on the same patient before finding one that yields any positive result. Space is insufficient to detail all the possibilities here.

When there is little or no improvement from various drug therapies, the doctor will often suggest that the couple try to improve the quality of the sperm sample by processing it (or "washing" it) in the laboratory and artificially inseminating the woman with it (IUI). Often to improve the chances of conception, the woman is first made "superfertile" through the use of Clomid, Pergonal, or Metrodin. If several attempts at insemination are unsuccessful, the next step is usually IVF (or sometimes ZIFT), a procedure that will allow the doctor to determine if the sperm are capable of fertilizing an egg in a laboratory dish. As part of an IVF cycle at a clinic equipped to perform ultrahigh-tech procedures, the doctor might also attempt micromanipulation of sperm and egg, in which the egg has its outer layer partially removed to make it easier for a sperm cell to penetrate and cause fertilization (partial zona dissection, or PZD).

What does it feel like?

No special comment needed for drugs taken in pill form. If taking an injectable drug, you will either have to learn to give yourself a shot in the upper thigh, or else receive a shot in the buttocks that your partner has learned to give. Whether or not your backside ends up sore will depend on how often your shots must be given and for how long you must remain on your injection regimen. The worst regimen (as far as local irritation goes) is probably Pergonal injections daily for eighty days.

Side effects?

That depends on the drug(s) being used. Some of the side effects of Clomid, Pergonal, and Parlodel are described in earlier sections discussing the use of these drugs in treatment of female hormonal disorders. Some men feel the side effects of drugs to be so severe that they want to give up treatment after a short time. Fans of the television series *L.A. Law* will remember the story of Stuart Markowitz and Anne Kelsey. After a short time on male hormone therapy Stuart broke out in sweats, was irritable and depressed, and never felt like making love to Anne when she told him it was "time." Stuart quit treatment, and he and Anne tried to adopt (with disastrous results), and then (typical TV ending) he got Anne pregnant despite his poor sperm count. The "it only takes one" theory of conception may be true, of course, but it should only be counted on by TV characters.

Effect on my life-style?

Taking medication that must be injected will constrain your travel and ability to go out at certain times, just as for women who receive shots. (See sections on women's injectables for some tips about traveling with needles and syringes.)

Questions and issues to discuss with my doctor?

Discuss effectiveness! Many doctors believe that male hormone therapies so seldom provide good results that it's not worth anyone's trouble to try them out. For example, Dr. Derek Llewellyn-Jones, in his book *Getting Pregnant: A Guide for the Infertile Couple*, says: "At present no specific, effective drug treatment is available to improve sperm count and to increase the chance of pregnancy. A recent Australian study compared the pregnancy rates of the wives of oligospermic men who had received a variety of treatments. In no instance was drug treatment more effective than no treatment" (p. 64). If your doctor disagrees with this conclusion, ask to be given copies of studies or articles from medical journals pointing to the value of the particular drug regimen he wishes you to follow.

Once you have decided to go forward with the drug approach, discuss how long you should stick with it before switching to another course of treatment or going to donor sperm. Also discuss the advisability of increasing your wife's egg-producing capability, using IUI to put a "washed" sperm specimen directly into her uterus, or trying a few cycles of IVF or ZIFT.

The second urologist I saw put me on testosterone. I asked my brother-in-law (who is a urologist in another state) about it, and he said, "Yes, it's done." I asked our infertility specialist about it, and he said "That's crazy." I tried it anyway for several months, but it didn't work. So I switched doctors. My next urologist recommended a series of beta-hCG shots. After six weeks my sperm analysis was at an all-time low, so I stopped taking it. We started IUIs (five total) and with each one the sperm counts went up. By the last cycle it was really, really good. The shots were supposed to help in three months or not at all, but it took five to six months to make a difference in my case. When we try to have another baby, I'm going to stick with the shots until my sperm count goes up.

Dan from Virginia

Testicular Cooling Device

WHAT IS IT?

A device that holds a cooling pack in place against a man's testicles to lower the temperature in the scrotal sac to below 94°F. I have learned of two different brands in use: one type is a jockstrap-like garment that contains a pack of "blue ice" (a special gel that retains its coolness for a long time after you remove it from the freezer); the other type uses water as the coolant, and includes an electronic box that is worn around the waist to control the rate of evaporation. In the first type the blue ice pack must be changed about every four hours; in the second type, cold water must be added to a small reservoir about every four to five hours.

How is it worn?

Both devices are meant to be worn all day, and removed only for sleep. The man can expect to wear the device every day for up to four months before seeing any improvement in sperm production.

Variations and combinations?

The man may use the cooling device while his partner undergoes treatment to boost her ovulation to increase the chance that the man's sperm will fertilize one of her eggs. He may also be counseled about changes in his life-style, such as decreasing the frequency or intensity of his exercise program, or changing from a job that puts him too close to a heat source (such as a bakery oven). Sperm quality of his semen specimen may be further improved by laboratory processing, after which it will be inserted into his wife's uterus (IUI) or used to try to fertilize an egg in a laboratory dish, as part of an IVF or a ZIFT cycle.

What does it feel like?

It's annoying, but as one respondent wrote: "You can get used to it." Condensation from the cooling unit will make your pants wet around the crotch from time to time, which can be embarrassing. You are better off wearing dark colors, or bringing a change of pants to work. You can *not* wear any rubberized or flannelized undergarment to try to contain or absorb the wetness, because that would decrease air circulation and increase heat—just the opposite of what you need. The device is also somewhat cumbersome and heavy.

Side effects?

Since the device is worn outside the body, it has no adverse medical impact within the body. The wetness and the bulkiness are certainly disadvantages, but they cannot be termed medical side effects.

Effect on my life-style?

You will be tied to a schedule of going to the freezer every four hours to pull out a new coolant pack, or going to the bathroom to refill the water reservoir of your device with cold water. It will be difficult to keep the fact of your infertility treatment confidential, unless your place of work provides you with your own private kitchenette and bathroom. You may want to keep several pairs of pants at work so that you can change when wetness becomes a problem. When traveling you must be sure you will have access to a freezer or a source of cold water (depending on which device you're using). It will take a good deal of commitment on your part to stick with the device long enough to tell whether or not it has helped.

QUESTIONS AND ISSUES TO DISCUSS WITH MY DOCTOR?

The device has been in use only since 1985, and so there are no long-term studies on its effectiveness; however, proponents claim that the pregnancy rate after use is more than 50 percent—"excluding those with the most severe degree of infertility."* It's difficult to know how to evaluate such a claim, without knowing much more about the men who made up the study group. Perhaps the most prudent course of action for the man considering wearing the device, would be to ask his doctor to provide him the most recent study, go over it with him, and help to make the findings intelligible to him in layman's language. You should also ask him about his own professional experience with the device. How many times in the past has he prescribed its use? How many pregnancies, if any, occurred afterward? If your doctor has never treated anyone with this device before, you are probably better off asking for a referral to a doctor who has.

You should also ask your doctor about the advisability of increasing your partner's fertility with ovulation-inducing drugs, and/or improving sperm count through laboratory processing of semen and IUI. If neither of these treatments helps to bring about pregnancy, you might consider IVF or ZIFT, possibly with micromanipulation of sperm and egg.

ABOUT REPRODUCTIVE SURGERY

Taking drugs, even the most powerful ones, to try to have a baby is one thing—but letting someone cut into your body to improve your chances of conceiving is something else again. If like most of us you want to

*Dr. Adrian Zorgniotti, quoted in *The Minneapolis–St. Paul Star Tribune*, "Doctors Take a Closer Look at Sperm to Treat Infertility," by Warren E. Leary.

Always Get a Second Opinion!

*M*y first doctor was so eager to find *the* reason for my infertility [this interviewee had already been seeing her doctor for a long time] that he mistakenly interpreted a mucus clog on the X ray for the hysterosalpingogram as a septum. I had surgery at ———— University Hospital with a specialist in resecting septums, and all they did was clean out a few spots of endometriosis.

*B*renda from New Jersey

avoid "going under the knife" unless it's absolutely necessary, then you must first take a few simple, prudent steps:

1. *Get a second opinion.* Unless two unrelated specialists agree that surgery is the best course for someone with your fertility problem, don't agree to it!
2. *Seek less invasive alternatives.* Go through every other plausible treatment for your condition with your doctor, one by one, and have him explain why each is not worth trying for a period of time in your case. If you do not find the doctor's explanations convincing, you should probably switch doctors.
3. *Call RESOLVE.* Call either the national office helpline or your local chapter, and ask for the name and number of a "contact"—that is, someone who has already been through the same operation you are considering undergoing, who can tell you just what it was like, and whether it worked, and if that person would repeat the procedure if given the chance, or would opt for some other approach (and if so, what?).

When you are finally sure that surgery is the right course of action for you at this stage in your life, then do it!

In this section I will provide general information about the types of infertility surgeries most frequently performed today, but will not go into detail about any one operation. If you are interested in the technical side of treatment, your surgeon can give you an exact account of what he will be doing, or you may prefer to buy a book written specially to help patients know what to expect before, during, and after any of the most commonly performed operations. Two such books are included in the Suggested Reading List at the back of this book. You may also want to check under the heading of your diagnosis in Chapter Four to see if there are any significant controversies surrounding the particular surgical procedure that you are considering (three examples of controversial surgeries would be those for varicocele and pituitary tumor removal, and the ovarian wedge resection for PCO disease).

I've had four surgeries [laparotomies for endometriosis]. It gets easier each time. The first time the pain medication afterward made me feel too "out of it." I was in the hospital five days. When I had surgery again, I tried to take as little pain medication as possible. I walked around afterward and I ate. It helped me recover faster and get home faster.

*C*arla from Texas

Types of Surgery

CONVENTIONAL

Conventional surgery is performed using general anesthesia. You are "put under," usually by an intravenous drug, an incision is made (if in the abdomen, the operation is called a **laparotomy**), and the doctor uses conventional surgical tools to accomplish his objective, then the incision is closed with stitches that must later be removed.

LAPAROSCOPIC

Performed under general anesthesia, laparoscopic surgery uses a much smaller incision than conventional surgery. The woman's abdominal cavity is first inflated with carbon dioxide gas. A small incision is made in or just below her navel; through this incision the doctor inserts a viewing scope with a light, called a laparoscope. Other instruments may be introduced through an equally small incision made just below the top of the pubic hairline. After the doctor has accomplished his objectives, he will close both incisions with no more than a stitch or two each. The patient usually will spend an hour or two in a recovery area,

COMMON REASONS FOR SURGERY

Female	Male
To remove uterine fibroid tumors or polyps	To repair a varicocele
To clear blocked fallopian tubes	To clear an obstruction in the sperm ducts or anywhere else along the path sperm travel during ejaculation
To remove scar tissue or adhesions from the uterus, ovaries, or elsewhere	To obtain tissue for biopsy
To repair a divided (septate) uterus	To insert a *penile implant*, a device that makes it possible for an impotent man to get and maintain an erection
To cut out or burn off endometriosis found on any of the reproductive organs or elsewhere in the abdominal cavity	To reverse a vasectomy (voluntary sterilization)
To reduce androgen-producing structures in the ovaries responsible for PCO disease	To remove tumors from the pituitary gland in the brain
To remove tumors from the pituitary gland in the brain	
To reverse a tubal ligation (voluntary sterilization)	

and go home to rest for the remainder of the day. Laparoscopy is used in the diagnosis of infertility, as well as the treatment of various conditions, including cauterization of endometriosis and correction of tubal abnormalities. The list of what can be accomplished through use of the delicate laparoscope is growing, as surgeons continually improve skills and develop new techniques.

Hysteroscopic

Hysteroscopic surgery will sometimes be performed in a doctor's office, using only local anesthesia. The patient is usually given a sedative beforehand to ease pain. The hysteroscope, a fiber-optic viewing scope, is inserted through the woman's dilated cervix into her uterus, which has first been expanded by injection of carbon dioxide gas or some other transparent substance. During hysteroscopy the doctor may remove adhesions, small polyps or fibroid tumors, or repair certain abnormalities, such as a partial septum (dividing piece of tissue in the uterus)—although patients who turn out to need more than minor repairs will have to have conventional surgery to accomplish the job.

MICROSURGERY

Microsurgery is performed with the use of a surgical microscope to allow the doctor to see and repair very fine vessels or tubes found in either the male or female reproductive tract. Common microsurgical procedures include reconnection of the vas deferens severed during a vasectomy, reconnection of the fallopian tubes severed during a tubal ligation, repair of any of the extremely fine tubules in the testicles.

LASER SURGERY

Lasers may be used during conventional, laparoscopic, hysteroscopic, or microsurgical procedures in place of a scalpel. Instead of cutting out the scar tissue or endometriosis or whatever needs to be removed, the surgeon directs the laser to the spot to burn it away (called *cauterization*).

BALLOON TECHNIQUE

Instead of cutting away or lasering through blockages, the doctor might use the balloon technique. With this technique, the surgeon threads an extremely thin wire through the affected tube. Attached to the end of the wire is a tiny balloon which, when it reaches the point of obstruction, will be inflated to open up the tube. This procedure may also be called *balloon tuboplasty*. In the female it can be used to open up a blocked fallopian tube; in the male it can be used to clear an obstruction in the sperm ducts, or isolate a varicocele. Though the technique is relatively new, it appears to be very promising, involving less risk of causing additional scar tissue than methods involving cutting and reattachment.

Questions to Ask Your Doctor About Your Surgery

When in my cycle/when in my wife's cycle will the operation be done?

When Your "One Day" Surgery Takes a Week to Get Over

*Y*our doctor tells you that your operation will be "minor." He may call it "in-out" surgery, or "one-day" surgery, or "same-day" or "Band-Aid" surgery, but all these terms are a way of saying that you will go home within an hour or so after the completion of the procedure.

This may lead you to believe that you will be able to go back to work, if not the same day, then the day after, or the day after that, and feel completely recovered when you do. WRONG! Nearly all the "minor" surgery patients I interviewed (except for a few outstanding stoics) reported taking much longer than the amount of time predicted by the surgeon to feel okay again. One woman told me that after her laparoscopy on a Monday she had planned to be back at her desk on Tuesday, but instead had to take off the rest of the week. Others went back to work within a few days, but still struggled with pain, soreness, and fatigue.

Lesson: Don't count on your doctor to predict your recovery time. If you have ever had any form of minor surgery (such as gum surgery or mole removal), use the recovery time from that experience to help you figure out your needed amount of time off. And don't schedule anything difficult in the following week if you can avoid it!

Any special preparations? Do I call to set up a presurgical interview with the anesthesiologist? Should I avoid eating or drinking anything a certain number of hours before the operation will start?

How much time will I need to take off from work?

Will you perform the actual procedure, or will you be supervising someone else (such as a resident or intern)?

Who else will be present? The anesthesiologist? Surgical nurses? Residents? Interns? Medical students? Other observers or participants?

How long will the procedure take from start to finish?

What type of anesthesia will be used? If local, will I be given a sedative beforehand, and if so, what is it? If not, should I take aspirin, ibuprofen, or acetaminophen beforehand?

Is this office equipped to deal effectively with an emergency such as a hemorrhage during the procedure, or a severe allergic reaction to the anesthetizing agent? (For in-office operations only.)

What are the risks of this procedure? What sort of complications have occurred in your patients?

How long will I be in the recovery room?

How is the incision closed? With stitches? staples? Will they need to be removed later, and if so, about how long after the operation?

How big a scar will I have after surgery? Where will it be? What are the chances that the scar will be thickened and raised (keloid scarring)?

Any special instructions to follow afterward? (Examples: Swab the site of the incision with alcohol before rebandaging; don't get the incision site wet until after the bandages have been removed; don't lift anything heavier than five pounds for six weeks after the operation.)

Will you prescribe a painkiller for me to take afterward, or is there a certain over-the-counter medication you recommend?

What warning signs should I watch out for after the operation? (Might there be bleeding, and if so, how much bleeding is considered abnormal? Fever, and if so, how high? Nausea? Headache? Abdominal cramping? Other signs?)

How long should it take for me to feel fully recovered? (See previous page regarding your doctor's reply!)

How soon afterward can I resume intercourse (or rather, how soon afterward will I feel up to having intercourse)?

What method is used to find out whether the operation was successful (e.g., sperm analysis, repeat hysterosalpingogram, repeat laparoscopy)?

What is your fee for this operation? (Check with your insurance company to find out if the surgeon's bill will be fully reimbursed.)

And most important: After recovery, what are my chances of conceiving/getting my wife to conceive, assuming the operation goes as it should?

*A*fter my laparoscopy I had incision pain for three days. A very helpful nurse suggested ice . . . and it worked!

*B*eth from Washington

Stacking Risks Against Benefits

You've asked the surgeon all your questions and have had a little time to think about the answers. You may have also done a little research on your own, reading books or articles about the procedure. You have sat down with your spouse or partner and have talked about how surgery would affect your sex life, your relationship, your future goals, and your budget. If, after all this homework, you have reached the following conclusions,

1. that the chance of "something going wrong" is minimal because the surgeon you have selected is highly skilled at this operation, and the hospital where it is to take place is excellent;
2. that the majority of patients who have undergone this operation performed by this surgeon have had significantly greater fertility rates than comparable patients who opted for a nonsurgical treatment, or for no treatment;
3. that the procedure is widely accepted in the medical community as the treatment of choice for a patient in your condition;
4. that there is no other nonsurgical alternative or ART that might be worth trying out for a few cycles first (such as IUI or IVF);
5. that your fear of surgery is not so great as to make this form of treatment seem a poor choice, even if, in purely medical terms, it appears to be the most effective solution to your infertility;

—then go ahead and schedule your surgery with complete confidence that you are making the best choice for yourself at this point in your quest to overcome your infertility.

CHAPTER SEVEN

ABOUT THE ASSISTED REPRODUCTIVE TECHNOLOGIES

The **ARTs** include a range of procedures, from the rather low-tech **IUI (intra-uterine insemination)** to the ultrahigh-tech micromanipulation of egg and sperm, and **cryopreservation** of embryos (freezing the human conceptus for later implantation). Most people who read the newspapers and watch TV news will know a little bit about two of the more commonly practiced ARTs: **IVF** and **GIFT.** You may or may not have heard of others: **ZIFT,** PROST, POST, TET, and ET. It's easy to become confused by this alphabet soup of names that doctors use to identify each new procedure they invent. After reading this chapter you will, I hope, be unconfused.

Before getting into what makes each ART different from the others, let's go over a few important ways in which they are all* similar:

1. *They are all incredibly expensive.* A single attempt at IVF, for example, could run you anywhere from $5,000 to $12,000, depending on your city and clinic. GIFT and ZIFT may be even more expensive.
2. *They all have discouragingly low "take-home baby" rates.* Even the most successful clinics treating the least-impaired couples with the most promising procedure, GIFT, report rates only in the mid-30 percent range. That means that over two thirds of the couples who invest their time and money in the procedure will go away with nothing. Some clinics have success rates of less than 10 percent, and a 12 to 20 percent success rate appears to be about average.
3. *All replace the sex act with a set of cold, clinical procedures designed to bring about conception.* The woman is given powerful drugs to regulate every phase of her egg-producing cycle, and the man is

*Except for IUI (intra-uterine insemination). IUI is included in this chapter because it is undoubtedly an assisted reproductive technology, though it is neither high-tech (since an internist or ordinary gynecologist can perform it) nor especially costly—and it is a reasonably effective method for many couples to achieve pregnancy.

told when and where to deliver his semen and whom to deliver it to. The fun is taken out of the baby-making experience, and a whole lot of new stress is added in.

4. *All involve certain risks.* The risks include multiple gestation (that is, getting pregnant with twins, triplets, or more); drug side effects, such as ovarian overstimulation or **hyperstimulation**; complications from the invasive procedures used in egg retrieval or insertion of an embryo, including bleeding, adverse reaction to anesthesia, and infection; and a higher than normal incidence of miscarriage.

5. *All involve tough decisions and big commitments.* These procedures should be considered only by couples who fully understand the low odds of success, who are in agreement as to how much time and money they will risk pursuing conception this way, and who for good reason have ruled out all other forms of treatment at this point in their lives.

6. *All raise certain questions of medical, legal, and social ethics.* How much (if any) tampering is morally acceptable in the aid of human conception and birth? How much research and medical resources should be directed to enabling the infertile to have biologically related offspring? What role, if any, should government play in regulating or restricting ARTs? What should the parents of a child conceived through an ART tell that child about the circumstances surrounding his or her conception? (These and other questions are the subject of an essay beginning on page 293.)

Having introduced my discussion of the ARTs with this series of negative remarks, let me now throw in a few rays of hope:

• Doctors are getting better at the ARTs all the time. Success rates at the best clinics continue to improve year after year.
• You can keep yourself from ending up someplace that is hardly ever successful if you will order the annual *Clinic-Specific Report* compiled by the Society for Assisted Reproductive Technologies (SART), which lists the success rates for the various ARTs for every clinic in the country that is a participating member of the American Fertility Society or any of its subgroups (of which SART is one). The report costs $30. For ordering information, contact SART at the address listed in the Resource Guide. If the doctors at your clinic are not members of the AFS or any of its subgroups, and have not agreed to adhere to AFS guidelines for responsible medicine, *you should find doctors who are AFS members.*

• Statistics can give only a very general idea of how successful a clinic is with an ART; the chance of success in your individual case could be much better than average—you don't know till you try. Thousands of babies are born every year in this country through ARTs. So they definitely *do* work for many people—and you could be one of them!

For each of the ARTs considered in this chapter I will answer four questions:

What is it?

What happens?

Who is a candidate for this procedure?

What are the issues and questions specific to this procedure that I should consider at the outset?

In answering the last question I will not repeat the six issues and concerns that I have listed above that apply to all of the ARTs; I will address only the additional issues and questions raised by the particular subvariety of ART under consideration.

In answering the first three questions I will provide only a generalized, patient's-eye view of each ART. There are good books by doctors available today that will describe in more precise medical terminology what goes on during each stage of each ART, and those who are interested in that level of detail should check the Suggested Reading List for recommendations of titles. I have taken the varying accounts given to me by my interviewees who have been through each procedure as the basis for answers to the questions posed.

THE ARTs

IUI-AI/H

WHAT IS IT?

The first set of letters stands for *intra-uterine insemination;* in the second set of letters the first two stand for *artificial insemination,* and the "H" signifies that you will be using your husband's (or partner's) sperm, not a donor's. IUI and AI are ways of referring to the same procedure, which, simply put, is a means to get sperm into the woman's uterus without sexual intercourse.

What happens?

The man first produces a semen specimen (as described under Sperm Analysis in Chapter Three) and delivers it to the lab for "washing." That means that the lab technician will run the sperm through several different steps, all designed to reduce the number of weak or unhealthy sperm, leaving a concentration of sperm of good shape and swimming ability.

When the sperm sample is ready, the woman goes in to her doctor's office and lies on the examining table as if for a normal pelvic exam. The doctor inserts a speculum to open up her vagina, dilates her cervix, and then threads a thin catheter into her uterus and injects the sperm. The whole procedure takes a couple of minutes. Some doctors will then insert a small sponge-like object into the vagina, to act as a plug and help hold in the fluid. The woman can then get up and go home, or back to work. About a half an hour after the IUI, the women can remove the plug by pulling on a string (just like removing a tampon).

Some doctors prefer a variation of IUI called ITI, or intratubal insemination. The catheter is threaded up through the uterus into the opening of one fallopian tube. The sperm sample is deposited inside the tube, and fertilization occurs there, as it would in nature. This procedure is more expensive, more uncomfortable for the woman, and requires greater skill on the part of the doctor, but may prove to bring about a greater chance of conception. The procedure is relatively new, so no long-term statistics comparing it to IUI for effectiveness are available.

Who is a good candidate?

The woman who has "hostile cervical mucus" in her vagina. IUI simply bypasses the vagina, leaving the sperm directly in the uterus.

The man who has a slightly or moderately low sperm count. Sperm "washing" will result in a concentration of the good sperm, and IUI places the sperm closer to the egg, so that they won't have so far to swim.

THE IMPORTANCE OF CHOOSING A SEVEN-DAY-A-WEEK CLINIC WHEN DOING IUI

*C*he first month on Clomid I ovulated when my husband was out of town. The second month I ovulated on a Sunday, and the clinic is not open on Sundays. The third month I had my first IUI—it was unsuccessful. The fourth month I ovulated on a Wednesday, which was my doctor's day off. The fifth month my doctor was out of town... [and after that, this patient switched clinics].

*B*everly from Iowa

The couple with "unexplained infertility." Testing may not be sophisticated enough to reveal all the problems that can occur after intercourse as sperm attempt to navigate through cervical mucus to find the egg. If the couple has been through several unsuccessful months of fertility-drug-assisted tries at conception through intercourse, they should consider doing between two and four cycles of IUI, before moving on to GIFT or another ART.

The couple with an identified hormonal problem, such as a luteal-phase defect, who have tried drug therapy for several months without success. Adding one or two IUIs to the treatment cycle could edge up the odds that conception will occur.

ISSUES AND QUESTIONS

When you're taking fertility drugs, it's bad enough being told by your doctor when to make love, but when you do IUI, it's worse than that: now you're told you *mustn't* make love just before ovulation, but must let the doctor handle the sperm delivery, too. You really have to be psychologically prepared to go this route, or else the husband will end up feeling like nothing more than a walking sperm bank, and the wife will end up feeling like an egg incubator. Talk all your feelings out with one another fully, and if one partner is hesitant while the other is enthusiastic, you may want to explore the benefits of counseling to help you come to a decision (see Chapter Nine for information about finding a counselor trained to deal with fertility problems).

Another thing to consider beforehand is the expense. IUI can cost anywhere between $200 and $1,000, and is frequently excluded from health insurance coverage. If you are already spending a few thousand a month for Pergonal, the several hundred extra for IUI might be seen as a way to decrease somewhat the risk of losing your original, larger investment.

In certain special circumstances you will also want to discuss the advisability of using frozen sperm. If the man is soon to undergo cancer treatment that will affect the health of his sperm, he can arrange to have several semen specimens frozen so that he and his wife will not have to delay their attempts at pregnancy (especially worthwhile if the wife is nearing the end of her reproductive years). The couple choosing this method of IUI must investigate extremely thoroughly the reliability and competence of the sperm bank where the husband's sperm will be stored. Poorly run sperm banks are unfortunately easy to find. Sperm mix-ups have occurred, sometimes with regrettable endings. A woman desiring to have a child with frozen sperm that had been banked by her late husband, a cancer victim, was given the wrong sperm sample and ended up having a child by an unknown man of another race. You can to a certain extent safeguard yourself against such sperm bank malpractice by dealing only with a sperm bank accredited by either of two medical societies, the American Fertility Society or the American Association of Tissue Banks (both of which require members to adhere to a strict set of standards and practices—see box on following page).

IUI-AI/D

WHAT IS IT?

The first set of letters are the same as in the above section; in the second set, the first two are the same, but the "D" signifies that donor sperm will be used.

WHAT HAPPENS?

First the couple must decide what form of sperm donation they want: totally anonymous (with or without a large degree of information about the donor), time-limited anonymity (meaning that the donor agrees that

Sperm Safety Alert!
Stay Away from Unaccredited Sperm Banks!

𝒟o not go to any sperm bank unless reliably assured that the bank adheres to all the safety standards set forward either by the American Fertility Society or the American Association of Tissue Banks. There are some small, quick-profit, quack-operated businesses out there, and you don't want to take the chance of becoming the victim of a fraud, a mix-up, or a deadly disease.

Responsible sperm banks will always

- test potential donors *twice* for diseases such as AIDS, hepatitis, syphilis, and other infections transmissible through semen. The testing must be done once upon initial screening and again, no sooner than six months after the first test, to be assured that the donor is not carrying a slow-incubating virus.
- screen out donors with health problems or dangerous habits, such as illegal drug use.
- get a complete medical history of each donor accepted and make it available to clients.
- set upper and lower limits on the age of donors.
- test sperm for fertilizing potential, and keep records of successful impregnations per donor, as reported by doctors.
- set limits on the number of children that may be fathered by the same donor, to minimize the risk that half-siblings fathered by the same donor might grow up and marry each other.

Be aware: The federal government does not *regulate the sperm banking industry, so it is up to you to watch out for yourself. Most Important Rule:*

- USE ONLY FROZEN DONOR SPERM. With fresh sperm it will be impossible to obtain complete assurance that the anonymous donor is free of AIDS. Yes, it's true that fresh sperm is somewhat more effective in causing conception than thawed sperm—but which would you prefer: improved chance at pregnancy, with increased risk of death for you and your child; or lower odds of conception that will be safe for you and your child?

his identity may be released when the child reaches eighteen), or open donation (the donor is known to the couple—he might, for instance, be the husband's brother, cousin, or close friend).

The first of the three forms of sperm donation is far and away the most common. There is a wide variation among sperm banks as to how much information is collected on donors. Nearly all will make the man's medical history available to the couple (this is important, in case the child later develops a hereditary disease). Most will also provide information on the height, weight, age, and ethnic background of the donor. Many will include information on his profession (medical student is very common), his religion, and his talents, hobbies, or interests. A few very specialized sperm banks will administer IQ tests, and then claim to offer sperm only from men who rank at the genius or near-genius level. The couple may need to investigate several sperm banks to find a reputable one that provides the range of choices they desire before making their selection.

Time-limited anonymity is a new concept being tried by one sperm bank called the Sperm Bank of California (in Oakland). In the past some children of sperm donors have complained of feeling uncertain of their identities, because they are forever blocked from contact with their biological fathers. Some sperm donors have also been left with a sense of loss and unfulfilled curiosity about the new lives they have helped to create. Allowing the grown-up child to get to know the donor will be psychologically healthier for both parties, according to proponents of this method of sperm donation. Those who choose this form of sperm donation who live distant from Oakland must make arrangements (through their doctor or by contacting the Sperm Bank of California directly) to make a selection and have the frozen sperm shipped by next-day air to the site of the insemination. It is also possible that other sperm banks across the country will soon be offering the option of time-limited anonymity to their clients.

A few couples will be interested in donor sperm only if supplied by a donor known to them personally. This may be a requirement of their religion (see Chapter Ten for discussion of this point), or simply a strong preference, to keep a "family line" from dying out (by using sperm from a brother or a cousin), or to ensure that the child will be accepted in a particularly tight-knit ethnic community. Many doctors disapprove of the use of couple-selected donors (thinking the practice can lead to emotional and legal turmoil over who the "real" father is) and will refuse to participate in known-donor inseminations. The couple may have to do some doctor shopping to find one to carry out the procedure as they wish.

It is also possible for women to perform the insemination on themselves, vaginally, in the privacy of the bedroom, following instructions that will be included along with a sperm sample purchased directly from a sperm bank. This method might be the first choice of the single woman who does not wish to enlist her doctor's assistance in her efforts to become pregnant (further discussion of this matter in Chapter Ten).

Once the donor is selected, the insemination is scheduled for the optimal day in the wife's cycle, and it proceeds exactly as described under AI/H.

WHO IS A GOOD CANDIDATE?

The man who has no sperm, or whose low sperm count cannot be sufficiently improved through treatment with surgery or drugs

The man who has tried treatment for a certain period of time but who is not willing to spend any more time trying to achieve pregnancy with his own sperm; the man who does not feel a strong need to have a biological link to his child

The single woman who does not wish to attempt to conceive a child through intercourse with a lover or male friend

ISSUES AND QUESTIONS

Form of donor sperm to be used

Information about donor the couple considers essential to make selection

Accreditation and reliability of sperm bank chosen (see box on page 263)

Availability of sample from same bank, same donor, for future use (so that the couple can try for a second child who will be a full brother or sister to their first donor-insemination child)

Cost per attempt and number of attempts couple is willing to try with same donor; total number of attempts couple will make before considering another course of action (such as adoption)

What they will tell the child about how it was conceived, and at what age they will do it

And of course, before going ahead, the couple should have sorted out their feelings about having a child that will be genetically related only to one parent, and they should feel confident that donor sperm is the best solution to the dilemma of male infertility.

IVF

What is it?

The letters stand for *in vitro fertilization*. *In vitro* is Latin for "in glass," referring to the glass lab dish in which fertilization will occur.

What happens?

The following is the usual sequence of events:

1. The woman has a baseline ultrasound (see Chapter Three for description).
2. She is given Lupron to put her ovaries at a state of rest, so that the doctor can choose the time to begin using drugs to stimulate her ovaries to make eggs.
3. She begins receiving injections of a fertility drug, usually Pergonal, a Clomid-Pergonal combination, or Metrodin—the dosage and frequency of medication as set by her doctor.
4. After taking the drug(s) for a number of days (five or six is typical), **monitoring** begins (see page 232 for description). Medication dosage will now be set during a daily phone consultation with the doctor.
5. After the ultrasound reveals a sufficient number of mature egg follicles and the blood test shows a sufficiently high (but not dangerously high) level of estradiol, the doctor tells the couple when the woman should have her **hCG** shot, which will "trigger" chromosome division of the woman's eggs, to make them fertilizable. (In IVF the hCG is not taken to cause ovulation, since the eggs are to be retrieved prior to their release from their follicles.)
6. Approximately thirty-six hours after the hCG shot the woman goes in for her egg retrieval (may also be called "egg harvest" or "ova aspiration"). Options for pain control during this procedure range from nothing, to light sedation, to general anesthesia. Be sure you know in advance what your doctor usually prescribes, and if you feel you are unusually sensitive to pain, discuss just

I had IV anesthesia during my egg retrieval, including a drug that was antinausea. It made me incredibly depressed for a day. I only had that particular drug one time out of my four egg retrievals. I found out what it was, and made sure I had something else the other times.

Ellen from New Jersey

how much extra pain relief you are likely to need. To perform the egg retrieval by the transvaginal ultrasound method,* the doctor inserts a needle through the vaginal wall, directing it toward the ovary guided by the image he sees of the woman's organs on the sonogram screen. When the needle reaches the inside of the follicle, all the fluid within the follicle, including the egg, is aspirated (sucked out) through the needle, down some tubing and into a receptacle. Then the needle is inserted into the next follicle and the process is repeated. After each mature egg follicle in the right ovary has been aspirated, the doctor goes through the same sequence on the left.

7. After taking some time to recover (as needed), the patient goes home. Meanwhile, the eggs are put into a special nourishing solution, or culture, in a lab dish (also called a petri dish).

8. Sperm that have been "washed" (processed in the lab to eliminate the weaker sperm) from semen obtained from the man are added to the petri dish.

9. The eggs are checked after thirteen to eighteen hours for first indications of fertilization.

10. Forty-eight hours after fertilization occurs, the two-celled, or four-celled, or eight-celled pre-embryos will be visible. Each is evaluated by the doctor and assigned a grade, according to how healthy it appears.

11. The woman returns to the doctor's office. The high-grade pre-embryos (generally to a maximum number of four) are loaded into a catheter, which is carefully inserted into the woman's uterus, and the contents injected.

*Though this is the method currently in most widespread use, some clinics still retrieve eggs via laparoscopy, an operation performed under general anesthesia. See Chapter Three for description. If you wish to minimize the number of invasive procedures you must undergo, you are best advised to seek out an IVF program that uses only the transvaginal ultrasound method.

THE EGG RETRIEVAL

Upon arrival I was given a shot of a drug, Versed, that made me feel drowsy and quite relaxed. Each time I had the procedure done, the length of time it took varied depending on the number of follicles I had, but before I knew it, I was in the recovery area. After the sedative wore off, I found that all my fears about feeling nauseous and dizzy were for nothing.

What I least expected, however, was to feel so uncomfortable about the fact that Versed is also an amnesiac and therefore I could not remember what had transpired, although I was awake and talking through most of it. For my third IVF attempt my husband (who is a journalist) got smart (he was sick of my endless questions about what had gone on) and brought a tape recorder and recorded the entire process, including his conversation with the doctor afterward. This was a tremendous help to me, and I listened to those tapes over again when I got home that night. Doing whatever works for you to feel in control is recommended during this time, when you might feel at the mercy of your doctor and your body.

Tandy Levine
Licensed Clinical Social Worker
practicing in Washington, D.C.

Tandy's tip for when you get back home: Pamper yourself! Arrange for your favorite food and have dinner in bed.

12. The woman lies still for anywhere between fifteen to forty-five minutes afterward. Then she goes home, and is advised to take it easy as much as possible for the next few days.

13. Often the woman will begin taking **progesterone** suppositories to build up her uterine lining, to maximize the chance of implantation occurring.

14. After a wait of about ten days after reinsertion, the woman goes in for a blood pregnancy test and finds out whether "it worked" this cycle or not.

WHO IS A GOOD CANDIDATE?

The woman with absent or completely or partially blocked fallopian tubes

The woman who has undergone treatment in the attempt to open her blocked or damaged tubes but has still not conceived after a period of time

The woman with endometriosis which is interfering with the movement of the egg from the ovary into the fallopian tube (and for whom surgery or drug therapies have been unsuccessful)

ISSUES AND QUESTIONS

After an extremely frank and thorough discussion with both your spouse and your doctor about the risks, costs, and chances for success, determine how many cycles you are willing to attempt, and what your next course of action will be if no pregnancy results.

If you are a woman age forty or over, ask your doctor to realistically evaluate your odds of successful IVF using your own eggs. If willing to consider the use of donor eggs, raise the subject with your doctor and discuss the pros and cons of that approach.

You should also consider the extremely critical question of disposal of *nonviable embryos*. These are embryos that have begun to develop in

ON USING OTHER PATIENTS AS A LEARNING RESOURCE IN IVF

After a few unsuccessful attempts that never got to the egg retrieval stage, I finally called some other patients and found out which drugs they took that had been successful for them. The next two tries I knew what to request. The second time I got the correct treatment, I got pregnant.

Sheila from Louisiana

the lab dish but do not appear healthy or normal, and so will not be transferred to the uterus. Clinics routinely dispose of these embryos or use them for research. Sometimes the patient consent form you must sign for IVF will tell you that any embryos produced but not implanted will become the property of the clinic, to be used as the clinic sees fit. However, if you strongly believe that "personhood" begins at conception, you will find such an arrangement unacceptable. In that case, you should certainly withdraw from that clinic's program and seek treatment at a clinic that allows you to determine the fate of the tissue created from your own body's cells. Alternatively, you might prefer to undergo only "natural-cycle IVF" (see box on page 272) to avoid the risk that an excess number of embryos could be produced.

Now for the equally critical question of disposition of unused but *viable* embryos. Let's say the doctor retrieves nine eggs from your ovaries, and eight of them fertilize and begin to develop normally. You don't want to risk having octuplets; it wouldn't be safe, either for you or for your offspring. The maximum number of embryos most doctors are willing to transfer to your uterus is four.* The following are your options:

If your clinic offers cryopreservation of embryos, you could have the extra four embryos frozen, to be implanted in subsequent IVF attempts, either after failure of this cycle, or after the birth of a first child. Cryopreservation is expensive, and you will still have to determine what to do with any leftover embryos after you have made your final IVF attempt.

If cryopreservation is not available (such a high-tech procedure tends to be available only at major fertility centers), but you consider it the preferred disposition of any leftover, viable embryos, you should switch to a program that offers it. If you live in a small town, that may involve a temporary move to a bigger city.

Or you could donate the extra embryos to the clinic, which would implant them in the uterus of a woman who could not produce her own eggs, allowing another infertile couple the chance to have a child. This means that your genetic offspring would become part of another family and grow up with no connection to you. Many couples find this option as unacceptable as they would giving up a newborn child for adoption; others find it comforting to know that their unwanted embryos can bring lasting joy to others. Before you enter an IVF program, be sure to find out what the policy of your clinic is on embryo donation.

---

*It would be highly unlikely for all four to implant; triplets, twins, a single baby, or failure of any to implant would be far likelier outcomes.

Some clinics even *require* that all unused, viable embryos be donated. If this is the case, and you are opposed to embryo donation, then you should immediately seek IVF treatment someplace with a different policy.

Or the unused embryos might be used for research or destroyed.

Since excess numbers of both viable and nonviable embryos are a common occurrence in IVF cycles, every couple undergoing IVF should be sure they understand their clinic's embryo disposition rules completely, and know what choices they would make under those rules.

GIFT

WHAT IS IT?

The letters stand for *gamete intrafallopian transfer. Gamete* means a reproductive cell—that is, an egg cell or a sperm cell. The whole phrase refers to the fact that the eggs are removed from the ovaries, combined with sperm, and then transferred to the fallopian tube, where fertilization (hopefully) will occur. GIFT is different from IVF mainly in the fact that the doctor does not try to bring about fertilization in a lab dish.

WHAT HAPPENS?

The GIFT cycle starts out like the IVF cycle, until you get to step 7. The patient does not go home after the egg retrieval, but instead is immediately prepared for the next step:

8. The woman undergoes a minor surgical procedure to put her previously retrieved eggs, together with her partner's "washed" sperm, into one of her fallopian tubes. The doctor may perform what's known as a mini-lap, which is like a laparoscopy but uses an even smaller incision. The mini-lap can be done under local anesthesia, with the patient given a sedative beforehand, or it can be done in the hospital, under general anesthesia. The doctor loads the eggs and sperm into a catheter, inserts it through the tiny incision in the woman's side and into the open end of the fallopian tube, where he injects the contents. (In some cases, both tubes will be used, requiring two incisions, one on each side.) The incision is closed and the mini-lap is over, having taken about forty-five minutes to perform.

IVF THE "NATURAL" WAY

*Y*ou are not required to take potent fertility drugs to go through IVF. These drugs will improve the odds of conception substantially, but there are reasons why a couple might prefer not to use them. The sequence for IVF in that case is somewhat abridged; steps 3 and 4 are omitted, and the woman's ovary is allowed to proceed in its usual fashion to develop a single mature egg, which is then retrieved as described, and the remaining steps are followed. IVF without fertility drugs is called "natural-cycle IVF," and it may be preferred over standard IVF for any of the following reasons:

1. The woman must avoid for safety's sake the increased risk of twins. Natural-cycle IVF carries no greater risk of multiple gestation than conception in the usual way.
2. The couple can afford only the much cheaper natural-cycle IVF. Use of Pergonal for a week or longer will generally add over $2,000 to the cost of each cycle.
3. The woman has had severe reactions to ovulation-boosting drugs and is advised to discontinue their use.
4. The couple object on ethical grounds to the disposal of any extra embryos that may be produced but cannot be inserted into the woman's uterus. Natural-cycle IVF very seldom results in more than a single viable embryo.

If any of the foregoing describes your situation, and your doctor has not suggested natural-cycle IVF as a possibility, you should certainly raise the question and discuss the pros and cons.

9. The woman may be instructed to take progesterone suppositories to maximize the chance that a fertilized egg will implant.
10. Twelve to fourteen days later, the woman may have a blood test to find out if she is pregnant.

WHO IS A GOOD CANDIDATE?

The woman with at least one fully functioning fallopian tube

The woman with ovulatory problems who has tried various fertility drugs and IUI without success

The woman over thirty-five with ovulatory problems who is seeking the most aggressive method to try to bring about pregnancy

The man with mild to moderate sperm problems, whose wife has already tried fertility drugs and IUI without success

ISSUES AND QUESTIONS

Be sure you have a realistic understanding of all the costs, the odds for success in your case, and the risks of multiple gestation or drug side effects.

If the woman is age forty or over, ask your doctor to counsel you about the chance of success using her own eggs, compared to the chance of success with donor eggs. If you're willing to consider donor eggs, discuss the pros and cons of that approach in your case.

Decide in advance how many GIFT attempts you are willing to make, and what you will do next if GIFT is unsuccessful.

A big problem I've had with GIFT is getting correct directions and information. No one ever talked to me about embryo grading. They froze two of my embryos, even though their quality was low and unlikely to result in a pregnancy (I only found out about grading by reading an article about it in the RESOLVE newsletter).

Also, I had used the wrong-gauge needle for my progesterone shots because the nurse neglected to tell me to use the larger needle to draw up the solution and the smaller needle to inject it. No one ever mentioned the option of using oral capsules or vaginal suppositories. No one ever explained why we needed to have the results of Jack's "hamster penetration test" before our GIFT procedure, when all his other tests were great. No one ever told me I'd wake up after the GIFT laparoscopy in pain and catheterized. In fact, I'd been told I wouldn't be [catheterized]. I've found the best information comes from women who've undergone the procedure before.

Beth from Washington

ZIFT

What is it?

The letters stand for *zygote intrafallopian transfer*. A *zygote* is a fertilized egg. ZIFT is like a cross between IVF and GIFT. Eggs are retrieved and fertilized with sperm in a lab dish, just as in IVF, but the resulting embryos are put back into the woman's fallopian tube, as in GIFT, rather than her uterus, as in IVF.

What happens?

Follow the IVF sequence to step 10, then:

11. Instead of putting the catheter containing the embryos inside the uterus, the doctor uses the same procedures described under GIFT (making an incision in one side of the abdomen, and inserting the catheter into the open end of the fallopian tube) to place the multicelled embryos directly in the fallopian tube.
12. As with IVF and GIFT, progesterone may be given to build up the uterine lining to maximize the chance of implantation.
13. After a wait of about ten days, the woman will go in for a blood test to find out if she is pregnant.

Who is a good candidate?

The woman with at least one fully functioning fallopian tube.

The woman with ovulatory problems who is over thirty-five and seeking the most aggressive program to become pregnant, but who has tried GIFT for several cycles without success.

The man with sperm problems, whose wife has open tubes but has failed to get pregnant despite use of fertility drugs, IUI, and/ or a few GIFT attempts. Many doctors will urge the man in this case to skip GIFT and go directly to ZIFT, since this ART allows the doctor to determine whether the man's sperm are capable of causing fertilization.

The couple who have tried GIFT for several cycles without success, and now would like to find out where their problem lies: in the inability of sperm to fertilize the egg, in the failure of the egg to develop normally, or in the failure of the embryo to implant in the uterus. ZIFT allows the doctor to observe and control several steps that are left up to nature in GIFT.

ISSUES AND QUESTIONS

Discuss the same issues raised under GIFT, keeping in mind that ZIFT will be even more expensive than GIFT, because more laboratory work (culturing the embryo and keeping watch over its development) is necessary.

If very poor sperm quality is the reason for considering ZIFT, discuss the advantages of proceeding directly to micromanipulation of egg and sperm, to allow the doctor the maximum chance to bring about fertilization in the laboratory.

Cryopreservation of Embryos and Subsequent-Cycle ET

WHAT IS IT?

Now we get into what sounds like science fiction to many couples. Embryos produced through IVF or ZIFT that cannot be put back into the woman's body in the current cycle may be frozen (cryopreserved), stored in special canisters, and then when desired, thawed, and placed in the woman's uterus or fallopian tube. The placement of the thawed embryo is called *ET*. No, you are not getting an "extraterrestrial"; you're getting an *embryo transfer*. When the thawed embryo is placed in the fallopian tube, sometimes the acronym *TET* is used—for *tubal embryo transfer*.

WHAT HAPPENS?

Follow the IVF sequence to step 10. If more than four healthy-looking embryos have developed, then the excess number will be prepared in the lab to undergo the freezing process, sealed in a special container, and kept frozen in liquid nitrogen under very carefully controlled conditions, until needed.

When would that need arise? Let's say you did not become pregnant on the cycle in which all those embryos were created. You might try again with thawed embryos in another month or two. Or perhaps dur-

ABOUT PROST AND POST
AND FUTURE ALPHABET
COMBINATIONS

*V*ariants of the different ARTs seem to crop up too fast to keep track of them. Two that seem to hold out some promise are PROST and POST. The first stands for *pronuclear-stage transfer;* the second, for *peritoneal ovum sperm transfer.* PROST is a form of ZIFT, the only difference being in the amount of time the pre-embryo is allowed to develop in the lab dish before being transferred to the woman's fallopian tube. In PROST, the transfer takes place as soon as the egg reaches the *pronuclear* stage—that is, has exhibited the first signs that fertilization has occurred. The theory behind PROST is that the sooner you get the pre-embryo back into a natural setting (the woman's body) the better the chances for implantation.

POST was born out of the observation that fertilization can also take place just outside the fallopian tubes, in the *peritoneal cavity* of the abdomen. POST proceeds like GIFT, but instead of placing the eggs and sperm inside the fallopian tube, the doctor leaves them just outside the opening of the tube, so that the fimbria, the finger-like structures at the end of the tube, can sweep down and pull the egg into the tube, just as would happen naturally, in the absence of medical intervention. Since sperm have had the chance the combine with the egg prior to its capture by the fimbria, the egg may already be fertilized when it begins its journey down toward the uterus to implant, or the sperm may swim into the fallopian tube to fertilize it there.

Is either PROST or POST more effective than ZIFT or GIFT? It's too early to tell. What other alphabet combinations will come along next to offer couples a chance of pregnancy? Is there a chance that the next ART will be easier to perform? less costly? have greater chance of success? be easier for the woman's body to tolerate? How we wish we had answers to these questions! (But maybe if we can just hang on a few years, we will.)

ing the cycle in which the embryos were created, the doctor found that your hormones were at the wrong level to allow implantation of an embryo. It often happens that the massive doses of fertility drugs needed to cause multiple ovulation will leave the woman's body poorly prepared to accept the implantation of any embryos. But if she waits a cycle or two until her hormonal levels have returned to normal, then conditions for implantation may be more favorable. A third scenario for use of the frozen embryos might occur when the woman has already had one child through IVF or ZIFT, and would now like to try to have a second one. Any child born from one of the frozen embryos would be the fraternal twin of the older sibling, in a sense, since both children were conceived from eggs and sperm produced at the same time—even though several *years* may have passed between the conception and the birth of the second child.

The chief advantage to cryopreservation and subsequent-cycle ET is that the woman does not have to undergo another round of fertility drugs or another egg retrieval to make a second attempt to have a baby. The doctor will simply monitor the natural progress of her hormones, and when the optimal point in her cycle has been reached, carefully thaw the embryo(s) and perform the tubal or uterine transfer. The chief disadvantage is that thawed embryos are more fragile than fresh ones, and will often become nonviable before the transfer can occur. And even when the thawed embryos appear healthy, the implantation rate is still less than that when fresh embryos are used.

The ET does not necessarily need to be done to the same woman who produced the eggs in the first place. When the transfer of the thawed embryo is made to the body of another woman, the situation is known as **host uterus** (see page 283). Under what circumstances might a woman need both cryopreservation and host uterus? If she has already had one baby through IVF or ZIFT, had the extra embryos frozen, but then finds out that she has, say, cancer of the uterus and must undergo a hysterectomy, ET to a host uterus can preserve her option to have a second child.

WHO IS A GOOD CANDIDATE?

The woman who has produced more viable embryos in an IVF or ZIFT cycle than can safely be implanted in that cycle

The woman who wishes to attempt to have more than one child through IVF or ZIFT

The woman who, after taking ovarian-stimulating drugs to produce the eggs needed for IVF or ZIFT, is left with hormone levels that create unfavorable conditions for successful implantation

ISSUES AND QUESTIONS

It is crucial for the couple to resolve at the outset the issue of disposition of frozen embryos that will not be used.* Let's say the woman produces five viable embryos. Four are implanted soon after their creation, and the remaining one is frozen. Suppose three out of the four implant and develop, and the woman gives birth to triplets. Now the couple has no wish to have a fourth child, but they still have an embryo "on ice"— and they must pay a regular fee for its storage. What should they do? Donate the embryo to another infertile couple? Allow it to be thawed and used for research? Have it destroyed? If they do not know in advance how they will deal with this set of circumstances, they could well end up in a state of emotional turmoil as they try to reach agreement on this very difficult question.

They should also discuss (although no one ever likes to) what they would do with their frozen embryos in the event of death of the husband or the wife. Would the husband want his widow to be able to continue to attempt to have his child posthumously? If the wife died, and the widower remarried, would she want his new wife to attempt to bear her child through ET? Equally difficult but necessary to contemplate is the subject of separation or divorce. Who gets custody of the embryos? Can one partner or the other have them destroyed? donated? or used to have a baby? Prudent couples who want to protect themselves legally will put their wishes in writing before embarking on a course of cryopreservation and ET. Those who like to be extra careful should consult an attorney with expertise in this area of their state's family law before drafting any documents. Due to past legal battles over ownership of embryos (for details, see the section Ethics and the ARTs), many clinics will now require the couple to sign a contract spelling out the rights of each partner in the event of a dispute.

You should also find out how each of you feels about making another

---

*Many of the legal, moral, and medical questions raised by the disposition of frozen embryos will be rendered moot when freezing of retrieved eggs becomes feasible. Though researchers have long been working on the problem, it is still not possible to freeze the egg so that it will still be fertilizable when thawed. Ultimately, though, this problem will be solved, and then the thawed eggs can be combined with thawed sperm to create fresh embryos that will have a greater chance to develop than frozen ones.

attempt at pregnancy through ART following the birth of twins or triplets from an earlier successful attempt. While contemplating what you would do if the hoped-for result occurs, you should also confront the reality that relatively few thawed embryos will successfully implant. Is the lower likelihood of pregnancy with subsequent-cycle ET worth the extra money it will cost?

Finally, you should consider the accessibility of this level of technology. If you live near one of the more sophisticated fertility centers, access will not be a problem. But couples from small towns or rural areas would very likely have to travel to a major city to find a clinic that could freeze and store their embryos safely. The couples would then have to return when the ET is desired.

*O*n my fifth attempt at IVF I had two frozen embryos thawed (they had been frozen in 1989) and transferred to my uterus, along with one fresh embryo created in that cycle [she had natural-cycle IVF]. The doctor said only one of the frozen ones looked good after thawing. He didn't think the other had much of a chance, though he transferred it anyway. Well, I got pregnant with twins [born in 1991]. One weighed six pounds, thirteen ounces, the other was seven pounds, fifteen ounces. You know, I think I can tell which one was from the frozen embryo. He loves the cold, and he loves ice cream. I call him my "Eskimo baby."

*K*athy from Tennessee

Micromanipulation of Egg and Sperm

WHAT IS IT?

The term *micromanipulation* can be used to refer to a variety of techniques the doctor uses when working with egg and sperm in the laboratory, viewing them through a microscope, and trying to induce the sperm to fertilize the egg. These techniques include *partial zona dissection (PZD), subzonal insertion (SZI),* and *microinjection.*

What happens?

The eggs are retrieved as described under IVF, and the sperm obtained and processed in the usual way. What the doctor can do with these cells to attempt to bring about fertilization is right now the subject of much research and experimentation. New techniques or improvements of earlier techniques may come along any day to make anything you read here obsolete. Partial zona dissection, or more simply "zona drilling," is most promising. The **zona pellucida** is the scientific name for the outer layer of the egg. The doctor makes a microscopic hole in it, which makes it easier for a sperm to penetrate and fertilize it. The doctor might also attempt microinjection: he will select a single sperm that appears to be healthy and normal and insert it through the microscopic hole he has made in the egg. There is still no way for him to be sure he has picked a sperm that is fertile. Much remains to be discovered about the conditions under which egg and sperm will fuse, and some of what we need to know may remain beyond our understanding for a long time to come.

Who is a good candidate?

The man who has a poor sperm count but still can produce a limited number of healthy-looking sperm.

The man whose wife or partner has undergone numerous IUI or other ART attempts with his sperm, without success.

The man who is willing to invest much time, money, and energy into the quest to have a biological child, rather than use donor sperm.

Issues and questions

Cost is the biggest hurdle most couples face when considering use of micromanipulation techniques. There is hardly an insurance policy in America written to cover this experimental procedure. Because the amount of skill needed for success at micromanipulation is so great, there are few doctors available to perform it, and scarcity leads (as it usually does) to high prices.

Availability is another problem. The couple living in a small town or rural area will probably need to move to a big city to find a fertility clinic with specialists able to perform micromanipulation techniques.

As with any ART, you should determine in advance how many attempts you will make, what you will do with any leftover embryos that are produced, and what you will do if after a certain period of time you still have no luck.

Soon—though not quite yet—couples going in for micromanipulation of their eggs and sperm may be faced with the question of sex selection of their embryos. Since the doctor can choose the individual sperm he will use, and since sperm are the carriers of the X or Y chromosome that determine a baby's sex, it is theoretically possible for the doctor to use only an X-carrying sperm for the couple who want a girl, or a Y-carrying sperm for the couple who want a boy. When the ability to select sex in the lab comes about, there will certainly follow an intense ethical debate as to whether the couple should have any say in determining their child's sex in advance.

Donor Egg

WHAT IS IT?

Pregnancy is the result of implantation of an egg produced by another woman, which has been fertilized by the husband's sperm.

WHAT HAPPENS?

First of all, a donor must be recruited. Sometimes the couple are responsible for finding the donor. They may place ads offering a certain fee to compensate her for the time and difficulties involved in using fertility drugs and undergoing an egg retrieval, or they may be able to enlist an unpaid volunteer, such as the wife's sister or close friend. Some clinics run anonymous donor egg programs, doing the recruiting, screening the potential donors to eliminate those with genetic diseases, drug habits, or other problems, setting the compensation, and presenting contracts to all parties in the attempt to prevent any future legal battles over custody.

Once the donor is signed on, she begins a program of ovarian stimulation with fertility drugs, as described under the IVF heading, ending with egg retrieval (step 6). The donor goes home, and if she retains her anonymity, she will play no further role in the conception, pregnancy, birth, or upbringing of her genetic offspring.

Once the donor eggs have been obtained, they will be combined with the husband's sperm in a petri dish, and any healthy embryos that result may be inserted into the wife's fallopian tubes via the ZIFT procedure, or placed in her uterus, via IVF. Embryos in excess of four may be cryopreserved for later implantation. The eggs may also be placed, unfertilized, in the wife's fallopian tube together with her husband's sperm, via the GIFT procedure.

If implantation should occur, then the woman should go on to experience a normal pregnancy and give birth to a child that is related genetically only to her husband and the donor. If donor sperm must be used, then the child she delivers will be no more genetically related to the couple than an adopted child—however the woman has still enjoyed* the experience of pregnancy and childbirth, and the couple is able to avoid the lengthy screening process and waiting period that most adoptive parents must go through before they receive a child.

Donor egg programs have been one of the most promising forms of treatment for women with severe ovarian dysfunction. Success rates at some clinics are identical to the rates for younger women attempting pregnancy through IVF using their own eggs.

Who is a good candidate?

The woman with poorly functioning or nonfunctioning ovaries, who cannot be helped by use of fertility drugs or surgery

The woman whose ovaries have been removed due to cancer or some other disease

The woman at the age of menopause, or past the age of menopause

The young woman who has experienced premature menopause

The woman with an inheritable genetic disorder, such as hemophilia, who does not wish to risk passing on the condition to her child

Issues and questions

As is the case when donor sperm is used, the couple must explore how they feel about the prospect of raising a child genetically unrelated to one of its parents.

*Some might question the use of this word.

They should discuss how they wish to recruit the donor, what sort of qualifications or characteristics they consider most important in the donor, and what, if any, compensation she is to receive for undergoing ovarian stimulation and egg retrieval. (Technically, she may not be paid directly for her eggs, since that would be considered the sale of a human body part, now forbidden by federal law. Although men have long been allowed to sell their sperm for money, and both sexes are allowed to sell blood plasma, the government has chosen to interpret the human egg as "irreplaceable tissue"—though most women have thousands to spare—thus justifying the ban on sale.)

The couple should talk to an expert (possibly a lawyer) knowledge-able in their state's laws regarding egg donation to find out how disputes involving compensation of the donor or child custody may be handled by the court system.

They should decide now what they would tell a child about its method of conception, and at what age they would first bring the sub-ject up.

As with all ARTs, they should be aware of their real odds for success; they should have determined how many attempts they will make (and whether or not to try to stay with the same donor for repeat tries), how much money they will spend, and what they will do if after a certain period of time they are unsuccessful.

They should ask if the same donor may be available some time later to donate again, so that a second child could be conceived who is a full brother or sister to the first child.

They should ask about the availability and cost of cryopreservation of extra embryos that may result from fertilization of the donor's eggs, and decide how they would dispose of any frozen embryos that cannot later be used by them.

Host Uterus

WHAT IS IT?

The host uterus procedure is the flip side of donor egg. This time the egg donor is the one who wishes to have a child, but while she is able to produce a healthy, fertilizable egg, she is unable to sustain a preg-nancy and give birth to her baby. The couple must then recruit a woman who will agree to have the couple's embryo inserted into her uterus; if she becomes pregnant, she must further agree to take care of herself during the nine months of pregnancy, have the baby, and then give it up to its genetic parents.

What happens?

First, the couple must find a woman to be the host. They may place ads seeking out a woman of the desired age, background, reproductive history, and character, and offer her a certain level of compensation for the time and physical rigors and risks involved in pregnancy, or they may contact an attorney specializing in facilitating such arrangements and leave the recruitment of the host to him. Alternatively, they could find an enthusiastic volunteer within their own families or circle of friends. Mothers have served as host uterus for their daughters; sisters have done it for sisters; and so have best friends. When the host bears the baby solely out of love, there will be far fewer questions raised about the legal and moral propriety of the arrangement than if the host is a stranger doing a job for wages.

Once the host woman has been chosen, the wife will begin the program of ovarian stimulation described under the IVF heading, until step 6, the egg retrieval.

At the same time the host also undergoes hormonal treatments to put her at the correct point in her cycle to receive a fertilized egg.

The retrieved eggs may be fertilized with the husband's sperm in the lab, and then cultured until healthy, transferrable pre-embryos have developed, which are inserted in the host's fallopian tubes (ZIFT) or uterus (IVF). Alternatively, the eggs may be transferred, unfertilized, to the host's fallopian tubes, together with the husband's sperm (GIFT).

If implantation occurs, then the host should experience a normal pregnancy and deliver a baby at the end that is genetically unrelated to her. She will then turn the baby over to its genetic parents.

In both the donor egg procedure and host uterus, the baby has, in a sense, two mothers: a genetic mother (the one who supplies the egg to be fertilized); and a gestational mother (the one who carries the baby for nine months in her womb). Which mother ends up with the baby is determined by the intent of the women involved. When the woman who wishes to raise a baby has a working uterus but trouble with her ovaries, then donor eggs will be used, and the woman who delivers the baby will be the one to keep it. When the women who wishes to raise a baby has working ovaries but a nonworking uterus, then a host uterus must be recruited, who must then deliver the baby to its genetic parents. The medical procedure, however, is identical.

Who is a good candidate?

The woman with uterine problems (poor shape, size, position, or internal abnormalities) but healthy ovaries, or ovaries that will respond to fertility drugs to produce healthy eggs

The woman who has tried to conceive through previous fertility treatments or ARTs, and is consistently able to produce viable embryos, but for whom implantation always fails to occur

The woman who for unknown or uncorrectable reasons has repeatedly miscarried or suffered stillbirths

The woman with severe endometriosis who has not been helped by drugs or surgery

The woman who, because of severe diabetes that cannot be kept under control with insulin, has been advised not to attempt to carry a pregnancy to term

The woman suffering from multiple sclerosis, severe hypertension, or some other serious illness or disability who has been advised not to attempt to carry a pregnancy to term

The woman who has uterine cancer, who is about to have a hysterectomy, or who has already had one but was left with functioning ovaries

Issues and questions

Choosing the host will be fraught with peril for nearly all couples (except for those who are able to recruit a trusted family member or friend). Who is this woman, and why is she willing to go through nine months of pregnancy with someone else's baby, only to give it away moments after it is born? Is she desperate for money? Is she emotionally unstable? Will she keep her side of the bargain? How will her family react to what she's doing? Will they pressure her to change her mind? Will she avoid drugs, cigarettes, and alcohol while pregnant? Will she expect to be included in events of the child's life later on?

No matter how airtight a contract you draw up, you will have no guarantees to the answers to any of these questions. If you can't cope with the thought of nine straight months of stress and uncertainty, then using a paid host uterus should not be your chosen method of resolving your infertility.

The couple should also thoroughly explore their feelings about the morality of this arrangement. You do not want to start a pregnancy in another woman, only to discover that you feel enormous guilt over the situation—so much so that you may even feel reluctant at the end to take away the baby that she has nurtured inside her body for the past nine months.

You should definitely seek the advice of an attorney knowledgeable in this area of your state's family law, to find out what steps need to be taken upon the baby's birth to establish the genetic parents' legal custody rights. It is a universal principle of common law that the woman who gives birth to the baby must be its mother. Technology has outpaced the law, and the genetic mother must therefore apply to the courts to legally adopt her own child—though the genetic father may easily be able to establish his paternal rights by means of a simple blood test. An attorney will also advise you whether a contract with a paid stranger who will serve as host uterus is legal and enforceable in your state, and if so, what should go in the contract.

If you are using an attorney to do the recruiting of the host woman, check that attorney out thoroughly! The CBS investigative news show 48 Hours ran a segment (August 5, 1992) exposing the shady practices of several professionals who advertised their abilities to bring infertile couples together with "carefully screened" hosts—women who turned out not to have been screened at all. Your local chapter of RESOLVE may be able to give you some guidance in finding a reputable go-between.

Be sure to discuss all the attorney's fees and other expenses that you will be billed for, *before* you start making any medical arrangements.

Be warned that there are few, if any, health insurance companies that will pay for any part of fertility treatment for a host uterus arrangement. If the woman you choose as host already has good health insurance, her maternity coverage should be assured; otherwise, count on paying for all her prenatal visits and hospitalization out of your own pocket, too.

You must also decide what level of contact you wish to have with the woman who will be pregnant with your child. Do you want to get to know her well? Do you hope to be able to watch "your pregnancy" develop? Do you wish to attend birth classes with her and be present in the delivery room? What will your relationship be like afterward? Will you keep in contact? Will she ever visit the child she helped to create?

As you can see, the host uterus procedure brings with it a large number of very thorny problems to be dealt with. Only those couples with great emotional fortitude, financial resources, and dedication to the goal of biological parenthood will be satisfied with the host uterus solution to their infertility. Know yourselves well before you embark!

Embryo Transplant

WHAT IS IT?

In some ways similar to donor egg, in some ways closer to *surrogate motherhood* (see next section for description), embryo transplant is an arrangement in which a woman is hired to be impregnated by sperm from the fertile husband of the couple, and then soon after implantation, have the embryo flushed out of her womb, retrieved, and reimplanted into the uterus of the wife, who has a healthy uterus. The wife then goes through nine months of pregnancy, and then labor and delivery in the normal way, giving birth to a child who is not biologically related to her but who is related to her husband.

WHAT HAPPENS?

As with egg donation, a suitable donor must be recruited. As in surrogate motherhood, the recruit must agree to become pregnant by means of artificial insemination with a stranger's sperm. Unlike in surrogate motherhood, however, she is not asked to give up the baby she has carried inside her for nine months; instead, she must agree that shortly after pregnancy is confirmed, she will undergo a procedure designed to remove the contents of her uterus, including the embryo, which will then be transplanted to the uterus of the wife. The embryo-removal phase of the process is known by the medical term **uterine lavage.**

Although Pergonal or Clomid may not be needed to cause a pregnancy in a normally fertile woman, it is often given to increase the chance that the woman recruited as the embryo donor will conceive within the first few cycles of artificial insemination. This part of the process is described in the section on IUI.

Before the embryo is flushed out of the donor, the wife's uterine lining has been built up with progesterone to help the transplant to take hold. The removal of the embryo from one woman and its insertion into the uterus of another is an in-office procedure, similar to the embryo-transfer stage of IVF, except that in this case the embryo was not created and cultured in a lab dish, but inside someone else's body.

WHO IS A GOOD CANDIDATE?

The same woman who would be a candidate for the donor egg procedure, but who, because of tubal problems, needs to have the embryo inserted into her uterus. Some doctors believe that conception becomes more likely when fertilization is allowed to take place naturally inside the fallopian tubes of the egg donor than if the eggs are simply removed from the donor's body to be fertilized in a test tube. Even so, the odds for success with embryo transplant are not very great (less than 20 percent at the average clinic).

A hired embryo donor might have to go through six or more cycles of ovarian stimulation, artificial insemination, and embryo flushing before success—and there are few couples that can afford the necessary (but nearly always unreimbursed) medical expenses, *plus* the price of compensation for the donor's time and physical toll. Even when the couple is willing and financially able, there are very few women willing to lend their bodies more than once to such a rigorous sequence of events, even when the payment is tempting.

For these reasons most couples seeking help from a third party in creating a child are advised to explore exhaustively other treatment options and ARTs first, before proceeding along this path.

ISSUES AND QUESTIONS

First, a general rule of thumb: the more difficult the procedure and the more outsiders involved in carrying out its steps, the greater the number of issues that must be raised, and the more troublesome those issues will be to resolve.

Take a look at all the issues raised in connection with donor egg. Now add to those many of the issues raised in host uterus, plus some of the ones raised in surrogate motherhood. Plus the usual lineup of stumbling blocks that accompany all the other ARTs: cost, poor odds of success, risk of side effects, and so on and so on.

It would be time well spent for any couple still seriously considering the embryo transplant route to sit down with a counselor specially trained to advise couples in infertility-related matters and go over the pros and cons, run through all of the emotional ramifications that would be involved if the procedure failed, and all the parenting questions that would be raised if it succeeded, and then come to a decision as to whether embryo transplant or some other resolution to their infertility might be the right choice to make at this time in their lives.

Surrogate Motherhood

WHAT IS IT?

When a woman can neither produce a viable egg to be fertilized, nor carry a pregnancy created with someone else's fertilized egg, she and her fertile husband may turn to surrogate motherhood to have a child that is genetically related to the husband, but not the wife. A fertile woman who is willing to be impregnated, and then carry the baby for nine months, and then give it up to its genetic father and his wife afterward, must be found to make the plan of action work. The recruited woman, usually a stranger hired at a set rate of compensation, is called the surrogate mother.

WHAT HAPPENS?

The most difficult step is finding a suitable surrogate. There are women who are willing to part with their eggs for a price, never seeing or missing the babies that will be created from those eggs; and there are women who are willing to carry the baby of another couple for nine months, not traumatized at having to give up a child to the couple whose egg and sperm created it; but it is another thing entirely to ask a woman to allow her egg to be fertilized by a stranger, then carry that stranger's baby for nine months, and give it up to him and his wife at the end. There are very few women willing to do all that for a price, and the ones who are tend to be either desperately poor or emotionally unstable. Neither type is someone you want to trust with your reproductive fate.

Yet despite the difficulties (made spectacularly public in the infamous and grueling "Baby M" child custody case*), surrogate motherhood arrangements still are made, and most of the couples who embark on this course do end up delighted with the babies that result.

---

*Which resulted from the refusal of the surrogate mother, Mary Beth Whitehead, to surrender her parental rights to the couple who arranged her pregnancy, the Sterns.

It is essential, however, for the couple seeking out a surrogate mother to find reputable go-betweens—preferably a team including a lawyer and a clinical psychologist or social worker—who will recruit the surrogate, *carefully* checking out her background to screen out anyone who

- is in desperate economic straits and will do *anything* for money
- has had episodes of depression or been hospitalized or detained for any mental illness, compulsion, or addiction
- has had an abortion and believes that by having a baby and giving it up she will be atoning for her past "sin"
- smokes, drinks to excess, or uses illegal drugs
- is in a relationship or marriage with a man who is strongly opposed to her participation in the arrangement
- appears (to the couple) to be conflicted, ambivalent, untrustworthy, or in any way suspect

Once a reliable, stable, fertile woman is found, the couple's lawyer will then draw up a contract specifying what each party's obligations are. Before you reach this stage, you may be informed that such contracts have been declared null and void by your state's law.* In that case, you have the option of looking for a surrogate in a state that has not outlawed the practice, or simply go ahead in your own state, knowing that if anything goes wrong, you cannot turn to the courts to enforce the deal you have made. After the contract is signed, the couple's go-betweens will then arrange for the insemination, a pregnancy test, a paternity test, and all prenatal care.

Perhaps as difficult as finding the woman to serve as surrogate is the task of finding a reputable, trustworthy, competent go-between with experience in the matter. Ask your family attorney or your local RESOLVE chapter for a recommendation. Even after you have been given a recommendation, find out from your state bar association whether the attorney has a clean record. Surrogate motherhood, unfortunately, has proved an attractive field for shysters and sharks who take advantage of all parties. See the section Host Uterus for an example of the kind of shady operator you will hope to avoid.

Once you have solved the problem of finding your surrogate, the rest is relatively simple. With a woman of proven fertility, there is no need for ovulation-boosting drugs, egg retrieval, or any of the rest of the expensive, high-tech show. The woman is instructed to keep track

---

*As of this writing, fourteen states have laws forbidding the hiring of a surrogate to bear a child and declaring invalid any contract written between the surrogate and the hiring couple.

of her ovulation, and when she is at the fertile peak of her cycle, she goes in to be artificially inseminated with sperm from the husband. If she is married, she must agree to abstain from intercourse with her own husband for a period of time before or after the insemination, or else be trusted to use a highly reliable barrier method of contraception, such as a diaphragm used in conjunction with a condom.

If, after several cycles, she does not conceive, she may try a mild fertility drug, such as Clomid, to increase the monthly chance of conception.

After pregnancy is confirmed, the couple must wait out nine anxiety-laden months, hoping that the surrogate does not change her mind and try to keep the baby. They must also trust that she will take good care of herself, keeping her prenatal appointments, refraining from drinking, smoking, or drug use, and avoiding transmissable diseases. After the baby is born, its biological father will take it home; his wife must then petition the court to allow her to adopt his biological child as her own, and the surrogate mother will sign papers relinquishing all her parental rights. There will follow a period of time (how long depends on the adoption laws of your particular state) in which the biological mother may change her mind and attempt to regain custody, before the adoption is made final.

WHO IS A GOOD CANDIDATE?

With all the other technologies available, it can be argued that no one is really a good candidate for this rather risky arrangement these days. The woman with neither functioning ovaries nor a functioning uterus could, for example, apply to an anonymous donor egg program, and arrange to have that egg fertilized with her husband's sperm, to be implanted in the uterus of a sister or female cousin, who would be willing to serve as host uterus. That way, nobody would be asked to give up a biologically related child, and the infertile woman would be assured that the woman bearing the child would be doing so out of love. Nor would there be a "natural mother" who might lay claim to the couple's child.

A single man who is set on having a biological rather than adopted child might turn to a hired surrogate mother for help—but a better choice might be to find a female friend or advertise to find a single woman who would like to share the responsibility for creating a new life, to give the child two parents to bring it up.

A gay male couple intent on raising a child together might also consider surrogacy, but they should expect to encounter difficulties in finding reliable professionals (lawyers and psychologists) to assist them in the endeavor. Further information on gay male couples' options is included in Chapter Ten.

ISSUES AND QUESTIONS

Is the couple absolutely certain that surrogate motherhood is the most desirable and feasible way for them to become parents? Has the couple had professional counseling about other options, including adoption and child-free living?

Once set to pursue surrogate motherhood: Is the attorney who will engage the surrogate mother honest, reliable, and able to oversee all the necessary arrangements within the bounds of the law? Is there a professional counselor or psychologist to evaluate candidates? How thorough is the background check? What kind of fee will be asked? Does the amount cover *everything,* or will other expenses be billed later or would there be any under-the-counter payments not included in the contract? Has the couple met the surrogate and been satisfied as to her motives and good faith in adhering to the terms of the arrangement?

NO SOAP OPERA HEARTACHE IN THIS SURROGATE MOTHER STORY

*I*f her life went anything like the plot of her TV show, you could bet that *Days of Our Lives* star Deidre Hall and her husband, Steve Sohmer, would not end up as the happy parents of a baby boy—but they did. The older couple (she's forty-four, he's fifty) had been unable to conceive a child together, and so they sought out and hired a surrogate (identified in the press simply as "Robin B.") to be impregnated with the husband's sperm. Everything proceeded uneventfully, and on August 23 in Los Angeles (according to *People* magazine, September 26, 1992) the surrogate delivered the eight-pound three-ounce baby for Hall and Sohmer to take home. Fans of the show will have to stick to the doings of Ms. Hall's psychiatrist character and her TV children for stories with sad endings and odd twists of fate.

How many insemination attempts will be made? If after a certain number have failed to produce a pregnancy, will fertility drugs be used, will a new surrogate be sought, or will the couple turn to some other means to resolve their infertility?

If a child results from the arrangement, what will the child be told about how it came into the family, and at what age? Will the child have any form of contact with its biological mother, such as an occasional exchange of letters or photographs, or even telephone calls? What custody arrangements would be made, in case of death of either the husband or wife during the surrogate's pregnancy? What arrangements would be made in case of divorce or separation during the pregnancy?

ETHICS AND THE ARTs: AN ESSAY

Whenever human beings start interfering with the natural processes by which other human beings are created, a wide range of ethical issues are raised. Some of these are questions of medical ethics—for example, is it right for doctors to select a specific sperm to attempt to bring about conception in the laboratory? Others are legal: should the government ban the sale of eggs or embryos as it does the sale of kidneys, eyes, and other bodily parts? But most involve moral choices that each of us must make in the privacy of our own thoughts.

If you don't consider and resolve to your own satisfaction the important ethical questions raised by the specific ART you are contemplating, tragic consequences may follow. You could end up like the Tennessee couple who, during their divorce proceedings, sued each other for possession of seven frozen embryos created during the wife's past IVF attempts. Or if you both died in a plane crash, as happened to a wealthy American couple who had traveled to Australia to undergo IVF, you could be leaving behind embryos that will be implanted in the bodies of strangers and brought up with no knowledge of you— and no right to inherit your estate. Or suppose you hired a host uterus, as did a California couple, only to find that the host, upon birth, was unwilling to part with the baby she had gestated for nine months. Would you take her to court to assert your contractual rights? And of course we all remember the heart-rending "Baby M" case, in which the hired surrogate mother, Mary Beth Whitehead, attempted to keep custody of the baby she had had by artificial insemination with the sperm of William Stern, whose wife Elizabeth was unable to sustain a pregnancy (Ms. Whitehead lost). Fewer perhaps will be familiar with the California case involving a couple who separated just as their surrogate mother was due to go into labor; after the baby was born the surrogate declined to give up custody to the father, who was by that time single. She sued, and won joint custody with the stranger who had fathered her child. The man's ex-wife ended up with no legal role in the life of the child she'd been so eagerly expecting to raise.

No one can promise that if you carefully think through and work out all the important questions of law, medicine, and personal responsibility that may arise in your chosen form of ART, you will then be able to avoid all conflict, whether emotional, legal, or social. But it is clear that to neglect to do so will leave you vulnerable to legal troubles, financial hardship, loss of privacy (if your situation attracts the attention of the press, as in the cases cited above), and unending heartbreak.

Most of us by adulthood have already formed a fairly solid set of values by which we judge what actions we believe to be moral or immoral. When it comes to new technology, even if unsure about the science involved, we can usually arrive at some sound conclusions by answering some basic questions, such as

Will anyone be likely to suffer as a result of the course we have chosen?

Is this procedure now widely accepted as ethical in the medical community when performed according to certain standards or guidelines?

Are those who will be involved in the procedure, whether doctors, lawyers, psychologists, or other facilitators, generally reputed to be honest, ethical, and respected in their fields of expertise?

After deep reflection, do we feel at ease with all aspects of the chosen ART, or does either one of us have disquieting feelings— of guilt, of apprehensiveness, of reluctance to continue down this path?

You probably will find that certain ARTs will meet your criteria for moral acceptability, while others do not, depending on how you view the relationships involved. For example, you might conclude that any involvement of a third party in your reproductive plans, whether as an egg donor, sperm donor, host uterus, embryo donor, or surrogate mother, violates your concept of the sacred bond of the marital relationship. Or you might draw the line at any ART that involves creating a new life inside an outsider's body, thus ruling out the use of a host uterus, embryo donor, or surrogate mother. Or you could conclude that of all the ARTs, only surrogate motherhood is to be avoided on moral grounds, as it is the only arrangement that requires a woman to conceive, carry, and give birth to a baby which she must then surrender to another couple.

However, you should also be aware that there are strong voices decrying the use of *all* of the ARTs. There are various philosophical justifications given for such blanket opposition, but the two most important schools of thought come from two diametrically opposite camps already known to the public by convenient (but probably inapt) labels: radical feminist and right to life.

Let's briefly consider the very different arguments that each group has put forward in support of the proposition that all ARTs are morally unacceptable. First, the radical feminist position.

Perhaps the most cogent and complete assault on ARTs from the feminist viewpoint can be found in *Ms.* magazine of May-June 1991, an issue devoted almost entirely to the topic of ARTs, under the overall heading "Women as Wombs: The Multi-National Birth Industry." Seven different writers in seven articles, one by one, took on the moral, legal, and social issues raised by ARTs, each time arriving at anti-ART conclusions, such as

ARTs are injurious to women's health

ARTs frequently result in the exploitation of poor women by rich men

ARTs serve the obsession of men to have offspring who will bear their names and pass on their genes

ARTs help to keep women defined solely as childbearers

ARTs are hugely lucrative procedures that enrich mainly male doctors, who induce their female patients to return for cycle after cycle of pain and risk, nearly always with no result

One of the *Ms.* articles raises the specter of a race of oppressed "breeder women" coming into being as a consequence of widespread recruitment of host uteruses and surrogate mothers. Men who do not wish to see their wives' figures enlarged and made "unsexy" in pregnancy will pressure them to abandon childbearing themselves, and turn to paid substitutes whose sole function is procreation. Another article expressed the fear that the coming technology for sex identification after test tube fertilization will lead to the routine destruction of female embryos by couples who have been societally conditioned to prefer sons. The writer pointed out that in countries such as India and China, amniocentesis is already commonly performed for the purpose of identifying and aborting female fetuses.

The right-to-life critique raises an entirely different set of alarms. ARTs do not serve to support the patriarchal system, the argument runs; rather, just the opposite is true: they help to undermine the traditional family, defined as the husband as provider and the wife as principal child caretaker. When childbearing is no longer a "natural" event, but is something that any woman can apply to have done for her in the laboratory, then why get married? Why even have a man around at all? All kinds of women who, in years past, would have been constrained from having children by their physiology if not by societal norms, may now become mothers: Lesbians, single women, postmenopausal women—all barriers are down.

Women during what used to be the normal childbearing years are then free to devote themselves exclusively, selfishly (according to this way of thinking) to their career ambitions, turning to medical science to make babies for them in their forties or even fifties, whenever they find it convenient.

More serious is the charge that all ARTs rely on the destruction of human life. In IVF and ZIFT procedures, "excess" embryos are often created only to be destroyed. Even a technology like GIFT, which does not involve laboratory fertilization, must be viewed as a product of research by doctors who routinely experiment with embryos to develop new techniques and hone their skills.

If embryos are not destroyed but frozen, that procedure is equally abhorrent to the right-to-life perspective. Two- or four- or eight-celled organisms are in moral terms "persons" who must not be deprived of their basic right to develop according to nature's plan. If it is unthinkable to put a newborn baby in a coma until such time as its parents feel able to have a child, then it must be the same to do so to a forty-eight hour conceptus.

Defenders of ARTs have attempted to counter both lines of attack. In their book *Tomorrow's Child: Reproductive Technology in the 90s*, three well-respected British feminists, Lynda Birke, Susan Himmelweit, and Gail Vines, effectively rebut many of the anti-ART charges lobbed by the *Ms.* writers and other feminist critics. ARTs have expanded the reproductive choices available to women, these authors contend, and are thus a positive development. Just as women need the freedom to choose when *not* to have a baby, they need the freedom to choose when to have one. No longer is childbearing limited to the young and those fortunate enough to have perfectly functioning organs and hormones.

As with any new technology, of course there are risks, but the authors remind us, women today are educated enough to evaluate the risks and are intelligent enough to come to their own conclusions. They do not need to be protected against new treatments, even if those new treatments are still largely ineffective, just as cancer patients do not need to be protected from experimental treatments that can save only a small percentage of lives. The patient in either case should be the one to say whether she considers the benefits of the desired outcome to be worth the risk.

As to the charge that men often pressure women to have children to keep up the patriarchal line, the authors cite research showing that it is most often the woman who wants a biologically related child. The woman who chooses fertility treatment tends to be an assertive, confident, and equal partner in her relationship, hardly the type to be pushed into doing something that goes against her wishes. Women decide how many cycles they want to attempt, and they decide when they are ready to move on to some other resolution to the problem of infertility.

As for the notion that ARTs such as host uterus and surrogate motherhood will lead to the creation of a race of "breeder women" having babies for a price for a ruling class that can't be bothered—that belongs to a far-out science fiction story, not to the reality of our times, or any times *we* are likely to be around to see. Far from seeking poor women to do their childbearing, virtually all women undergoing fertility treatment in fact yearn to experience pregnancy and childbirth. It is only those few who are physically unable to do so who must (reluctantly, in most cases) enlist an outsider's cooperation. Besides, there is hardly a doctor in the country (patriarchal conspirator or not) who would arrange a host uterus for a patient who simply didn't like the idea of being pregnant.

But even if you had a vast conspiracy of male doctors pushing for host uterus in every situation, and even if you had a large number of women who were looking to have someone else carry their babies for them, you still could not end up with very many children created by this method, because the technology is simply too limited. The time and expense of the procedure put it out of reach of large numbers, and the poor success rate means that most of the couples would go away disappointed. Technology is not moving fast in this direction, either.

Just the opposite: it's moving in the direction of enabling more and more women who were previously thought incapable of sustaining a pregnancy to conceive and to bring their babies to term.

More and better ARTs will mean women will have more control over their reproductive lives, an end the authors believe that all feminists should welcome.

As for the right-to-lifers' charge that ARTs have enabled women to delay childbearing to pursue careers, to the detriment of the traditional family structure, an interesting retort may be found in the 1991 best-seller *Backlash: The Undeclared War Against American Women,* by Susan Faludi. Her investigation of infertility statistics exposes the myth that infertility is a "career women's disease." In fact, she notes, infertility rates are rising far faster among poor women with little access to health care than among middle-class professional women. Citing the U.S. National Center for Health Statistics, she concludes, "Women in this age group [30 to 34] had a mere three percent higher risk of infertility than women in their *early* twenties. In fact, since 1965, infertility had *declined* slightly among women in their early to midthirties—and even among women in their forties. . . . As usual this news made no media splashes." Yet groups hostile to abortion rights and full sexual equality have continued to promote the misinformation that having a medical abortion or delaying childbearing until one's thirties will frequently lead to infertility—and the mass media have generally reported such statements without further investigation.

As to the argument that the availability of ARTs has contributed to the decline of the American family by enabling Lesbians, single women, and other "unsuitable" types to become mothers, one need only take a glance at the figures from the Bureau of Labor Statistics to see the insignificance of the relationship. Only slightly under 21 percent of American families still conform to the traditional pattern of breadwinner-father-and-stay-at-home-mother. Of the remaining 80 percent, only a tiny fraction are families composed of unmarried women who have availed themselves of medical technology to have children. Obviously, other societal factors must be far more important in the decline of the traditional family structure than the development of a few ultrahigh-priced and statistically unimpressive laboratory-fertilization procedures.

Now considering the relationship of ARTs to abortion: It must be pointed out that in nature the union of sperm and egg is a most commonplace event, happening (as some researchers speculate) nearly every time that fertile sex cells come into contact with one another. However, pregnancy is far less frequent an occurrence, because of the far lesser likelihood of implantation following fertilization. Thus, millions of hu-

A PATIENT DESCRIBES THE MORAL DILEMMA SHE FACED AFTER A SUCCESSFUL IVF CYCLE

While everyone at the IVF clinic was caring and informative, there were some things no one ever mentioned to us. All too often the moral and ethical issues are ignored because the success rate in IVF is low. I had sixteen well-developed eggs retrieved, and twelve of them fertilized. The doctor transferred four embryos to my uterus and all four of them implanted. I was pregnant with quads. You can imagine how I felt. Here I was praying for a child for seven years and now I was going to have four! I'm of small build and there was no way I could have carried them to term without endangering the entire pregnancy and my health as well.

I was advised by many physicians to undergo a pregnancy reduction to reduce the pregnancy to twins. I went to an expert and had the procedure done. It was to be the single most horrible experience of my life thus far. [This patient goes on to describe in detail how the doctor had to locate the heart of the two "excess" fetuses within her uterus and then insert a needle filled with a substance to stop those two hearts beating. The whole process was long, emotionally wrenching, and physically painful.] I took the pain and almost wanted more pain to somehow assuage my guilt. Anyway, in January of the following year [1990] I gave birth to twins, both six pounds and healthy. . . . When I look at my boy-girl twins, I can't imagine life without them. But I can't help but also think, "What if it had been Danny that I had injected with poison, what if it had been Amy?" The thought is horrific. No one ever told me that there was a possibility of this happening.

I also have four embryos frozen and I have been feeling increasingly uncomfortable about that. They have been frozen for three years now and although they are strong, I don't know if they would survive thawing. I am torn between wanting to donate them and destroying them to free them from their frozen state. . . . Now I have great respect and gratitude to the ———— Clinic for helping to create my family, but I do wish I could have been more informed of these moral dilemmas *beforehand*.

Jeanne from Alberta, Canada

man conceptions will be lost, or "aborted," at the two-, four-, or eight-celled stage. Such loss is no more significant in the natural scheme of things than is the loss of trillions of sperm or egg cells that die unfertilized every day. If you view the pre-embryo not as a person but as a mass of undifferentiated tissue that *may* (given a vast number of favorable conditions) turn into a baby in time, then a program involving disposal or freezing and storage of that tissue can be seen as an acceptable moral choice for the infertile couple.

CHAPTER EIGHT

"IT DOESN'T WORK!"

ABOUT DOCTOR-SWITCHING AND CLINIC-HOPPING

After you have been in treatment a while you will come to know and dread that moment when you look down in your underwear and see the first tiny telltale brown spots, the sign that your period is coming. You have endured all the rigors of your program for the past several weeks . . . you have done everything *exactly* as your doctor ordered . . . you have paid all that money . . . and for nothing!

You may even get this sinking feeling after failing to conceive on your very first cycle of treatment. Others may not start to feel let down until after the second, the third, or even the fourth or fifth month. But by the sixth month at the very latest, most couples will be feeling terribly discouraged.

By this point, if not sooner, your doctor (unless he is not really tuned in to your feelings at all) should have called you, suggesting that you come in and talk about your treatment plan and where it's going. Maybe you will do better trying a variation on your treatment for the next few cycles. He might also give you reasons why you should stick with what you've been doing for a little while longer.

If your doctor has *not* suggested such a consultation after six unsuccessful months, you should call up and make an appointment for one, regardless. You *need* to talk. However the consultation comes about, you will get more out of it if you come prepared to do more than just sit and listen. Jot down your questions and ideas on a notepad, and be an active participant in choosing the next step. Be sure to ask the following:

What is your best guess as to why the treatment has not worked so far?

Do you think it possible that my diagnostic tests failed to pick up some additional factor contributing to my infertility? Would it be worthwhile, in your opinion, to repeat any of the tests? Perform any new tests?

Is there some simple variant of the treatment I've been on that might increase my odds of conception? (Examples: If on Clomid, try an hCG shot on the day that ultrasound reveals the presence of mature egg follicles; if on Pergonal, try varying the day on which the first shot is given, or building up the dosage more slowly; try IUI).

Don't be afraid to ask the doctor about techniques you have heard about from other patients, from RESOLVE meetings, from books, magazine articles, and TV news reports. If the technique you bring up is not right for you, your doctor will tell you why.

One thing I have learned from talking to other patients who have been successfully treated: keep your ears open—you never know when you might hear of something that could be of value in your case. Some doctors *do* resent it when their patients follow medical news, thinking that they are trying to play doctor when they aren't qualified. Women patients especially have reported to me their doctors' condescending reactions to mentioning new medical techniques—reactions such as, "Don't worry yourself about *that*, dear," and, "I'm the doctor—let me handle it." Though your doctor may react unenthusiastically, persist. My interviews were filled with stories like these two:

I suggested adding progesterone to my treatment. My doctor said I really didn't need it, but finally agreed to let me try it. I became pregnant the next cycle.

*A*nne from Washington, D.C.

I'd been on Clomid for a while, but kept ovulating rather late (past Day Seventeen) in my cycle. I heard about women starting it earlier than Day Five, and I asked my doctor if he thought that might help. He agreed to let me move up the starting point to Day Three, and it did bring my ovulation forward a little.

*R*obin from Maryland

But what if you have a doctor who never listens to your ideas, never takes the time to explain to you why he thinks a technique you've brought up is unsuitable, and doesn't seem to notice your growing frustration at your inability to be heard about matters affecting your own body? Then it's time for a new doctor!

In the emotion-laden business of trying to make a baby, you need to have someone you know you can talk to, someone who cares what you think. You will be more satisfied with your treatment, whatever the outcome, if you end up feeling that you had the best possible help in your struggle, an ally who respected you and was really rooting for your success.

Continual condescension, failure to listen, gross arrogance, and general insensitivity—these are all reasons to look for help elsewhere. You might also start thinking about switching if your doctor has done any of the following:

- consistently forgotten your name or your spouse's name (one or two slips may be forgiven)
- mixed up your file or case history with someone else's more than once—for example, the doctor has asked you repeatedly when were you coming in for your egg retrieval, when you are only doing Clomid
- seldom returned your phone calls, or had the nurse handle all telephone contact with you, even when you had questions that only the doctor could answer
- seemed uninterested in your case; has been consistently aloof or impersonal; has treated you as if you were a collection of tubes and organs, not a whole human being
- prescribed a drug that carries an FDA warning about dangerous side effects for patients like you, but couldn't or wouldn't satisfactorily answer your questions about whether it was safe for you to take
- performed a procedure that he said would cause only "minor discomfort" but which put you in severe pain—pain that he dismissed, refusing your request for a prescription painkiller
- made no attempt to assist you in your dispute with your health insurance company; refused to list procedures using accepted insurance company terms; consistently described procedures that might be covered using terms you have told him your insurance company associates with policy exclusions; refused to write letters or notes to substantiate your valid claims for reimbursement

- maintained limited office hours, resulting in your missing out on necessary tests or treatments, because the proper timing for those tests or treatments coincided with weekends or holidays or times of the day when the clinic was closed
- couldn't be reached in an emergency (and you could not reach one of the doctor's colleagues, either), such as a threatened miscarriage or severe drug reaction; or when reached by telephone, scolded you for bothering him over what turned out to be a minor problem, or simply directed you to go to the emergency room of the nearest hospital without phoning ahead to arrange your swift admission, or failure to come to see you during your hospital stay
- failed to follow the normal procedures and precautions that you have learned are standard practice through your talks with patients of other doctors or counselors at RESOLVE—you have asked him why he is not doing such and such, but his answer didn't make sense to you
- turned out to be lacking in the skills needed to diagnose or treat your problem properly, or has diagnosed your problem correctly, but lacks the ability to treat it with the most effective means
- turned out to be someone you simply don't like (Yes, this *is* a valid reason for switching doctors! Not for all patients—some will feel, "Well, he's tops in his field, so what does it matter if he's not Prince Charming? It's not like I'm going to bed with him!" But if you are the type to want more from a doctor than mere competence and trustworthiness, if you feel a true need for warmth and empathy before you can open up and work comfortably with someone on problems of your intimate life, then for you sociability is a must.)

Dialogue Overheard in the Clinic's Waiting Room

First patient: Dr. R. seems so stiff, so cold. I'm really having difficulties talking to him.
Second patient: Really? You think *he's* cold? I switched doctors because my last doctor was *really* cold. Dr. R. is Mr. Personality compared to Dr. D.!

Can't Get Through to Your Doctor? Lose Your Temper!

*B*etty from Iowa tried for four straight days to get hold of her doctor on the phone. She had a simple question about the development of her follicles. She needed an answer by Thursday, because her husband would be going out of town on that day, and if she would be ovulating around that time, she would make plans to go with him on the trip, so that they could try to conceive that month. When she didn't hear from the doctor by late Wednesday afternoon, she finally lost her temper with the receptionist. "I told her I felt I had wasted a couple of thousand dollars if I could not get an answer when I needed it," Betty writes. "Within one hour of losing my temper, the doctor returned my phone call."

Some patients will take six months to realize their discontent with their doctor's work style. Others will know right away that it's time for a change. If you're not sure, think of how you've been dealing with your doctor regarding phone calls or the scheduling of appointments: Do you often put off calling the doctor, or try to postpone your appointments until the last possible moment? Do you dread going in to see him, or have trouble telling him what's going on? If you do, then by all means, find someone you will feel more comfortable with.

Once you have decided to make the switch, *do it!*

Don't be put off because you are embarrassed or feel guilty about it. It's not a divorce, and you haven't failed at being a patient. Quite possibly it's no one's fault—it's just one of those things. There is nothing to be gained by agonizing over your decision once you've reached it.

Don't feel you have to give the doctor some long, drawn-out explanation, either. Nor do you have to apologize. Keep your statement simple and to the point. You might say:

"I have decided it would suit my schedule better to see a doctor closer to my home [or work]."

"I have decided to take some time off from treatment—I'm not sure how long."

"I've been feeling kind of anxious about how my treatment is going, and I think I'd feel better getting a fresh perspective on my problem, so I have scheduled an appointment with Dr. ———. I'd like to see how it goes with her for a while."

The latter two reasons for switching will leave you the option to return, if you later decide that your first doctor was better, on the whole, than your second.

After your doctor learns of your decision, he may well want to talk it over with you, to find out what, if anything, he has done to make you dissatisfied with your care. That is a good sign, and it could well be that the doctor only needs to be made aware of your reason for unhappiness to become more attentive to your needs. It's entirely up to you whether you want to stay with him to see if things improve, or move on just the same. Resist feeling pressured to stay if what you really want to do is leave.

When You Suspect You've Been Seeing a Quack

Leaving a doctor who has abused your trust or your body should be handled very differently from leaving one who has simply failed to live up to your expectations. In that case you will want to spell out on the record exactly what the doctor did that you believe was wrong. That means you must put your complaint in writing.

Don't phone the doctor or call his staff to tell them why you are leaving, but send the doctor a clear, nonangry letter that step-by-step describes exactly what he did, and on what dates, that violated accepted principles of good care. Examples of malpractice include

- unclean handling of instruments
- careless prescribing of drugs; failure to monitor the use of Pergonal or Metrodin
- lying to you or your spouse about any aspect of your diagnosis or treatment
- fraudulent representation of credentials or medical experience
- personal impropriety, such as sexual advances, joking about your sexual parts or practices, or any other form of harassment, whether by word or deed
- any violation of the confidentiality of the doctor-patient relationship; any talk about your case outside his office with anyone—unless expressly authorized by you to do so

If any of the above has occurred, make sure you save all documentation that might substantiate your claim. Keep all bills to prove that you were in the doctor's office on the dates you said you were; take note of names of nurses or other staff members who were present and might be witnesses; try to recall if you had complained at the time to any third parties (such as a coworker or neighbor) about the doctor's behavior in your case, and keep all written instructions, empty prescription bottles, and any other materials you may have received from the doctor or his staff.

Whether you are able to substantiate your claim with hard evidence or not, it will still be worthwhile to forward a copy of your letter of complaint to your state's medical board. If you suffered unnecessary pain or incurred additional medical expenses because of the doctor's misconduct in handling your case, you will probably want to consult a malpractice attorney as well. To find one who is knowledgeable in the standards of care for fertility patients, you might try asking your local RESOLVE chapter for a referral.

While the vast majority of the infertility specialists today are competent and responsible practitioners, there *are* some quacks out there, so you should try to stay alert to any behavior that strikes you as out of the ordinary or unprofessional in any way.

A frightening but cautionary tale might be in order here. It's the story of Dr. Cecil Jacobson, who for twelve years ran a booming fertility practice in a northern Virginia suburb of Washington, D.C. He was once one of the most respected members of his profession, being the first practicing OB-GYN in this country to perform amniocentesis. But after the use of amniocentesis became routine among other gynecological practices in the mid-1970s, his patient referrals from other doctors fell off sharply, and he turned to the fertility field to attract more business.

Soon he had a full appointment book, and was taking in over $400,000 a year. Between 1976 and 1988 he treated hundreds of women for infertility, some with drugs, some with IUI, using what was supposed to be their husbands' sperm, and still others with what was supposed to be fresh (not frozen) sperm from donors. Only it turned out that Dr. Jacobson had *no* donors. After the patient arrived for her insemination and handed over to the doctor twenty dollars in cash, which he said was "for the donor," who was "waiting in the next room," he would excuse himself, disappear for a few minutes, and then return with the sperm sample—his own—which he inserted in his patient's uterus. In some cases, when the husband delivered a sperm sample to be used to inseminate his wife, the doctor simply substituted his own sperm and performed the insemination. When the doctor's fraud was finally exposed, prosecutors charged that up to seventy-five children were believed to have been fathered by this man.

But that was not the only form of quackery that he practiced in his clinic. Another equally heartbreaking deceit involved the deliberate misreading of sonograms and pregnancy tests to make infertile women believe they were pregnant when they were not. First he would treat his patients with a series of hCG shots. Then he would have them come in for a pregnancy test. The type of test he used works by detecting the level of hCG in the patient's urine—which of course would be positive, since the patient was already pumped full of the hormone by artificial means. After the patient had been "pregnant" for a few weeks, he would then tell her to come in for a sonogram, to get a look at her "fetus" on the monitor. While the patient watched happily, he would point out dark, blobby spots on the grainy screen and say that this is the heart beating, or that's the baby's head, or "identify" other body parts in this way.

When, after some more time passed and the patient got her period, she would return to the doctor, who would explain to her that she had experienced a form of miscarriage in which her fetus was somehow "resorbed" into her body. There was no dead tissue to remove through the **D and C** procedure (dilatation and curettage) that is usually performed after a miscarriage, because the fetus just wasn't there anymore.

His patients grieved for their "dead" babies, but many of them kept coming back to him for further treatment. One woman was told she was pregnant *eight* times, and that every time the fetus had been "resorbed." When some patients began to wonder whether they should seek a second opinion, Dr. Jacobson emphatically warned them not to. Other doctors didn't "understand" his revolutionary techniques, he said. If patients wanted to have babies, they should just trust him and stick with him. He even told some of his patients, "God doesn't give you babies—I do."*

But eventually some of his patients, after many "miscarriages," did go to other doctors and ask what was wrong. Each one would then learn that it was highly improbable that she had ever been pregnant. She had simply been hoodwinked, strung along for months, or in some cases, years. Eventually, too, someone alerted a local television station, WRC, to the fraud that was being perpetrated.

After WRC's investigative team ran their TV exposé of Dr. Jacobson's

*Quoted from the federal indictment

practices, a flood of malpractice suits was unleashed. The quack was forced by his insurance company to shut down his practice. The FBI began its own investigation, and in 1991 he was charged with fifty-three felonies in an eighty-six-page indictment. In 1992 he was convicted of multiple counts of fraud and sentenced to five years in prison and a $116,000 fine.

The case raises many crucial questions for fertility patients today: How could such medical misconduct have gone on undetected for so long? Why weren't Jacobson's patients put on the alert earlier, when he told them not to consult other doctors about his unusual treatments? Shouldn't there have been some form of regulation or government oversight on the use of donor sperm? And why didn't any of the doctors who first saw some of Jacobson's "recurrent miscarriage" patients report their findings to the state medical board?

EIGHT IMPORTANT LESSONS YOU CAN LEARN FROM THE CECIL JACOBSON CASE

Lesson 1: If your fertility doctor ever compares himself to God, get out of that man's office *now*!

Lesson 2: If you suffer more than two miscarriages under treatment from the same doctor, make an appointment to see a specialist in recurrent miscarriage. The specialist should review your records from your first doctor, and search for the cause of the problem, and if possible, treat it. If you should become pregnant again following treatment, you should be classified as a "high risk" pregnancy from day one, and follow a program designed by your specialist to increase your odds of retaining the fetus until it can safely be born. "Resorption" of a miscarried fetus into a woman's body is a relatively rare event, and if told that is what has happened to your fetus, immediately seek confirmation in the form of a second opinion.

Lesson 3: If your doctor ever tells you *not* to get a second opinion, beware! Good doctors don't feel threatened by second opinions, *but all quacks do*!

(continued)

Lesson 4: If you have an ultrasound performed to confirm that you are pregnant, ask the sonographer to "take a picture" of the fetus for you to take home. The modern ultrasound machine is capable of freezing an image and duplicating it on the spot. If you later suspect there is anything amiss with your doctor's handling of your pregnancy, you can show the ultrasound picture to another doctor to find out how he views it.

Lesson 5: Talk to other patients in the doctor's waiting room. Find out their experiences. Are any back trying to have a second baby with the same doctor? That's an encouraging sign. But if more than one or two tell you any stories that give you pause, you might want to start talking to patients of other doctors, to do some comparison shopping and to find out if yours is doing anything weird.

Lesson 6: If it feels weird, it is. You should leave a doctor who does anything at all that "gives you the creeps." Macabre "jokes," offensive language, pelvic exams without a nurse present are all examples of suspicious behavior, and you should not wait around to see if anything worse will occur.

Lesson 7: Fresh donor sperm is *not* safe! The doctor may promise that you will conceive faster if he uses only fresh sperm, but what good will that be if you get AIDS in the process? A reputable doctor will use only donor sperm collected, frozen, and stored according to guidelines established by the American Fertility Society or the American Association of Tissue Banks.

Lesson 8: MOST IMPORTANT! Don't see any one doctor for an unlimited period of time. Always set a timetable at the outset. For example, if you are a woman age thirty or younger, you could decide you will see this doctor for a maximum of three years from the date of your first consultation. If you are between thirty and thirty-five, two years; if over thirty-five, one year to eighteen months. After that period is up, change doctors—even if you think your first doctor was doing the best job possible. You need a fresh perspective. Any really good doctor will think that switching under these circumstances is reasonable. In fact, a really good doctor *won't let* you go on cycle after cycle doing something that seems to be going nowhere. A really good doctor may even counsel you to start again with someone new, or perhaps start looking into other, nonmedical options (such as adoption, or the child-free lifestyle).

There is plenty of fault to spread around in this case—not just to the perpetrator, but to the patients as well, for being naive and too trusting; to our government, which imposes all kinds of regulations on our foods and drugs but not on the commercially salable sperm that may be inserted into our bodies; and to other doctors for suspecting that something was not right about Jacobson's clinic but taking no action to protect their patients.

But while the blame in the Cecil Jacobson case falls to many, the case clearly shows that you, the patient, must be alert and protect yourself from becoming a victim of a similar medical criminal.

The Couple Who Saw a Quack

One of the most troubling stories I heard in the year that I spent researching this book came from a couple, Vera and Alex, who live in Hawaii. After struggling and failing to get the treatment they needed from the free military health care facility available to them through Alex's Army service, they decided to pay for treatment by a private doctor out of their own pockets. They chose a fertility specialist, Dr. L., who supposedly had a great reputation.

Alex had been diagnosed with a poor sperm count. The first thing the doctor suggested he do was drink a lot of pineapple juice "to improve semen quality and increase vitamin content."

After some months had passed and the couple still had not conceived, Vera mentioned to Dr. L. that the stress of infertility was taking a toll on their sex life. The doctor then told her that she needed to "learn to seduce your husband," and he even went so far as to advise her to have a talk with a prostitute for ideas on "how to get his juices flowing"!

If that wasn't bad enough, when she had pelvic exams, he would have her wait for him to come into the room with her legs already up in stirrups. Vera writes, "I *refused* to wait for the doctor in that position!"

Toward the conclusion of her long and moving letter Vera writes, "Dr. L. made me feel very uncomfortable with my body . . . dirty for the first time in my whole life. We now have a sexless marriage partly as a result of worthless treatments received under Dr. L.'s care."

INTERVIEW QUESTION: WHY DID YOU DECIDE TO SWITCH DOCTORS OR CLINICS?

I left ——— Clinic because it was impersonal, also inconveniently located, and they seemed to be mostly interested in making lots of money by cutting down on your time with the doctors and even the nurses.

*R*ita from Maryland

I was very bitter about my experience with ——— Clinic. There was no consideration of my individuality. They had a plan and they put you through steps X, Y, and Z, and you could bet that no one gets to step Z until they've done steps X and Y.

*E*llen from New Jersey

*W*hen my husband's sperm count came back high, my doctor said, "I guess it's your fault then." He also made a crass remark about my occupation, that my blood pressure was high due to job anxiety. [After that, this couple began searching for more considerate and compassionate treatment.]

*C*laire and Jerry from Texas

*A*t my OB-GYN's office I was referred to (quite loudly) as "the infertility patient" in front of a roomful of expectant women.

*S*heila from Louisiana

*M*y first doctor misjudged my time of ovulation and then tried to convince me that he hadn't, even though my hormone levels clearly showed otherwise. I really resented being treated as if I knew nothing. It seemed the office was only in it for the money a procedure would get them. . . . My main criticism was that the same technique was employed again and again, even though it wasn't working. I understand that a progressive clinic tries a technique for a certain amount of time, then moves on to another. That wasn't done, and that's why I switched practices.

*S*andra from New Jersey

(continued)

I stopped going to my first clinic because I felt I was being rushed there into major medical intervention, and I got a recommendation for another doctor. At first I was pleased with my new doctor, but then a major problem developed. My doctor couldn't remember that my periods ranged from 30 to 75 days. He gave me a dosage of Pergonal/Metrodin that caused a hyperstimulation response. It took me a few months to recover from the experience, and I am still very angry at his near-malpractice.

Judith from Washington, D.C.

My first doctor was paternalistic and condescending. He talked to my husband rather than to me. When I saw him alone, he wouldn't answer my questions. The nurses were uncomprehending of the emotional side of treatment. Nobody ever remembered who you were or what your history was. It was a cattle call.

Sharon from Washington, D.C.

At ——— Clinic after six months of almost daily treatment the doctor still did not know our names, and although he'd done my laparoscopy, he asked me if I had blocked tubes!

Dorothy from New Jersey

Trying to reach the doctor with questions over the phone was quite difficult. I continually had to go through assistants or nurses. Finally, on one occasion, my husband and I sat down and wrote out all the questions we had and dropped it off at the doctor's office. We subsequently were asked to set up an appointment (they called it a conference meeting) to sit down with the doctor (for which we were charged a fee of, I believe, $50). The doctor answered our questions but in a technical way. We had to ask for clarification several times. . . . Another frustrating aspect was how many hours I was spending waiting at the doctor's office. I was in a Ph.D. program and ended up missing classes because I would have to wait so long—up to two to three hours—for the doctor to take me.

Mary from Illinois

Five Ways to Make Sure
Your Phone Call Is Returned

The number two complaint of my survey respondents (after "The doctor is insensitive") is that it's nearly *impossible* to get the doctor on the phone when you need him.

The best approach to this problem is to find out the doctor's return-call policy before you sign on as a patient. If he takes and returns phone calls only between certain hours, then make sure he has the phone number to reach you during those hours, and you just stay put till he calls. If you just can't manage to be at one number for a block of time during the day, then consider renting a pocket pager (a beeper) or a cellular phone for the week or for the month.

What if your doctor does not have a regular time to take patients' calls? Then you need some way to make your call stand out in the mind of the person who takes down the message, and in the doctor's mind when he reads it. Here are a few things you might say that should send off alarm bells in the doctor's head (and hopefully get him to give you a quick call back).

1. "The doctor said I was to let him know immediately if such and such occurred."
2. "I am having a strange reaction [to medication, or to a procedure that was performed] and I'm not sure what to do."
3. "I've been given contradictory instructions. Nurse X told me to do one thing and Nurse Y told me to do something else. I need the doctor to clear this up or I could end up taking the wrong dose."
4. "If I don't get the answer I need by [deadline] I'm going to switch to a practice that is more responsive to patients' needs."
5. "This is an emergency!" [Of course, you should save these words for a true emergency, such as severe pain, bleeding, blacking out, etc.]

Choosing Your Next Doctor or Clinic

Now you are determined to make a change, but how do you know that your second doctor will be any better than your first? After all, you followed all the right steps the first time around, didn't you? You got recommendations from knowledgeable sources, you investigated statistics, you asked all the right questions—and it still didn't work out. So what should you do differently this time?

I asked this question of many patients who had switched doctors, and here's what I learned. Once you have been in one program, you have a much clearer idea what you're looking for, because you already have a standard against which any new clinic can be compared. The questions you ask while second-time doctor-shopping may be the same, but now you are much better equipped to evaluate the answers you receive. You are better attuned to pick up on small things that you didn't catch the first time around: how abrupt or how courteous the staff members sound when they pick up the telephone; the look on the faces of the other patients in the waiting room (this time it may be easier for you to tell who looks anxious or frazzled, now that you've felt that way yourself); and the tone the doctor takes when he tells you about his practice. And now when you hear him talk about LH surges, spinnbarkeit, HSGs, and EMBs, you can follow along without feeling swamped.

This time around you will also know far better what weight to assign to different factors. Perhaps convenience of clinic location didn't seem like a big thing when you were looking before—but after spending an hour and a half in your car to get there, for ten or twelve days out of every month, location is now practically your number one consideration. Perhaps you thought it wouldn't bother you to discuss the frequency and quality of your bedroom activities with a male doctor, but now you realize that you could talk more freely with a woman.

Time and experience lead to many such changes in perspective, so you would first do well to sit down and organize your thoughts. Take a moment to jot down the answers to these questions:

What are your bottom-line requirements for your new clinic?

What are some other desirable features you are seeking? Rank them in order from ten (top) to one (bottom).

What did you most dislike about the clinic you are leaving? List in order of importance.

What, if anything, did you like about your old clinic?

Which, if any, unpleasant aspects of your medical care do you believe will remain the same, regardless of which clinic you choose?

After you have set your priorities for what you want, you are ready to begin the information-gathering process. This time around you probably already know quite a few other couples who have been in treatment elsewhere. You have met other patients in the waiting room of your first doctor, and they have told you about other doctors they have seen; or you have joined RESOLVE and have been able to chat with patients of other doctors at meetings and get-togethers. Call these friends now and tell them about your desire to change. Let them know exactly what you're looking for, and see how they think these other clinics measure up against the criteria you've laid out.

It's still important to check out success rates as described in Chapter Two. It's still *essential* to find a place that is properly equipped and open for business at times that will serve your needs. It's wise to read all promotional materials and brochures skeptically, relying on their representations far less than on the evidence of your own eyes and ears. And of course you will still be looking for a clinic that has at least one doctor who is board-certified in the fertility subspecialty relevant to your case.

But most important of all remains the gut feeling that you get from your "look-see" consultation with the doctor. Let her know at the outset that you were once a patient of Doctor So-and-so. Describe that doctor's handling of your case, including anything he may have done that you weren't happy about. Listen carefully to this doctor's reaction. If she immediately starts defending her colleague or belittling your version of events, take that as a warning that you may not be too happy with this doctor either. A fair-minded doctor will usually say that she needs to review your records before she can comment on your past treatment by another doctor. A sympathetic sort will accept your complaints as valid (after all, it was *your* experience), even if she has no objective evidence in front of her to substantiate your claim.

One thing you will be likely to discover: your new doctor will be very reluctant to criticize (or second-guess, as she might put it) whatever treatment your first doctor had prescribed. Yes, doctors do tend to stick up for one another—but don't let that bother you too much if you are otherwise favorably impressed with the doctor's demeanor. Doctors also tend to like to be able to show that they can succeed where others have failed. Your new doctor will thus have extra incentive to do her absolute best to bring your case to the conclusion you desire.

At your look-see visit you should also be sure to ask the doctor all the same questions you asked while doctor shopping the first time around (see page 96 for suggested question list).

Beyond those questions, you should also ask this doctor what additional tests (if any) she would be likely to perform, and (assuming that your first doctor's diagnosis was correct) what she considers to be your best treatment options at this time.

If you have already made up your mind that there are certain tests or treatments that you would not consider, say so plainly, and give your reasons why. If you intend to play an active role in choosing and evaluating the progress of your own treatment (and I strongly recommend that you do), it's best to let the doctor know of your attitude up front. And if she reacts with disapproval to the idea that you might be an equal player on the team that is working to solve your infertility problem, then you should probably keep looking for another doctor to be the captain of your team.

GET YOUR RECORDS!

*W*hen you do find a new doctor who strikes you as good, make sure that doctor is given access to all your medical records from your previous doctor. I can't stress this too strongly. Without your records to review, your doctor will undoubtedly have to order repeats of tests you have already undergone, wasting time and money and causing you needless discomfort. There's no question of embarrassment at having to call your old doctor and explain why you want the records sent, since all you should have to do is sign a release form for the new doctor's staff to send in to the old doctor's office. If your new doctor does not offer to obtain your records for you, you *must* bring the matter up. Beware of the doctor who says he does not need your records to treat you effectively. A doctor who is not interested in your past medical history or who will not help you to get your records is not a doctor you want to be dealing with. Keep looking!

One last reflection on doctor-switching: Fertility treatment is by its nature an iffy business. Some doctors "get lucky" and succeed on the first try—even with some very tough cases. They are not necessarily better doctors. Others are doing everything right and just can't seem to get anywhere—even when your problem may be considered mild. But your failure to conceive after a set number of treatment cycles does not prove that your first doctor was no good. Still, the frustration of trying and trying and never succeeding can begin to drag you down after a while, and even though you know it's not the doctor's fault, can make you start looking to make a switch.

Patients Give Tips on Finding a New Doctor

Use your time in the waiting room to your advantage. Get to know the other patients. Talk to them about their experiences with whatever other doctors they have seen, either at this practice or at other clinics. You can learn a lot by finding out what's working and what's not working for others like you.

Anne from Washington, D.C.

The criteria I looked for in selecting a new program:

1. Office open 365 days a year for blood work, ultrasounds, and procedures (my former program was closed Sundays, so if you ovulated and needed IUI on Sunday, the whole cycle was wasted)
2. Staff of reproductive endocrinologists with a sympathetic team approach and proven track record
3. Prompt call-backs and test results
4. A primary physician who respected my feelings and did not discourage independent decision-making

Marcia from New Jersey

Author's comment: An excellent checklist! I'd recommend this list to anyone searching for a clinic, either first time around or later on.

We chose our last doctor with great care, after some years of experience in infertility treatment. We chose Dr. ———— because he was affiliated with an excellent program, and only after I had interviewed two other doctors in the field as well. His reputation was excellent, but so were the reputations of the others I had seen in the past. Because I've learned that even doctors of great reputation can make what I consider to be mistakes, I went to three doctors with my records, explained my history, and asked how they would proceed. I chose Dr. ———— because the tests he suggested made sense to me. Also, it was clear that he planned to move carefully, but quickly, as well.

Cathy from New York

That's perfectly okay, and a common thing to do. Ex-patients tell me, "I just felt if I switched I might get lucky with somebody else." It may even be the doctor himself who tells you, "I'm sorry this doesn't seem to be working out for you. Maybe if somebody else took over for a time you might get a different result."

A startlingly high proportion (84 percent) of the patients I surveyed had consulted more than one doctor for their infertility. The vast majority were glad they did. Even when the second doctor was not able to do any better with the case than the first, at least the patient knew her lack of pregnancy was not simply the result of one doctor's unhelpful approach. Switching doctors at a time of unbearable stress and frustration, if nothing else, appears to serve as an excellent coping mechanism.

ABOUT BREAKS IN TREATMENT

Stepping Back to Think

Sometimes when you think you have had all you can take of treatment, you don't need to switch but simply take a break. You need some time alone with your partner to rest awhile and reflect. Of course, many older patients who feel they have only a very limited time to try to get pregnant (perhaps as few as two or three more years) will resist this idea. Why give up even one cycle that you could be using to try to conceive? Here are just a few sound reasons:

- Treatment generally takes a toll on the body. Cycle after cycle of drugs or invasive procedures not resulting in pregnancy may leave your body less likely to conceive. Some studies suggest that women who don't conceive after the first few cycles have a greater likelihood to do so if they give their bodies at least a few months to recover.
- Knowing in advance that you will take a break at a certain point will make you better prepared psychologically to continue treatment than if you were to commit to consecutive cycles. For example, you could say that you will do four cycles of X, then rest, then decide whether to continue X, or move on to Y or Z.
- When you return from your break you will be more relaxed, feeling less stressed—and it's a proven fact that reducing stress improves the odds of conception.

- A break gives you an opportunity to recharge your batteries, to do something pleasurable, to get away on a much-needed vacation.
- A break gives you some time to settle your thoughts, reevaluate your priorities, and/or read up on other options (whether for different treatments or for nonmedical alternatives).
- A break eases the strain on your pocketbook.
- A break lets you concentrate on some critically important aspects of life that you may have let go by the wayside: your relationship with your partner, your career, hobbies and interests that you used to pursue, or perhaps just time to be alone with your own thoughts.

Once you decide that a break is what you need, how do you know *when* to take it? This varies, naturally, from patient to patient, but the following questions might be helpful to you as you try to decide if you need to take your break anytime soon:

- Do you feel tired of treatment? Have you been feeling discouraged or depressed?
- Have you tried out more than one form of treatment without success?
- Have you been more than four months on any one form of treatment?
- Have you suffered a miscarriage after what you had thought was a successful treatment cycle?
- Is treatment interfering with any plans you would like to make—to travel, to attend some special event (a family reunion, a wedding, etc.), or just to get away during your normal vacation time?
- Is treatment causing increasingly severe side effects (such as cumulative weight gain, an increasing number of ovarian cysts, worsening hot flashes, or any other symptoms you would dearly love not to have for a while)?
- Would you simply like not to have to think about treatment for a period of time?

If you answered yes to two or more of these questions, you'll probably benefit from some time off.

Is there any time of year when a break might do more for you than at other times? Yes! Patients tell me they feel so much better leaving treatment temporarily around the end of the year. You can enjoy Christmas or other holidays, and all the family gatherings and parties so much more when you're not worrying about taking your medication on time, or getting up early the next morning for your monitoring appointment.

August is another recommended time to skip treatment. Oftentimes clinics will be short-staffed, as doctors, nurses, and other personnel go on vacation. Your own vacation time might be due that month, and you don't want to have your travel plans constrained by the cycles of your reproductive organs.

Talking with Your Doctor About Your Break

You don't have to involve your doctor in your decision-making about your break if you don't want to. All you really need to tell him is when you're taking off, and if you know it in advance, for how long. But there are circumstances in which you might prefer to get medical advice before you decide to take your break, including

- if your physical condition or age make it advisable for you to stick to a certain treatment schedule
- if you are not sure how a break would affect your chances for success after treatment resumes (for example, if you're not sure whether your PCO disease or endometriosis would worsen during your time off, beyond the point at which future treatment would be able to reverse the damage)
- if certain specialists, equipment, or special clinic hours would no longer be available by the time you return
- if you have become so accustomed to involving your doctor in every phase of your reproductive planning and have so close a relationship that it seems to you unthinkable not to seek his advice in the timing of your break.

Keep in mind that good doctors will generally understand and support their patients' decisions to take breaks. If your doctor seems hostile to your announced time off, find out why. If the reason given does not strike you as important, then it just could be that his annoyance at your absence has more to do with the loss of billing for that time period than concern for your reproductive future. (You see, BMW payments do not take a holiday, just because a patient does.) You will probably be better served in the future if you switch to a doctor who is more sympathetic to your need to take some time away from treatment.

But let's say you decide to stick with the doctor who is not keen on your break—then be firm in your decision to take off when you feel you must. There is nothing to be apologetic about. It's *your* reproductive system. I know I have made this point before, but it bears repeating. In the hustle-bustle of the infertility business, it's so easy to get caught up in the anxiety of trying to do everything right that you end up blindly following medical instructions for months on end. You may tend to fall into a mindset that you must follow the doctor's timetable, rather than asking the doctor to work within a timetable that suits *your* physical and emotional needs. Yet you are the one to experience the discomforts of treatment, so you must be the one to say when it's time for a rest.

How You Can Use Your Time Off

Most patients like to get away and think about treatment as little as possible when they're on a break. It's good to spend at least the initial period of your time off just clearing your head (if you can).

After a while (how long depends entirely on you) you should feel ready to start planning for what you want to do after your break. Listed below are some ideas for actions you might want to contemplate during the calm of your time away from treatment:

Draw up a list of issues and concerns to discuss with your doctor, so that when you return to treatment you can work to iron out any difficulties you have had in your doctor-patient relationship.

Look into the pros and cons of other treatment methods.

Draw up a timetable for what treatments you are willing to try, in what order, and for how many cycles after your treatment resumes.

If unhappy with your current doctor, investigate the success rates of other doctors or clinics.

Work with your spouse or partner on stresses in your relationship caused by your infertility.

Work with your spouse or partner to sort out your conflicting views on what alternative to pursue if treatment ultimately does not work for you. Now is the right time to come to an agreement on what nonmedical form of resolution (adoption, child-free life-style, or "partial parenting") would be your new goal.

Look into professional counseling to help you deal with the stresses and strains you have experienced during treatment.

Come to the conclusion that life without treatment is really so much better for you that you decide to make your break a permanent one.

How Many IVF Attempts Is Too Many?

The scandal of the infertility business is that there are far too many doctors willing to subject patients to IVF cycle after cycle without success. The patients keep at it, despite the pain, the cost, and the low odds of success, because the doctor encourages them to believe if they will just give it one more shot, maybe *this time* it will work. They live on false hope. Studies have consistently shown that the odds of conceiving on an IVF procedure peak after four to six cycles. Only about 3 *percent* of IVF patients who conceive do so after the sixth attempt. The same statistics hold true for other ARTs, such as GIFT and ZIFT.

Yet there are women whose doctors have performed ten, fifteen, even *twenty* IVF procedures on them, to no avail. Why? When you consider the fact that doctors make thousands of dollars every time a patient does IVF, it's not hard to guess the answer: it's greed, pure and simple. There is no other, more favorable interpretation to put on the doctor's behavior in most cases of overuse of IVF.

How can you protect yourself? It's fairly simple: after your sixth unsuccessful attempt, give it up! If you wish, find another doctor to discuss why (if any reason can be found) the procedure did not work for you, and perhaps suggest something different that just *might* improve your pregnancy odds (say, use of donor eggs), but on no account should you go ask your new doctor to start doing the same procedure that didn't work for you all those previous attempts. For most couples, the time has come to seek another way of dealing with infertility. Yes, it's sad to have to stop believing that technology will make your dreams come true, sad to have to admit that all the money already spent has gone for nothing, but how much sadder it would be to keep deluding yourself, to keep on throwing money away, all while you could be aggressively pursuing adoption, or teaching yourself to enjoy your child-free life.

Breaks: How Long and How Often?

These questions, as with the question of the right time for a break, are highly individual matters. However, some commonsense rules may apply:

- *If you don't feel ready to go back, then don't.* Even if you told the doctor that you would only be taking a month off, but it turns out a month is not long enough for you to feel better about starting treatment again, then take two, three, or more months, as it suits you.
- *Take at least as long off as it takes for your body to feel completely freed of the side effects from your last treatment cycle.* When that bloated feeling is gone, and you have no more headaches, nausea, or hot flashes, and your ovaries have gone back to their normal size, then your body may be ready to go through another round of chemical alteration.
- *The partner who is ready to go back first should refrain from pressuring the other (or even subtly nudging the other) to go back.* Until *both* partners are ready, it's best to sit out another month.
- *The length of your break may be set by certain events of the calendar.* Let's say you took off at the beginning of July. You may find that Labor Day is a convenient marker to use as your starting point for renewed treatment. Or let's say your break started a few months before your anniversary. You might decide that you will celebrate that event, just the two of you, and worry about what you will do next to increase the size of your family after the celebration is over.
- *The length of your break may be measured in the woman's cycles.* You may for instance decide you will go back to treatment after three more menstrual periods have occurred.

The one whose body is undergoing the most impact may be accorded the chief responsibility for picking the date of return. If the man has to wear a testicular cooling device all day, then let him be the one to say when he's ready to put it on again. If the woman has been getting daily shots and spending her early-morning hours being monitored at the clinic, then wait for her to tell you that she wants to try another round.

As to the problem of intervals between breaks, you might want to set up a regular pattern of treatment-break-treatment-break. It might go something like this: four tries of Clomid, break, followed by four tries of Pergonal (first without IUI, then with IUI), break, then move on to GIFT—two cycles—and then, after a much longer break, decide whether to resume with one or two last tries, this time of ZIFT, and then finally quit treatment for good.

If you think you would find such a schedule constraining, you might feel more comfortable taking your breaks whenever you find the need arising. You would certainly want to take some time off after any particularly discouraging event, such as a miscarriage or ectopic pregnancy, or after an emotionally wrenching experience unrelated to your infertility, such as the death of a parent, or after any cycle that caused excessive side effects, pain, depression, or other deep emotional upset.

One caution: if you get to the point at which you seem to be spending more time off treatment than on, and by the end of each break you still dread going back, then even a very long break won't be enough to get you feeling good again about your pursuit of parenthood through medical means. Take such feelings as a sign that you are now ready to arrive at some other, nonmedical resolution to your infertility. (See Chapter Nine to learn what these alternatives are and how to help yourself discover which one is right for you.)

Without exception, the couples I interviewed who had stopped treatment after a certain number of years without success were all extremely satisfied with their decisions. Each then went on to build a life for themselves (with or without adopted children) that lived up to or even exceeded the expectations they had had of what life would be like had their medical treatment worked out according to their highest hopes.

CHAPTER NINE

COPING WITH STRESS

PREPARE AS FOR WAR

No matter where you are in your quest to have a baby—whether you are just starting out or you've been through years of fruitless treatment—*you* will *feel stress*. It may come in different degrees at different times to different people, but however and whenever it comes, you will be able to cope with it more easily if you are prepared for it.

Stress is the one thing that all my interviewees had in common. For one woman it struck hardest when she had to be around other women who were pregnant or had just given birth. Baby showers were such torture for her that she faked illnesses rather than attend. Another couple almost broke up because the wife wanted to adopt, but her husband was only interested in having a biological child. Many couples told me of problems in communication: *she* says he doesn't really listen to her when she talks about her feelings; *he* says she's become so obsessed with her infertility that she hardly ever talks about anything else.

Most frequently described by IVF patients was a special variety of stress known as the "roller coaster syndrome." You start out looking forward to the beginning of your treatment cycle, and then as monitoring begins and you daily watch the developing follicles on the sonogram screen, your hopes slowly start rising. Up, up, up you go, till you reach a high point on the day that you learn that some of your retrieved eggs have fertilized in the test tube. After the eggs are transferred to your uterus, your mood starts to level off. You glide along for a while, waiting, but with a slowly heightening anxiety. Did it take or didn't it? Are you pregnant or aren't you? And then one morning your doctor calls to say that your pregnancy test came back negative. All at once you're plummeting down, down, down—maybe with some screaming and crying along the way, because you know your cycle is over and you've ended up back where you began, only a lot poorer for the cost of the ride. Still, a short time after it's over, you may be right back to try it all over again.

No matter what form your stress takes (or if it comes to you in many different forms), you need to know that you *can* cope. You know you can because many others have been there before you, and perhaps have even gone through worse than what's happening to you (more failed ART attempts, more miscarriages, even the loss of newborn babies) and they have still survived with souls intact. You can learn from them what works best to prepare you to deal with the stresses of treatment.

At the end of this section (page 328) you will find a list of fifteen strategies to help you cope, compiled from the suggestions of former infertility patients. Following the list will be a section explaining each of the fifteen strategies—but the first three are most important. These make up the basic elements of what I call the "infertility battle plan."

I use the term *battle plan* because in some very important ways, going through infertility treatment is like going to war. You start out with a goal you feel is worth taking risks for, and you know the struggle will be a costly one. You also start out somewhat fearful—will you come through it okay?—but then as you begin to get involved in your training for your chosen method of attack, you build a sense of confidence, and even start to look forward to taking some action at last. But nothing ever happens as fast as you want it to. There may be weeks or even months when nothing seems to be going on, when you're just sitting around, with your anxiety level rising the whole time. But, as is the case with soldiers waiting for combat to begin, there is also camaraderie with the other patients you meet in the waiting room or in your IVF prep-aration class. You may form deep friendships that will last far beyond this time of crisis in your life. And along the way, you will probably discover an inner strength and courage you never knew you had, for in facing the reality of infertility (somewhat as in facing the reality of death in war) you will come to realize what truly matters most to you: whether your love for your spouse, your religious faith, your sense of dedication to your work, or whatever it is that gives meaning to your life. As with war, too, when you're in the thick of it, it's hard to imagine that one day you will return to normal life. But some time from now you, too, will be a veteran, and can sit around telling stories of what the struggle was like. One day this present hell will be distant memory. Whatever the outcome, you will be able to take pride in know-ing you gave the best you could give under extremely trying circumstances.

Finally, as with any war, your chances of success will be improved if you go into it knowing what you intend to do and what strategies you can try if things don't immediately start going as you'd hoped. My fifteen recommended strategies are as follows:

1. Formulate a plan that suits your needs and capabilities.
2. Have a fallback position.
3. Enlist the support of strong, dependable allies.
4. Don't worry about "who's to blame" for your infertility.
5. Use positive imaging to keep your outlook optimistic.
6. Take comfort in small things.
7. Avoid mental booby traps.
8. Use your religion or guiding philosophy to help see you through.
9. Keep your outside interests up.
10. Make time for your spouse.
11. Arm yourself with knowledge.
12. Harness your creative energies.
13. Release your anger at the right target.
14. Use your experience to help others.
15. Use humor to help see you through.

Your Infertility Battle Plan

For any battle plan to have a chance to succeed, it needs to be based on solid intelligence. First, you must take into account the physical facts. Consider what you know about your body's reproductive functioning and attempt to discover which medical approach yields the best odds of success. Study what has worked for others like you before you proceed. As in war, morale is also a critical element: you should reflect on what is involved in carrying out your chosen method of attack and whether you have the stamina to go through with it. Then consider what you might do if your first chosen method of attack on the problem does not succeed.

When you have taken all these factors into account, you are ready to draw up your plan. A plan may be extremely specific, as in this example:

1. Clomid—maximum of four months
2. Clomid with hCG and IUI—three months
3. Pergonal or Clomid-Pergonal combination with IUI—four months
4. If conception does not occur, take a three-to-four-month break, after which (if still willing) . . .
5. GIFT or ZIFT (as doctor recommends)—three cycles
6. If conception does not occur, begin investigation of nonmedical alternatives

Or a plan may be very generalized, as is this one:

1. Medical intervention as recommended by doctor for a maximum of two years
2. If no success, seek advice from a second doctor for one additional year
3. Begin seeking a nonmedical resolution

You might also decide on a two-pronged plan of attack:

1. One year of drug-only therapies
2. One year of ARTs, during the last six months of which we will begin the process of applying to adopt

Time limits are an essential element of your plan. Without knowing how long you will stick with any one part of the plan, it is all too easy to get bogged down at one stage and end up spinning your wheels. But if you establish at the outset how much time you will devote to each form of treatment, you will avoid the feeling of being stuck and instead will always maintain the sense that you are moving forward, on track toward a goal. So give the greatest care to this aspect of your formulation of your plan.

Also keep in mind that a good plan is a flexible one. A good plan allows for a change of course whenever new information is uncovered that points you in a different direction. A too-rigid adherence to a pre-set formula may cause you to miss opportunities for improved odds of success. So plan—but always be ready to revise and update your plan to keep abreast of your changing situation.

After you have drawn up your plan, the next thing you should undertake is to formulate a fallback position. That is the position you will adopt if after a set period of time you fail to conceive. Why plan for failure? Because even the most brilliant general and best-trained and best-equipped troops can't win a war fought against overwhelming odds. You never can tell how bad your situation may turn out to be, but whatever happens, you will find security and peace of mind in knowing in advance that there is something else you will do if the best medical efforts aren't able to bring about a pregnancy and birth.

Your fallback position may be any of three nonmedical alternatives: adoption, *partial parenting,* and the *child-free life-style.* (These last two terms are explained in the sections beginning on pages 361 and 358, respectively. Also, later on in this chapter will be some discussion aimed at helping you discover which one might best suit your needs.) It is not necessary in the early stages of your planning for you and your partner to be in accord as to which fallback position you will choose; but it *is* important that you both recognize that there are other ways you can achieve your goal of having the kind of family you want.

The third component of your battle plan is to get help from a strong, dependable source. No one should ever go through infertility alone. But if you look to the wrong person to help you through the crisis, you could end up receiving not the comfort and support you had sought, but wrongheaded advice and insensitive remarks, such as

"Don't spend all that money on treatment—just relax and it will happen naturally."

"With all the homeless children in the world, why don't you just adopt?"

"If nature is preventing you from conceiving, maybe you just weren't meant to be a mother."

So choose your ally carefully! The following are four of the most likely candidates to play the role of your confidant(e) and emotional mainstay:

1. your spouse or partner
2. a good friend (usually of the same sex), who has been someone you've been able to depend on during past troubles in your life; may also be a sibling, cousin, or other relative
3. an outsider with expertise in the emotional fallout of infertility: may be a professional, such as a clinical psychologist, psychiatrist, or MSW (master of social work), or a nurse-therapist; may also be a nontraditional therapist, such as a meditation instructor or yoga teacher, or a religious counselor (minister, rabbi, or priest), the person's credentials being less important than his or her experience in working with others who have suffered from the stress of unsuccessful infertility treatment
4. leaders or other members of a RESOLVE support group (or any other self-help group formed to help ease the stress of infertility)

A table listing the pros and cons of relying on each of the above choices can be found on pages 332–333.

OTHER STRATEGIES

We've covered numbers one, two, and three on the fifteen-point list. Forming a treatment plan, deciding on a fallback position, and knowing whom you will count on when tough times set in—these are actions that I recommend for *every* couple, in every situation. Of the next twelve strategies for coping, you may want to pick and choose which ones you think might work for *you*.

4. Don't get into "Whose fault is it?"

Infertility is neither a character flaw nor a marital failure. You should think of it as an illness—which it is. The body is simply not working as a healthy body was designed to do. If you or your spouse were to get a brain tumor, you wouldn't talk about fault then, would you? There are, of course, two major differences between being infertile and having a brain tumor: (1) doctors have a much better chance of success against infertility than against brain tumors, and (2) brain tumors are often fatal, but infertility never is. When feeling down sometimes, you might find it helpful to remind yourself that compared to a brain tumor, infertility isn't quite so bad, after all.

5. Use positive imaging.

This is a technique that has been developed for sufferers of other chronic or even terminal conditions. Positive imaging teaches a series of mental exercises to promote an optimistic outlook and reduce the patient's fear and stress. The basic idea is that you focus on how you want your body to respond to treatment and on what you expect your life to be like after treatment has been completed. You remove yourself to a quiet room for some portion of each day, lower the lights, and put on some relaxing, nonjarring instrumental music. Then, if you are a woman, you might

- talk to your eggs, telling them to grow and be ready to be fertilized
- talk to the embryos that have been returned to your body after an ART cycle, welcoming them to your uterus, and asking them to implant and make their home there
- imagine the embryonic cells dividing, and a new person coming into being; talk to the person you hope will become your child

CONSIDERATIONS FOR CHOOSING YOUR CONFIDANT(E) AND CHIEF EMOTIONAL SUPPORT IN TIME OF STRESS

	Pro	Con
Spouse	Your spouse knows your worries and fears as well as or better than anyone else, and so is in a unique position to give comfort and support. You and your spouse are going through this together. You don't like the idea of involving any outsiders in your problems.	Your spouse is under stress from treatment, too, and may not be able to help you cope with yours. Males and females usually react differently to the stress of infertility and will need different types of emotional support to help them cope. Sometimes being too close to someone prevents that person from being able to see a problem in proper perspective and recognize solutions.
Friend, Sibling, Parent, or Other Relation	You have already built up an intimate relationship with each other, are used to hearing each other's secrets. You have confidence that this trusted person understands your feelings and won't say or do anything hurtful to you. The person may not know a lot about infertility treatment right now, but would read any books or articles that you offered in order to become a more informed and helpful confidant(e) to you.	Unless the friend, sibling, or relation has been there, that person can't really know what you are going through. If the person already has children, you may feel envious when in her or his company. If the person does not have children, she or he may not fully understand the depth of your desire to have children. Older family members (parents or grandparents) will sometimes find it hard to comprehend the high-tech nature of treatment. They may be dubious of the necessity for the treatment, be shocked at what you are paying for it, or be discouraging of your chances for success.

(continued)

	Pro	Con
Professional Counselor	The professional counselor is experienced in dealing with the very real, sometimes serious, problems encountered by those in infertility treatment, such as depression, sleeplessness, panic, hostility, inability to concentrate, loss of libido, marital tension, and other symptoms of stress. If the counselor is an MD or works in conjunction with an MD or works in prescribe drugs if necessary.	Professional counseling is expensive! Counselor's bills may not be covered by your health insurance. Counseling is also time-consuming—do you want to have more appointments on your calendar? It can be difficult to find a good counselor-patient match. You may need to see several counselors before finding one who can really work productively with you to solve problems.
RESOLVE	At general meetings and small group gatherings you will meet others in your situation. You can find support through group activities or seek to make friends with one or two individuals who seem particularly understanding. You might also learn things of practical value, such as new drug combinations that you can ask your doctor about. You can participate in RESOLVE with or without spouse, and usually find subgroups composed of members with your particular interests.	Attending meetings is time-consuming. You may not like the idea of talking about your problems with strangers, even those whose problems are similar. If your infertility treatment is still low-tech and your RESOLVE group is made up mainly of patients involved in IVF, GIFT, and other very rigorous programs, you might think that others won't take your situation seriously.

INTERVIEW QUESTION: WHO HAVE YOU TURNED TO FOR EMOTIONAL SUPPORT?

My family and friends have been my best support. I had to educate them at first. I would suggest [to other people undergoing fertility treatment] to be patient with friends and family. Most people have no idea how to react or what to say to an infertile person. I photo-copied material for my family to read. . . . I did hear at lot of "advice" from people. I usually give a set response. It angers me at first, but I realize most of the time they are trying to show me they care when they give advice. I try to educate people that my problem has nothing to do with relaxing, that it is a medical problem.

Nicole from Texas

My clinic recommended an LCSW [licensed clinical social worker] with years of experience in infertility. Seeing her helped me a lot! Talking doesn't get me any closer to a baby, but it has taught me some coping methods. My husband attends sessions when I want him to or when he feels he wants to.

Linda from Maryland

Yes, the counseling [offered through her IVF clinic] was helpful, but frankly, I got a lot more out of the RESOLVE support group I attended. Not only support, but information, answers to quest-ions, etc.

Ellen from New Jersey

Therapy helped change my mental/emotional state from passive, helpless, hopeless, to an attitude of "I'll give it all I've got, do my best, and see what happens." I took charge of my treatment, sought a second opinion, and had my baby.

Karen from Texas

If you are a man, you might

- imagine your sperm as little explorers going out to seek a treasure
- tell one sperm that he must be the leader, and must break through all the barriers until he gets inside the castle, where he will find and drink a magic potion of renewed life

Be careful not to go overboard with positive imaging. Don't get so caught up in your imaging fantasies that you start naming your eggs or sperm or planning for their college education. Keep your images at the fairy-tale level. If you know you would feel silly thinking up fairy-tale stories, then simply focus on positive feelings and calming thoughts. If you have ever taken meditation lessons, recite your mantra, or use any other relaxation techniques that you have learned.

The Suggested Reading List includes a recommendation for a book explaining what positive imaging is and how you can use it to help you.

6. *Take comfort in small things.*

A silly superstition, a catchphrase, or an odd coincidence can be used to help you get a handle on your stress. Do you have a lucky number? If your LH surge or egg retrieval happens to fall on the date of that number, take that as a good sign. Infertility treatment is something of a gamble for most couples, and it helps to have a gambler's insouciance about luck. When you're eating in a Chinese restaurant and your fortune cookie predicts "You will have many descendants," save that slip of paper and treasure it. Read your horoscope on the day of your IUI. Take along your lucky penny or whatever special talisman you own. My own personal comforting ritual: After each treatment cycle, I would go out and buy a new outfit. If the treatment failed, then I would at least have some new clothes to enjoy. If it worked, I knew I certainly wouldn't mind being unable to fit into my new dress because I was pregnant.

7. *Watch out for mental booby traps.*

The worst mental booby trap is hopelessness. If you find yourself thinking "I'll never be a parent," turn that thought off right away! You must also be on guard for the opposite trap: too much hope. Couples who start acting as if any minute they will be parents, who pick out baby names, buy baby products, or even decorate a nursery while in treatment, are bound to be much more miserable than they would otherwise be when treatment doesn't work out. Another common but perhaps less obvious trap is *codependency*. The term is usually reserved for those who let a spouse's dependency (on drink, drugs, or whatever) rule their lives. In infertility cases, the trap is becoming a codependent of the doctor. The patient becomes obsessed with her relationship with the doctor; she calls him all the time; she looks to him as to a miracle worker who can make everything turn out okay. If you feel yourself being drawn into such a pattern, you could probably benefit from some counseling to help you put your doctor's role in proper perspective. You may also find it necessary to switch doctors so that you can start off your relationship with your new doctor in a more realistic and productive way.

8. Use your religious faith or guiding philosophy to help you cope.

Each of us needs to discover within ourselves what basic beliefs we hold to help us make sense of a confusing situation. For some, a philosophy of acceptance is the key. You do not question why you have been unable to conceive but simply take each day as it comes, doing what you can when you can, not thinking about it when you can't. Others prefer to view their infertility as a challenge, an adversary that must be actively opposed. Still others find comfort in the idea of the mysteriousness of the universe. So many things in nature are random, unknowable, beyond our comprehension. Our difficulties of the moment are insignificant when considered against the vastness of time and space. There is no intrinsic fairness in nature, so there is no point in being angry or feeling punished by our inability to conceive.

If you are of a religious nature, you will certainly find sustenance in prayer and in the rituals of your faith. But be a little cautious in bringing up your infertility with the leader of your church or other religious institution. Sometimes well-meaning but uninformed clergy can be more hurtful than helpful. If your clergyman knows little about the physiology of conception, he might be less than understanding of the necessity in your case of leaving fertilization in the hands of a doctor working in a lab. A few patients I interviewed were even made to feel guilty by their congregation leaders for spending money on medical technology instead of taking in an unwanted child through adoption—or worse, made to feel as if they were committing adultery by seeking conception through the use of an outsider's sperm or eggs (for more detail on what is permitted and forbidden by four major religions, see Chapter Ten).

So before you go to your religious leader for counseling, find out what you can about his or her attitude and extent of knowledge about problems of infertile couples. Perhaps you might raise the subject theoretically before you confide any secrets about your life. If you sense a negative or judgmental reaction, then consider seeking out a spiritual guide who has expertise in this regard. RESOLVE members of your local chapter may be able to aid you in your search. RESOLVE news-letters in the past have also included special prayers and sermons about infertility written by ministers, rabbis, and other religious leaders who have had experience with the problem.

9. Keep your outside interests up.

Don't let infertility be the only thing in your life. You were an active, vibrant person before you discovered your problem: no need to stop being who you are just because your reproductive organs aren't func-tioning well. Don't put your life on hold. Do all the things you used to enjoy and more. Do them *now,* because if you do have a child, it will be so much harder to do them then. Go dancing, take up a new sport, learn to fly a plane, start a collection of something, join a club, do something you've always been a little afraid to try. If infertility treatment seems to leave you no time to spare, *make time.* You must have some-thing to do that takes your mind completely away from your infertility for a while, or you will drive yourself nuts.

10. Keep your romance alive.

As important as it is to make some time for yourself, you must also make time for your spouse—and more than just around the fertile time in the middle of the wife's cycle. Spend a weekend at an intimate little inn, have candlelit dinners at home, take a long walk by moonlight, give each other back rubs and massages, buy each other little surprise gifts, and most of all, make love forgetting about the calendar whenever and wherever you can!

11. Arm yourself with knowledge.

Make sure you understand everything that is happening to your body in treatment. Ask every question that occurs to you—no questions are too stupid. If you let things happen that you don't understand, you will quickly come to feel out of control, manipulated, resentful, and abused. But if you keep yourself aware and informed, you can be sure that you remain the chief decision-maker over your own body and your own future. Women may find it harder to be assertive than men. One thing I have noticed at every lecture or group meeting on infertility that I have attended: though the audience will be divided fifty-fifty between

I remember how close to homicide I felt when on the day of the insemination we were stopped at the door by someone from the financial office because of a $30 balance we were told we'd have to pay first. Many a time we have felt our veneer of politeness and civility was worn down to the grain.

Allen from Massachusetts

the sexes, men ask 70 to 80 percent of all questions. Women, speak up! Only by getting the answers to your questions can you make yourself into a smart decision-maker and combat your irrational fears.

12. Harness your creative energies.

Know that whatever happens—whether you end up having biologically related children or not—you will still leave a lasting imprint of yourself in this world. For most of us a significant part of our urge to procreate springs from a need to leave behind some kind of legacy, to prove we were here, and that our lives made a difference in the world. Having children who will in turn have children and so on is one way to satisfy this need. But you can also channel this procreative energy in other ways that can be equally meaningful to you. You could create a poem, a song, a picture, or some other form of art; plant trees; work to bring back life to a river that has been killed by pollution; become an activist in any cause that stirs your soul. Or you may not need to go beyond your own office to find the lasting good you can do (or if you can't find anything of lasting value in your job, then perhaps you should consider changing careers to do something you find more satisfying).

13. Release your anger at the right target.

Being an infertility patient can make you mad! Sometimes when people say insensitive things, or when the nurse calls to give you bad news, or when your own body won't respond to drugs the way you thought it would, you just feel like exploding with rage. It's normal and healthy to want to yell about something as unfair and upsetting as being infertile. But just be careful not to yell at your spouse, or yell at anyone else

> $\mathcal{I}$f IVF is not covered by insurance where you live, write your legislature, your congressmen/-women, and people in the insurance lobby in your statehouse. You may be embarrassed at first [to make a public issue of infertility], but it's really not embarrassing, if you're not embarrassed about it. It's like people with cancer, diabetes, or any other physical problem. By educating people about it, you'll be accomplishing something, if not for yourself, then for those after you. There will always be infertile people.
>
> $\mathcal{M}$ichelle from Ohio

who isn't to blame. Yell at your doctor if your doctor has treated you badly—that's constructive anger. Yell at the driver in the car in front of you whose attempt to make an illegal left turn is making you late for your morning blood test—that will help get your tension out. But if there is no one around who is a deserving target of your anger, then shut yourself in your room and just let yourself pour out all the anger you feel. That way when you see your spouse again, you'll have gotten your anger out of your system and can be loving and understanding.

14. *Use your experience to help others in your situation.*

Whether you conceive as a result of treatment or not, some good will come of it if you put what you have learned to use. Become active in your local RESOLVE support network. If there is no chapter in your area, organize one. Meet other infertility patients and tell them what you wish you had known before you started. Work for fairness in insurance laws or lobby for federal funding of research into human reproduction.

15. *Keep your sense of humor up.*

You know you've been in treatment too long when you no longer can find anything funny about it. You start getting touchy about everything; you see offense in friends' innocent remarks about their kids; you react with anger to strangers' polite inquiries about your family. You need to laugh! If you're thinking right now, "Infertility is nothing to joke about," then you should consider that by making fun of something bad, we can usually keep ourselves from feeling frightened or anxious. Death scares us, so we laugh when a cartoon coyote runs off a cliff and falls a thousand feet down into a canyon, emerging annoyed but alive. Surgery scares us, so we enjoy watching a TV sitcom like *Doogie Howser, M.D.,* that tells us that a wisecracking teenager can be a better doctor than an adult.

Infertility itself isn't funny, but the things we do to try to overcome it are often hilarious, or at least absurd. There's a movie called *Funny About Love* that is full of comic scenes familiar to couples in treatment. At one point the hero, played by Gene Wilder, is instructed to produce a sperm sample in the bathroom of his wife's gynecologist's office. As he's behind the locked door, a long line of pregnant women who are dying to empty their bladders forms outside. When he finally emerges, disheveled and with collection cup in hand, the women break into applause, and the hero slinks sheepishly away.

I have heard similar stories—though not quite as extreme—from men who had to produce their samples under less-than-conducive circumstances, and many couples told me about the funny things that happened that threatened to call a halt to their lovemaking during the "compulsory sex" phase of their treatment cycles.

I have also heard a few infertility jokes, which I hope will give you a chuckle when you need it most:

Why does my bottle of Clomid always come with a childproof cap?

What should Mr. and Mrs. F. name their fertility treatment daughter? Ivy.

What did the OB/GYN say when asked how he was able to successfully deliver so many sets of twins and triplets? It's a GIFT.

What song does a labworker sing while combining sperm and eggs in a test tube? ZIFT-i-dee-doo-dah, ZIFT-i-dee-ay.

What song should you sing to let your husband know that your ovulation test stick was positive, and it's time for you to make love? "Love Is Blue."

Why do fertility doctors make so much money? It's easier than making babies.

Why did the fertility doctor cross the road? Because there was an affluent childless woman over thirty on the other side.

How many fertility doctors does it take to screw in a lightbulb? None: they don't put them in that way—they use IUI.

Make up your own jokes, too!

To Hell and Back; or,
Surviving the Last Two Weeks of Your Cycle

The worst part of the treatment cycle, most patients agree, is that two-week period that occurs between your ovulation and your next menstrual period. It's the uncertainty that's so unnerving. Am I pregnant or not? Every little twinge in your body must be analyzed to death. Do my breasts feel any heavier? Are my nipples getting just a little darker? What was that spasm in my lower abdomen—could it have been an implantation cramp? Or was it a preperiod miscarriage—the movement of the fertilized egg out of my uterus and into oblivion? You can go crazy trying to decide if what you're feeling is a reaction to the drugs you are taking or maybe something worse—an ectopic pregnancy or a developing fibroid tumor.

These feelings are hell for most women and the men who love them. But the following are seven strategies that I hope will be helpful to you as you go through this especially difficult portion of your treatment cycle.

1. *Don't expect to recognize the signs of pregnancy before it's time to take a pregnancy test.* Despite what you may have heard from your mother or your friend about how soon they knew that *they* were pregnant, few if any women can feel the moment of implantation or have breasts so sensitive that they begin to change color or shape just days after conception has occurred. Stop feeling your body parts and stop looking at yourself naked in the mirror. It will be at least two weeks after your ovulation before you will know for sure. So when your thoughts turn to the subject, immediately start thinking of something else. Find something absorbing to do. Don't you have at least one closet that needs to be cleaned out and organized?

2. *Don't start altering your life-style on the assumption that you are pregnant.* If you ordinarily have a glass of wine with dinner, don't go depriving yourself two weeks out of every month out of fear that you will "hurt the fetus." Don't give up drinking diet sodas or using haircoloring for the same reason, either. The chemicals in these products are only to be avoided after pregnancy has advanced far

enough for the fetus to be attached to its mother's blood supply through the placenta—and that's not until well after pregnancy has been confirmed. In the meantime you will find life easier if you will just try to live the way you normally do.

3. *Keep yourself busy during this time.* You no longer have to go in to the doctor's office daily for monitoring or other treatments, so now's the time to catch up on some of the work you may have missed during the first two weeks of your cycle. But don't work so hard that you become stressed out over *that*. Balance your work with other, more enjoyable activities, keeping your days full, but not overloaded.

4. *Refrain from certain strenuous activities.* Not all activities are equally good as ways to divert yourself during this time. Arduous physical challenges, such as mountain climbing, running long-distance races, long bicycle trips or other extremely competitive events are best avoided, because of the added stress, both physical and mental, that they entail. Pick activities that allow you to occupy your mind while relaxing your body. Getting caught up in a long novel, going out to concerts or listening to music at home, seeing movies, and going on a nature walk are all recommended. Swimming, stationary bicycling, and doing low-impact aerobics are all beneficial forms of exercise.

5. *Pamper yourself.* It's great to schedule a massage or a facial or go out and buy yourself something special during this time. Yes, you need to save money now, what with the burden of treatment on your budget, but you don't want to cut *all* luxuries out of your life. Better to borrow and pay back, putting off the financial pinch until later, than suffer from your infertility and from your tight financial straits both at the same time.

6. *Think ahead to what you'll be doing two to three weeks from now.* Don't fixate on this particular part of your cycle. If it's going to work, it's going to work, and nothing that you can do now will change that. Think ahead to what your treatment plan calls for in the coming month. If you already know about what day you'll begin your new cycle, pencil it in on the calendar with the date on which your next round of medication or doctor's appointments will begin. Focusing on what you will do when pregnancy does not occur will keep you from becoming overoptimistic that this time it will happen, and too disappointed when it does not. You may also want to create some nonmedical event to look forward to. You might want to plan a dinner party for the weekend after you expect to get your period. That way, when the period comes, you'll be too wrapped up in the

SOME OBSERVATIONS AND ADVICE ABOUT STRESS FROM FORMER PATIENTS

The fertile world tends to be pretty dense about infertility.

Frank from Washington, D.C.

I heard all the comments: "Relax, you'll get pregnant," and "How much fun you must have trying . . . " Getting three shots a day and waking up at four A.M. to make it to the hospital for ultrasounds and blood work, and *years* of scheduled sex, are *not* "fun." Neither are surgeries, hot flashes, and depression.

Nora from Ohio

Isolation is the worst aspect of infertility. It's important to reduce the self-blame we all seem to feel. "Relaxing" does *not* get you pregnant.

Carol from New Jersey

I've found the emotional support I need through family and friends, but also through keeping a personal journal.

Marjorie from California

My husband has two children from a previous marriage. I often felt angry and resentful that he had children and I didn't. I used to think I shouldn't have these feelings. I've since realized that I was expecting too much of myself. It was really okay to dread his kids coming over and calling him Dad. We must try to be good to ourselves and not expect ourselves to be martyrs. Allow yourself to feel the pain—that is how we heal.

Mary from Illinois

At first we were in shock and denial about our infertility, and the whole clinic idea seemed sort of weird. But we plodded along and now the infertility clinic seems like a normal (but still awful) part of our lives. Once you learn more about infertility, it *does* get easier, especially once we developed a good relationship with our doctor.

Alice and Mark from Arizona

The prolonged treatment [four years] put a major strain on my marriage. It was only when I began going to ———— Clinic that I entered support group therapy, which was extremely helpful in offering reassurance and information.

Beth from New Jersey

arrangements for your party to take much time to grieve over not having conceived.

7. *Get away together during this period, if at all possible.* A weekend at a country inn, a camping trip, or a visit with friends you haven't seen in years might be just the thing to make the time pass quickly and happily.

SEX AND THE INFERTILE COUPLE

When you and your partner first met and fell in love, you probably viewed the procreative side of sex as a nuisance, something that interfered with your pleasure in bed. You (the woman) had to fumble around in the bathroom trying to put your diaphragm in right, or you had to squirt yourself full of messy foams, or you had to remember to take your pill each day. You (the man) had to keep a supply of condoms on hand, and then they didn't slide on easily or they reduced the sensation of your lovemaking too much. You naturally thought: When we start trying to have a baby, won't things be great! No birth control hassles, no worry—just sex, whenever and however we feel like it.

And now . . . it's work, work, work. It's compulsory sex on Days Fourteen, Fifteen, and Sixteen. But no sex allowed on Days Twelve and Thirteen. That postcoital test which the doctor scheduled for first thing Monday morning means that you *must* make love after midnight Sunday or before six A.M. the next morning. A semen analysis means you can't have sex for three days beforehand, and then you've got to be able to "do the job" into a little plastic cup, off in a dingy unused lab room in the clinic, the walls decorated with warning signs about infectious waste disposal and AIDS prevention techniques.

A month of two of this routine is almost enough to turn any couple off sex for good—and sometimes, sadly, it does.

Is there some way to keep infertility treatment from ruining your sex life and maybe even your marriage as well? There is no magic formula, but according to former patients I interviewed, there are some things to try that just might help.

Fifteen Ways to Please Your Lover

1. On days when you're not constrained by doctor's rules, *do exactly what you feel like doing*. If you don't feel like having sex on your "off days," don't feel you have to. If you both do feel like it, then do it, and try not to think about pregnancy or fertility treatment.

2. On days when you have been told not to have intercourse, *sex substitutes are okay*. Try the kind of heavy petting that used to turn you on in high school. Take a shower together. Try mutual massaging. But if either of you is worried about ending up feeling frustrated and unfulfilled by these activities, then don't feel you must engage in them.

3. When having sex on days when you are "supposed to," work to *get the mood just right*. Turn off the ringers on your phones, unplug the answering machine, dim the lights, have some champagne, maybe relax a little first by watching an erotic movie together— do whatever you and your partner find most stimulating and pleasurable to get things going.

4. *Vary time of day* if possible. When you both get home after a long day at work, maybe after a hot, crowded commute, you're most likely to be tense and fatigued. Then to remember that you "have to do it" tonight can seem a burdensome thing. You'll find the prospect far more inviting if you try to get away at lunch time, or come in late so that you can have the morning to yourselves, or leave work early enough to get home with energy to spare.

5. *Vary place.* If it's not too much of a financial strain, you might find it worthwhile to book a room in a nice hotel for the night. Have a room service dinner, then put out the Do Not Disturb sign, and enjoy!

6. *Foreplay is more important than ever.* The woman needs to show her man that she doesn't just view him as a sperm-delivery system. The man needs to show his woman that she's more than just a womb waiting to incubate a fertilized egg. So don't rush—take

all the time you need to do the things your partner finds the biggest turn-on.

7. *Use fantasy* to create the mood you need. When the day you have to "do it" comes along, and you find yourself feeling out of sorts and unsexy, try using your imagination to turn your mood around. Pretend you're an actor filming a scene in a steamy movie with an actress you've always found irresistible. Or pretend your husband is a total stranger, someone you've just picked up for a thrill, and you don't even know his name. There are thousands of fantasies you can use. If you pretend well enough, you just might find reality becoming even more exciting than your fanstasies.

8. *Avoid blame or guilt* for those days when you are supposed to "do it" but you can't. Don't keep trying when it's not working for you—you'll only end up feeling worse. Just kiss and go to sleep, and maybe you'll feel more like it when you wake up the next day. Keep in mind that *everyone* has these problems from time to time during infertility treatment. You are not impotent, or frigid; you're just under too much stress. And if you miss out on the whole fertile period, don't kick yourself. There's always next month.

9. *Try new and different techniques in bed.* If there's something you've always wanted to do in bed, now's a good time to try it out—as long as it doesn't prevent the man from ejaculating inside the woman at the end. Couples who hope to conceive through one of the ARTs don't have to worry about how their sexual position affects their chance of pregnancy, since fertilization is no longer linked to sex. They should feel freer than ever to explore different sexual techniques. If you'd like some ideas about what to do, try flipping through a good sex manual, such as *The New Joy of Sex* (see Suggested Reading List for additional titles).

10. *Develop your intimacy in nonsexual ways, too.* Talk about what's important to you. Tell each other your secrets and stories from your childhood. Make an extra effort to really *listen* when your partner is talking about her day at work, or anything at all. The better you get along out of bed, the more relaxed and ready you will find yourselves when you are in bed together.

11. *Be more tolerant of each other's flaws.* Now is not the time to complain of all the little things that bother you about your partner. Don't yell at him for not picking up his dirty socks. Don't argue with her when she gives you unsolicited directions while you're driving. Does it really matter so much? You don't want to let slow-

simmering anger and irritation work their way into your sex life where they can do much damage.

12. *Change yourself for the better.* Look out for the little things that you do that annoy your partner. Since I've just told you to stop complaining so much about each other's flaws, make it easier by giving the other person less to complain about. Pick up your clothes when you know it bothers her to see them left on the rug. Don't give him directions if he's told you he doesn't need or want them. Your partner will find you far more desirable when you are not playing the role of nagging parent or critic.

13. If, despite the foregoing advice, you still find yourselves arguing constantly over little things, and neither of you seems able to change your behavior, *consider whether counseling might help.* Strengthening your day-to-day relationship can only help your sex life, too.

14. *Keep your appearance up.* I know it's hard to feel desirable when you've gained eight pounds on Pergonal, and you feel bloated and tired and are having hot flashes. And it's hard to feel like Superstud when you know that the only reason you are having sex tonight is because the doctor said you have to. But you will both feel a lot sexier if you take care of yourselves, inside and out. Get some new clothes you know your partner will like. Exercise and trim off some of your unwanted fat. Try a new hairstyle. If you're able to treat yourself, consider getting "the works" at a trendy salon.

15. Don't forget to *say the words.* Say "I love you," and "you look terrific," and "you're so sexy"—use whatever pet phrases you like to let your partner know how desirable you find him or her. When under the stress of doctor-directed lovemaking, it can really help to let your partner know that your love and desire are as strong as ever. It must be, because it takes a strong love and passion to survive the rigors of fertility treatment.

TO TELL OR NOT TO TELL

Nosy people are everywhere, but you probably had no idea how many were out there until you had been married for a while without having had children. Then the questions started coming: "When are you two going to start a family?" "Don't you want kids?" "Is something wrong?" "Aren't you worried about trying at your age?" Even worse than the questions is the unsolicited advice: "You don't want to wait too long, dear. I had my kids early so I'd have them out of the house and still be young enough to enjoy life," and "You don't really know what unselfish love is until you've had a child." Infertile couples hear it all, no matter how rude, intrusive, and thoughtless the comments may be.

And not just from your mother and your Great-aunt Edna, from whom you expect it. It's the next-door neighbors, your boss at work, the guy who comes to fix your dishwasher, the cashier at the checkout line, and total strangers that you meet at the bus stop. Nosiness from all quarters, couples report, is a major source of stress.

If you expect to keep your sanity, you need to have a ready response to these kinds of remarks. Different personalities will prefer to take different approaches to the problem. There are those who will be unhappy having to divulge any part of their reproductive plans to *anyone,* even their closest friends. Others will feel just the opposite: they won't be comfortable trying to conceal anything from anyone, even the most casual acquaintance. There are endless gradations in between, but you should be able to find your approximate place on the five-part scale on the next page.

Now show the scale to your spouse or partner, without revealing your own ranking. Are you both at about the same point? If not, how far are you apart? If only one step apart, you will have little conflict over this issue. If two or more steps apart, you should start doing some work on this problem to keep it from becoming a sore point in your relationship for the duration of treatment.

Here are three possible ways you could work out your differences.

1. *Defer to the more private party.* Since it's usually easier for the more open person to keep a matter confidential than for the private person to open up, the compromise should be toward the privacy side. You should sit down together and decide which (if any) questions you will answer and who (if anyone) will be allowed to ask them. To prevent continued inquiry from those you have decided not to tell, have a prepared line that you will both use to turn questions aside. Being firm tends to work best. Say simply, "We do not discuss these personal matters with anyone." In most cases, you will receive a fast apology from the questioner. If you don't, that person is not someone you want to have continued social dealings with.

2. *Both of you move toward middle ground.* This is the way to go when the more open partner has a strong need to talk unrestrictedly

Private ←——→ Open

Most Private	Private	Midpoint Between Private and Open	Open	Most Open
Will not discuss infertility with *anyone* but spouse or partner.	Will discuss infertility in limited way with close family members, best friends.	Will discuss some infertility treatment details with certain family members and selected friends. Limited information given to colleagues and extended family members. No discussion of subject with casual acquaintances.	Will discuss infertility with family, friends, colleagues. Will limit details with casual acquaintances.	Willing to discuss infertility, including treatment details, with anyone who wants to know.

about feelings engendered by infertility and will feel frustrated and unhappy if forced into silence. Then the more private person should work on relaxing his or her sense of inhibition. (Incidentally, my researches indicate that it is far more often the woman who wants to talk openly about infertility, and the man who wants to keep it private.) Very private persons might try some mental exercises to help them move toward the center. Remind yourself regularly: "There is nothing wrong in what we're doing." "One in six couples in this country are infertile." "Infertility is a medical problem like any other medical problem." "Friends and family ask us questions only because they care so much about us." When the more private person feels ready start talking about his problem with others, she or he should first sit down with her or his partner and together draw up a list of who it will be okay to tell, and just how much detail may be divulged.

3. *Agree to disagree.* It's okay for each partner to respond differently when asked about their childlessness. The more private partner may choose not to respond at all, while the more open one is free to tell whomever he or she wishes. This strategy works best when the man and woman tend to move in different circles. His friends and colleagues don't know; hers all do—and the two groups never interact to discuss the subject behind their backs. When the couple share friends and colleagues, the strategy is a little trickier to pull off. The more open one must stress the point that the news must be held in confidence, and that the listener must be trusted not to inform other friends and colleagues of the news, or even let on to the other infertile spouse that she or he has learned anything about their infertility or its treatment.

But what if one or both of you is unsure how you want to handle this issue? If you have not yet started treatment, you may not be able to predict how it's going to affect you. You may be surprised to find that you need a shoulder to cry on, when you had assumed you would want to keep everything to yourself—or you may find just the reverse.

One question that I asked all my interviewees was, if you had to do it all over again, would you still be as private (or as open) about your infertility as you were? Most couples said they would take the same approach, but of those who said they would do things differently if given the chance, more of those who had maintained secrecy said that they would be more open than the other way around. Why? Couples felt they expended a lot of psychic energy keeping things hush-hush, and that tensions built up that might have been released if they had

OPENNESS VERSUS PRIVACY

Reasons to Be Open	Reasons to Maintain Privacy
1. Gets it off your chest	1. It's nobody else's business
2. Puts an end to speculation about your childlessness	2. Preserves dignity, avoids opportunities for embarrassment
3. No longer have to invent excuses for absences from work to see doctor or to avoid going away on a business trip	3. Won't have to answer a lot of nosy follow-up questions, such as "Whose fault is it?" and "Are you pregnant yet?"
4. After painful tests or disappointing treatment cycles, you won't have to hide it if you are feeling bad	4. No danger that erroneous third-hand versions of your treatment will circulate
5. Confiding in your family and friends shows them that you trust them and count on their love and support	5. Having a shared secret strengthens the special intimate bond of marriage
6. Allows others to play supportive roles	6. Protects you from moral judgments of others about "interfering with nature"; keeps you out of arguments about the Baby M case, or about how far science should go
7. No anxiety that someone has guessed or discovered what you are doing	7. Preserves separation between home and work, sets precedent for preventing boss or colleagues from involving themselves in aspects of your family life that are not relevant to your job

simply told people straight out what they were doing, instead of inventing elaborate excuses for absences necessitated by their treatment schedules.

If you are unsure as to how you come down on the secrecy/privacy question, see the chart above, listing some pros and cons to consider as you make up your mind.

INTERVIEW QUESTION: WERE YOU OPEN ABOUT YOUR INFERTILITY, OR DID YOU KEEP IT A SECRET?

We kept much secret early on. Isolation made the pain more difficult to bear. It's important to share with those who have the capacity to listen and empathize. As my infertility lasted for eight years, I gained the skills necessary to seek support from others. I grew more candid toward the end, more involved with RESOLVE, and more aware of myself and my feelings.

Karen from Texas

I told everyone about our infertility, and I wish I hadn't. Most people say the wrong thing or try to joke about it. Or else they act like they care and want a moment-to-moment update. . . . It's really difficult working full-time, though, and not having the people around you know, especially if you have to do an ovulation test while at work.

Alice from Arizona

I felt that not talking about it would work against us. We needed information! My husband was reluctant to talk about it, but at my urging finally began to tell people. We did get some interesting information from concerned friends. We also learned that some friends were infertile—which we'd never known.

Betsy and Jim from New Jersey

We told one sister-in-law who had infertility problems herself. I did tell my boss and was forced to tell coworkers because we have such a small office, and my personality was very affected while I was on the drug [Clomid caused her to become irritable and even occasionally irrational]. I have no regrets about keeping it secret from my parents, who live out of town. It made my life easier not to have to worry about their feelings when I wasn't in the mood to talk about it. I feel that only people who have experienced infertility can really understand how we feel.

Polly from Illinois

(continued)

I now think I should not have been so secretive with friends, because I now have nobody to offer me sympathy or understanding of why for these past few months I have been "incommunicado" with my friends, avoiding them. [This patient had to be hospitalized twice due to a dangerous reaction to fertility medication.] If I had told them, it might have eased my own burden of healing somewhat. It still would have been a hard road, but I have made it harder, trying to be stoic.

Dana from New York

At first I was very open about my infertility. Then I couldn't handle all the "free advice" I was getting—so I clammed up.

Kate from Connecticut

I discovered two other friends who are going through the same thing. This made us closer. Most of your fertile friends don't want a play-by-play description of your menstrual cycle! What a relief to have some friends who truly understood everything. (My husband only told a few of his friends. This is something that men don't seem to talk about.)

Diane from Indiana

KNOWING WHEN IT'S TIME TO QUIT—AND WHAT YOU'LL DO NEXT

How do you know when it's time to stop counting on medical science to make a baby? When is the right time to start searching for another way out of the infertility maze? When do you say, Enough is enough! and move on?

Here are four possible ways you might arrive at the decision to take a nonmedical approach:

1. *Your doctor tells you it's time.* A truly caring doctor won't *let* you keep trying, cycle after cycle, when the odds for success appear to be too low. But how low is too low? What your doctor sees as very poor odds, you may think is still a worthwhile long shot. In that case you would probably be well served finding another doctor to review your history. If a second, independent doctor says it's not worth going on, believe him.

2. *You "just know."* Many patients don't need to wait to be told when it's time to stop treatment. It just comes to them one day (or it comes gradually over several days or weeks) that they do not want to subject themselves to further medical measures to have a child. A common problem is that one partner will get this feeling ahead of the other, and they will disagree as to when the time has come to stop treatment (suggestions for ways to resolve such conflict can be found on page 364). When the feeling first hits you, it's important to look back on your treatment and ask yourself if your desire to stop might be the result of a particularly bad but one-time experience, such as a recent miscarriage or a complication from surgery, or whether the feeling might have arisen during a drug-induced mood-swing. You may need to take a break of a few months to be able to evaluate your experience more objectively and sort out your complex feelings. If during your time off you feel no desire to go back and "give it another try," then you can be sure that stopping treatment was the right thing to do.

3. *Try counseling.* A trained professional could give you the help you need in examining your record and weighing the choices according to criteria that you lay out. Experienced infertility counselors may be located through RESOLVE. You may need only a session or two to point you in the direction that's right for you.

4. *You never really make a cut-and-dried decision to stop.* You may start pursuing another approach—for example, adoption—while at the same time preparing for your next GIFT cycle. Or you might stop rearranging your life to suit your doctor's treatment schedule and decide you will begin enjoying your child-free life-style, although you never formally announce to each other that that's what you're doing. You may keep trying to have a baby without medical help, though you now find quasi-parental satisfaction in being a Big Brother to a boy in need of a male role model, or in being god-mother to your nieces and nephews.

THREE NONMEDICAL APPROACHES

This is a book about being a fertility patient, but I firmly believe that you will have a better experience as a patient if you are prepared ahead of time to deal with the situation in which medical intervention proves

DECIDING TO QUIT

*W*hen it appeared [after eight tries] that IUI was not going to work out, our doctor recommended going straight to IVF/GIFT. We knew we did not want to do that, and decided to stop.

*M*aureen and John from Washington, D.C.
(parents of an adopted girl from Central America)

I feel like I'm not going to torture myself. I would never go through an IVF cycle again. When I decided to quit, it was as if the sun came out. I stopped agonizing over my cycles. I smiled for the first time in three months.

*P*olly from Illinois
(now pursuing private adoption)

of no avail. Though it may seem difficult to see it now, other couples attest to the fact that there are more ways to make a happy family than by giving birth to babies. You can have children through adoption; you can choose to consider your family complete as just yourself and your spouse, adopting what has been called the "child-free life-style"; or you could choose to play the parental role for a limited period of time, or in limited ways, such as by foster-parenting, being a godparent, or being a mentor or role model to children through an organized program such as Scouting or Big Brother/Big Sister (I am calling this last option "partial parenting").

The key word here is *choice*. You don't simply give up on the kind of life you've dreamed of having just because medical science hasn't worked to give it to you. You change your vision of your future life to suit the reality of your present circumstances, and then you work to make that future unfold the way you want. Along the way you will discover a whole new set of joys you never dreamed existed.

Which is the right future for you? As adoptive parents? As a child-free couple? As partial parents? Each choice needs a book in itself to cover the pros and cons adequately, so I advise you to turn to the Suggested Reading List for recommendations of titles that treat each of the options in full. The sections that follow will be limited to outlining the most common questions and concerns raised by each.

Following the sections on nonmedical options will be a discussion of what to do if the partners are in conflict as to which alternative is best for them to pursue.

Adoption

It was unanimous. *All* of the couples I interviewed who had given up treatment and adopted said they were thrilled at the outcome, and could not possibly imagine loving any child more than the one that had come to them in this way. Many added that they wished they had stopped treatment earlier and begun the adoption process sooner, so that they could have begun enjoying parenthood that much quicker, freeing themselves from additional months of treatments' discomforts and stress. Couples who had adopted struck me as every bit as happy as couples for whom medical treatment had worked to bring a baby.

This doesn't mean, of course, that adoption is the right route for everyone when medical efforts don't work. But I did learn that it was fairly commonplace for couples to initiate the adoption process while having some doubts about their own suitability as adoptive parents; yet all of these couples reported a fading of such doubts by the time they first held their baby in their arms. Adoption works for many couples who never thought it would.

Whether you start out wholly enthusiastic or at least partly ambivalent, it's wise to think through all the major issues raised by adoption before you initiate the process.

First of all, what kind of adoption are you interested in pursuing? These days would-be adoptive families have many choices: Domestic or international? Infant only, or would you consider a toddler or an older child? Would you consider a child of another race, or one who is biracial? Does the child's religious or ethnic background matter to you? Do you hope that your child would be completely healthy, or might you be willing to give that extra measure of care to a child born with a disability, illness, or impairment? What sort of process would you use to find your child? The traditional adoption agency that acts as a buffer between the woman who is giving up the child and the couple who will adopt it? Private adoption, arranged by an attorney? "Open adoption," in which the couple meets the biological mother and perhaps even visits her regularly during her pregnancy and is present at the birth?

Then there are questions about yourselves that you should be prepared to answer readily, if you decide to pursue adoption through an agency. How do you and your spouse fit the specific criteria (such as age, duration of marriage, employment, religion, etc.) set by the adoption agency for prospective adoptive couples? Are you familiar with the "home study" process used by the agency to screen adoptive families, and are you comfortable with being investigated? Is there anything in your background or family history that you worry might disqualify you from consideration as adoptive parents? Do you think you could discuss your feelings about adoption constructively with the social worker assigned to your case?

And finally there are those questions that you must first confront in the privacy of your own thoughts. Do you feel able to love (or to learn to love) a baby born of another's body as you would one born to you? Do you have inner fears that an adopted baby might turn out to be a "bad seed"? Would you always wonder whether the baby's biological mother drank alcohol or ingested harmful drugs during her pregnancy? Are you worried that your parents or other relatives might not be able to accept the adopted child as a full-fledged member of the family? Are you frightened by the prospect of the biological mother returning to claim her child sometime before the adoption has gone through? Do you think if you conceived a child naturally after the adoption of a first child, that you might end up favoring "your" child over the adopted one?

Don't rule adoption out automatically, just because you don't feel you can give the "right" answer to all these questions. But do go slow, and give yourself ample time to sort out how you feel.

You may not be able to decide definitively how you would respond to many of these questions without some guidance from people of experience and good judgment. Fortunately, help is available from many sources. There are many excellent books on your library or bookstore shelves today, both on the general topic of adoption as well as on the many specialized types (e.g., cross-racial adoption, international adoption, private adoption, etc.). Books may provide an introduction to the subject, but if you wish to pursue it further, you will certainly want to talk to others who have already successfully adopted. RESOLVE is an invaluable resource in this regard. Most chapters will put on special adoption lectures, group meetings, and/or seminars at various times of the year. You will be able to ask questions of experts, meet other adoptive parents, and learn what agencies and private adoption attorneys handle cases in your area and how they are generally regarded. If you are still not sure whether you should go ahead after you have asked yourself the right questions and met with knowledgeable people, then you might want to consider seeking the advice of a professional counselor to help you sort your feelings out. RESOLVE again will be useful

ON CHOOSING ADOPTION

*Y*ou need to loosen the grip of a mindset that often occurs that says "because a child is genetically linked to us, he or she will look like, act like, and of course, be like us in some critical ways." For adoption to work for me I have to be able to place a premium on and appreciate difference rather than sameness. Oddly enough, thinking about it this way was a big relief—a lifting of expectation—as well as a challenge to appreciate and love what would be unique about an adopted child. I realized that my relief was due to my feeling that I had never really fulfilled my father's expectation of me to be more like him. And so, perhaps, I could escape repeating the same pattern with my child.

*A*ndrew J. Geller, Ph.D.
Clinical psychologist practicing in Boston

in helping you to find someone with experience in working with couples who are uncertain about adoption as the resolution of their infertility.

Child-free Life-style

Many couples who are trying to have a child have complex feelings about their goal. They are not simply aiming at becoming parents—they have very specific hopes and dreams of what their child will be like. They need to know that the child grew out of them, and that after they are gone, there will be that continuing genetic piece of them that will live on, as long as their children have children. They just aren't sure they could bond to a child who comes to them without this biological link.

There is nothing wrong with any of these feelings. Indeed, it would be wrong of a couple to pursue adoption if they seriously doubt their own ability to love a child born to someone else. If you don't feel that the way to happiness for you is through bringing an adopted child into your home, then you may prefer to make your own route to happiness without children. Look at how you and your spouse have lived so far. If you think that on the whole your life together has been a good one (even though you often feel it would be better if you had been able to have a baby together), then your best alternative might well be to pursue making your own lives as rich and complete as possible, just the two of you.

To *choose* to get the most out of life that you can, without children, is not to be child*less* (that term implies that you are missing something); instead you have decided to live *child-free*.

But how do you know this life-style is for you? The following are some of the questions you and your partner should ask yourselves:

Do you have serious doubts or fears about adoption that lead you to lean against it as a solution to your infertility?

Do you believe that your life with your partner now is basically a happy one, providing you with ample love, emotional support, interest, and attention?

Do you occasionally or frequently wonder if having a child (whether biological or adopted) might take something away from your special relationship with your partner?

Do you sometimes or often doubt whether you have the right temperament to bring a child up satisfactorily? Do you wonder whether you will be able to set a good example, control your temper, make necessary sacrifices for the child's good, make needed adjustments in your habits, hours, work practices in order to devote enough time to a child?

Are you afraid that traumatic incidents in your childhood or troubled relationships with your own parents might affect your relationship with a child, if you had one?

*W*hen I realized I needed IVF to have a child, I wanted to die. Why me, why me? Anything but this! I went through all five stages of grieving: denial, anger, bargaining, depression, and acceptance. It takes time (in my case almost eleven years), but eventually you realize that you're not going to die if you don't realize your dream of bearing a child. Life compensates. I have a wonderful, smart, handsome, funny husband that I almost forgot how much I loved.

*M*olly from Ohio

Do you have interests and activities that give you the sense that what you're doing with your life is satisfying, important, and worthwhile?

Is your job fulfilling? Are you ambitious in your chosen career?

Do you think that if you had children (whether by birth or adoption) that you might miss some of the freedom that you now enjoy? Is the ability to do things spontaneously, to go out whenever you feel like it, or take a trip without much advance planning, very important to you?

Do you think if you never had children that you would be able to make satisfactory arrangement for needed care if you should become aged or infirm, and your spouse had predeceased you?

Do you think if you never looked into adoption and you reached the age after which adoption becomes difficult or impossible, that you would not feel regret for your lost opportunity?

Do you think if you didn't adopt, that you could still see your friends and relatives who had children and not feel envious or full of yearning and regret?

Do you think you could cope with the highly child-oriented nature of society? With continuing pressure from relatives and friends to have a child?

If you answered yes to all or nearly all of these questions (one or two nos or I'm-not-sures are okay), then you will probably find the child-free life-style your preferred nonmedical solution to your infertility.

If you had more than two nos or I-don't-knows to these questions, then the child-free life-style might still be right for you, but you need to investigate your feelings further. Begin by sitting down, you and your partner together, and talking the subject out between you, exhaustively. Talk about your visions of your future life, your true goals. List all the reasons why you had hoped to have children, and all the reasons why you're not sure you really want them. Make up pro-and-con lists on your feelings about adoption, and then compare them. Not all reasons will be equally important, so rank them on a point scale from ten down to one. If the score for not having children is far greater than the score for having them, then forget all the other suggestions below—you can already see clearly that you would be happier being child-free.

If after the above exercise, you are still not certain, then talk to a counselor. You probably do *not* want to use one affiliated with an adoption agency—they naturally tend to be encouraging of the adoption route and may downplay your negative emotions. Through RESOLVE you may be able to get a referral to a professional who has experience working with infertile couples who have chosen the child-free life. Also through RESOLVE you might learn of seminars or group meetings for couples interested in finding out about the child-free option and how it has worked out for others.

As you are pondering this alternative, keep one thing in mind: it's one of the more reversible of decisions you can make about parenthood. If you gave birth and then changed your mind about parenthood, you aren't allowed to send the baby back, and adoption is likewise a commitment that will last at least until the child reaches adulthood; but you can always decide you will give up your child-free life. Adoption *does* become more difficult to arrange as you pass forty—it's true—but it is still possible to become parents to a child (though maybe not a perfectly healthy, newborn baby). There are older children in need of loving parents, as well as children with problems that present a challenge that perhaps you are the right person to meet. There are children from poor countries in which the number of couples able to adopt falls far short of the number of children who need homes. For this reason many couples who cannot easily reach agreement on which nonmedical alternative to pursue may wish to try the child-free life-style for a specified period of time, and see how well it suits them. (More on other methods of conflict-resolution later.)

Partial Parenting

Partial parenting means that you take on some of the responsibilities and benefits of parenthood, but you do not commit yourself to twenty-four-hour-a-day care from infancy through adulthood, the way you do when you adopt or give birth to a child. Foster parenting is one form of partial parenting in which the child comes to live with you only for a limited period of time—a few weeks or perhaps a few months. God-parenting is another form; in this case you make an enduring commitment, but the amount of time you spend with the child may be limited to a few hours per week or per month. "Role modeling" is yet a third form. You build a strong relationship with a child, or a group of children, generally through your involvement in an organization such as the Boy Scouts, the Girl Scouts, Campfire, 4-H, Boys' and Girls' Clubs, or a Big Brother/Big Sister program. Those not interested in joining any organized group could also form a role model relationship on their own with a neighborhood child in need of tutoring, for example, or could serve as mentor to a young protégé(e) on the job.

You may also become a partial parent without going out and choosing the role. You may marry into the status, or acquire it through your relationship with your partner who has children from a previous marriage. If you reach the decision that you will make no further attempts to have a baby through medical intervention, you will then be free to focus on your relationship with your stepchildren and work to build that into the central parenting experience of your life.

As you can see, there are many ways to play a parental role without becoming an adoptive or birth parent. Why take this road? The possibilities include the following:

- You've considered adoption and have concluded that it is just not right for you.
- You've considered child-free living, but you know that you would regret not forming a strong, emotional bond with a child if you chose that life-style.
- You would like to keep control over the amount of time you will commit to your relationship with a child or children. You know that if you sign up to be a Scout leader, for example, that you will spend so many hours per month with your kids—just the amount that suits your schedule.
- The part of parenthood that appeals to you most is the teaching of a fresh young mind, and hearing the child's thoughts, and knowing that you are there when that child needs a loving friend to talk to.
- The part of parenthood that appeals to you least is the care and feeding of infants and toddlers. You really don't relish the idea of waking up to the sound of crying four times in the middle of each night, and changing dirty diapers, and cleaning up a floorful of mess after every meal, and all the other inescapable chores that come with having a baby.
- You have always enjoyed being around kids, you know you have much to contribute to a child's life, and you feel a need to put your parental energies to good use—though not on a full-time basis.

How can you be sure that partial parenting is the best nonmedical alternative for you to pursue? Just try it! This is one option that requires little soul-searching or investigation before you start. And it's 100 percent reversible.

But do be careful not to get in over your head at the outset. You don't want to apply to become a full-time foster parent to a child with a severe disability after just one chat with a social worker. It's better to get involved in slow, logical steps.

If you have a special interest in any of the well-known organizations that work with kids—say you look back with great fondness at your years as a Scout—then check out that organization first. If you know about farming, try volunteering with 4-H; if you're a great tennis player, try calling your city's recreation department and see if they could use someone like you in an existing summer sports program, or ask whether you could help to set one up. Follow your own creative thoughts.

You might also look into youth programs put on by your church or religious organization. There may be a service to match children from single-parent families with adults who are willing to give moral guidance and emotional support.

Your city's social service agency will probably offer an orientation course for adults interested in learning what is involved in foster parenting. Without committing yourself to anything, you can learn what kind of children are usually placed, and for how long with each family, and what financial support the city provides for the child's foster parents.

But you do not have to work through any outside organization. Your good friends, siblings, or other relatives might come to you and ask you to play an important role in their children's lives, to promise to take care of them should they be orphaned, and to take an interest in their development, introduce them to new activities and experiences, and offer them comfort and wisdom in time of trouble. This nature of this relationship may be spelled out by your religion (as godparent-godchild) or it may be set down according to law (as in a will naming you legal guardian in case of the parents' death), or it may remain informal, existing simply as an understanding between you and the parents of the child.

Although you probably don't need to do much preparation to get

*Y*ou have to be at peace with yourself. There are so many things you can do [besides having children]. You can cherish your friends' kids.

*T*ina from California

involved in a partial parenting relationship, you might enjoy reading a little about it before you begin. The Suggested Reading List has information about books on stepparenting, foster parenting, and other forms of partial parenting.

WHEN THE COUPLE CANNOT AGREE

He's ready to adopt but she's uncomfortable with the idea and would prefer to live child-free.

He has a child from his previous marriage and can't understand why his wife is not content with her stepparent role; she wants to adopt.

She's got a protégé at the office and is also a doting aunt to her sister's three kids; he says he wants a child of his own to raise.

I've described scenarios such as these to experts, and the answer I get back is invariably counseling, counseling, counseling. And yes, counseling is often helpful, especially when the relationship is in danger of falling apart over disagreement about alternatives to continued infertility treatment. But many couples don't like to leave their intimate problems in the hands of outsiders—and they shouldn't have to, unless the strategies suggested below will not work for them.

First Strategy: Take an Analytical Approach

Each of you should first write a list of the reasons why you favor or disfavor each of the three nonmedical options. Writing things down tends to crystallize your ideas, helping you to focus on what's really important to you. Try to separate your firm belief from any passing notions or vague fears you may have. Rank your reasons in order of priority. Then sit down with your partner and compare lists, searching for points of agreement. Try to identify where the "give" is in the other person's list and in your own list. If each of you eliminates the least important of your listed considerations, what are you left with? You may well be able to identify an area of overlapping sentiments by the time you finish this process.

The following example illustrates this strategy. As his number one reason in favor of the child-free option the husband writes, "I really love you so much just the way you are, that I'm a little worried that by adopting a child you might change, and our wonderful relationship might change, too." As her number one reason in favor of adoption the wife writes, "I feel that if I go through all of life never experiencing motherhood, I'll end up feeling miserable, envious of others, and resentful of you for not wanting to adopt." After he sees what she has written, he realizes that his number one priority is really for the two of them to be happy together—but she cannot be happy without a child. Therefore, logically, neither will he. They begin to explore the adoption alternative.

Now let's take an example from a very different couple. She writes that she isn't ready for adoption, and wonders if she could ever really accept a child that another woman has given up. He writes that the genetic link is unimportant to him, and that he would feel the same joy of fatherhood for any baby, regardless of how it came into the family. He wants to stop delaying and start working toward becoming adoptive parents now. After each has studied the other's words, they might come to see that adoption could work for them both—though not just any form of adoption. A privately arranged, open adoption might be the answer, so that the wife can meet the pregnant woman and come to understand why she needs to let another family raise her child. The wife can then get past her guilt over "taking someone else's baby," as she sees that she will actually be helping a woman out of an unfortunate bind. As the pregnancy draws to a close she can feel she's bonding with the baby and feel confident that when she takes it home, it will truly be hers. The husband, meanwhile, will have his need to "get moving" met by not surrendering the search process to an adoption agency and then just waiting passively until selected to receive a baby. By placing ads, interviewing adoption attorneys, and looking for leads among friends and acquaintances, he can take charge of his own case, and by doing so, probably speed up the process by months or even years.

If, on the other hand, you each write down your priorities and after thorough analysis find no common themes in your lists, then you might consider implementing one of the three other strategies below.

Second Strategy: Let the Strongest Emotion Prevail

The one who is less adamant about the preferred option should yield to the one cares most intensely. But don't get bogged down in an argument over who feels more deeply than the other. If it's not immediately clear which of you has the strongest feelings, then perhaps counseling is in order to sort the matter out.

Third Strategy: Stick with the Status Quo

If neither partner has intense feelings about which way to go, then don't go anywhere. Keep your life as it is. Let's say the wife is leaning toward adoption but says she could see living a child-free life-style, while the husband leans toward the child-free option, though might under some circumstances consider adoption: perhaps a trial period of child-free living is the right course. They agree to a two-year period in which they devote themselves to enjoying their own lives together. If at the end of that time they feel they're missing out on anything, then they still have time to pursue adoption by one means or another. But if they were to adopt now, and then discover their discomfort with that solution, it would be too late to go back.

Fourth Strategy: Trial and Error

When one partner wants to adopt but the other is uncertain about it, have a trial run at child-rearing by foster parenting. Social service agencies may be able to place an infant in your home for the short term (babies whose parents are temporarily unable to care for them because of illness, unemployment, or other unforeseen circumstances). You should consider this plan only if you are able to take in a child who does not need special nursing care or therapy. When you're not sure if you're equipped to deal with the average baby, you don't want to test your limits by taking on too much of a challenge. If both you and your spouse act on this strategy, and you quickly find yourself falling in love with the child who will soon leave, or if you find yourself thinking, "I'll be sorry when my time as a foster parent is over," then you should take your reaction as a sign that you are ready to begin the adoption process.

And when you do, you will find that you now rank much higher in the eyes of adoption agency workers because you have had the experience of being foster parents and handling a baby on your own. On the other hand, if you find yourselves reacting to the experience with thoughts such as "This is harder than we thought it would be," or "I'll be glad when this is over," then you might conclude that adoption is not for you.

If none of the four methods of conflict resolution outlined above helps you to arrive at the nonmedical alternative that works for you both, then by all means consult a professional counselor.

CHAPTER TEN

FERTILITY AND THE NONTRADITIONAL PATIENT

When you read other books or magazine articles about couples in fertility treatment, or you watch TV news reports or hear interviews with couples on radio call-in shows, you may be struck by one thing: the couples are always alike. They are all middle-class—married, of course—and healthy (except for their infertility), ranging in age from the late twenties to early forties, trying to have a first baby, and not constrained in their choice of treatment by the laws of their chosen religion.

But what if you don't happen to fit this description? What if you are

a single woman

a single man

a partner in a heterosexual relationship, but you're not married

a partner in a gay male relationship

a partner in a Lesbian relationship

a postmenopausal woman

disabled or seriously ill

already the parent of one child but you have been unable to conceive another

a practicing member of a religion that restricts or forbids some forms of infertility treatment.

These are some of the questions that may be going through your mind:

Can I be helped?

Will it be hard to find doctors willing to work with me?

How do I go about finding the help I need?

What are my main options for treatment?

Are there any considerations special to my situation that I should bear in mind?

A discussion of each of these five questions will follow for each of the types of patients listed above.

The Single Woman

CAN I BE HELPED?

Yes, there's no reason why you couldn't receive treatment for problems interfering with conception, just the same as any other woman who desires to become a mother.

WLL IT BE HARD TO FIND DOCTORS WILLING TO WORK WITH ME?

Not in big cities, where you have a good amount of choice among doctors and programs. About half of OB-GYNs (according to *Harper's Index*) said that they would be willing to help a single woman become pregnant. So if the first doctor you see expresses any reluctance to take you on, or appears in any way judgmental or disapproving of your desire to have a child, keep looking. Try to get a sense of what the doctor is like over the telephone before you set up a consultation. If he sounds patronizing or starts to lecture you about morality, then you know you don't want to spend any money on a look-see visit. But even with sympathetic doctors you may have to put up with a certain amount of questioning about your motives that married couples are never asked: "Are you sure you want to do this? Can you afford it? How does your family feel about it? Have you thought about childcare?" If you can't give your doctor firm, well-thought-out answers, you may not be ready to face the world as a single mother.

HOW DO I GO ABOUT FINDING HELP?

You can check out fertility clinics and doctors just as recommended in Chapter Two, but when asking the doctor questions during your look-see visit, add a few to the standard list. Ask whether the doctor has treated single women before. Discuss the method by which you will attempt to be impregnated (for options, see below). If it is important to you to keep your treatment confidential, discuss how you would prefer the doctor's office to contact you during working hours, so as best to preserve your privacy.

You may find valuable advice on starting your quest to conceive by contacting a national support group of women who have made the same decision as you, called Single Mothers by Choice (see Resource Guide for address).

OPTIONS

Your choices for treatment of reproductive-tract problems are the same as for any married woman—it all depends on what your problem turns out to be. Where choice comes into play is in your selection of the method by which you intend to acquire the sperm to fertilize your egg. Basically, there are four ways to go about it:

1. Artificial insemination by an anonymous donor (AI/D)
2. Artificial insemination by a donor known to you (usually a close male friend) who has agreed to provide the sperm
3. Sexual intercourse at the fertile peak of your cycle with a man who understands and supports your desire to become pregnant
4. Sexual intercourse at the fertile peak of your cycle with a man you have not informed of your desire to become pregnant

There are medical, emotional, practical, legal, and ethical consider-ations involved in choosing any of these options. The table on page 370 spells out some of the most important ones for you to consider when making this life-altering decision.

SPECIAL CONSIDERATIONS

In addition to the questions raised in the table you should consider the following four issues:

*   *Financial.* Can you afford treatment? Two incomes are often nec-essary to be able to handle the bills when IVF or other ARTs are involved. Unless you are a high-level earner, you will probably need to find a health insurance policy that provides the broadest possible coverage. Check carefully to see if the policy contains any restrictions about infertility based on marital status.

SINGLE WOMEN'S CHOICES FOR SOURCE OF SPERM

CONSIDER-ATIONS	AI/D—Anonymous Donor	AI/D—Known Donor	Sexual Inter-course—Informed Lover	Sexual Intercourse—Uninformed Lover
Medical	Donor sperm is carefully screened—no risk of AIDS or other venereal diseases.	Volunteer donor should agree to be screened for diseases and have fertility potential analyzed.	Lover should agree to be screened for diseases; possibly have fertility potential analyzed.	No sure way to find out if lover is fertile; no sure way to rule out AIDS and venereal diseases.
Emotional	May always wonder who donor is. Child may grow up feeling uncertain of identity, heritage.	May be difficult to find man willing to provide sperm. What role, if any, does father expect to play in child's life. What will child be told about father?	Does lover actively want to father a child or is he simply continuing to have sex with you, even though you told him you will no longer use birth control? If pregnancy results, will relationship be damaged?	You may feel guilty that you tricked your lover into fathering your child. Ambiguous or negative feelings about the father may lead to similar feelings about the child you have had by him.
Practical	Easy to arrange. No need to search for willing male. Easy to preserve privacy.	AI sometimes requires several tries before it works. Is donor willing to keep	Easy to arrange if already in ongoing sexual relationship. All you may need to do	Requires deception to keep lover from finding out that you are trying to become

(continued)

CONSIDER-ATIONS	AI/D—Anonymous Donor	AI/D—Known Donor	Sexual Intercourse—Informed Lover	Sexual Intercourse—Uninformed Lover
		on providing sperm?	is simply stop contracepting.	pregnant. Keeping track of lies can be complicated.
Ethical	Is it fair to child to intentionally bring into single-parent situation? What about child's right to know paternal relatives, family history?	If child eventually is told who father is, but father has not agreed to support or help bring child up, will child feel rejected by father?	If you and lover have agreed to bring a child into the world, consider marriage (even if you think it will be short-lived) to spare your child the stigma of being called "illegitimate" by an intolerant society.	Nearly everything about this method of becoming pregnant is ethically questionable.
Legal	No possibility of custody conflict with biological father—nor any possibility of getting child support or sharing child's upbringing with child's father.	Potential for custody conflict if father decides to press for parental rights. Sperm donor should sign legal agreement with you to spell out what child support, if any, will be paid, and what role, if any, he will play in child's life.	Of all sources of sperm, this presents greatest potential for custody conflict, because intimate relations with your partner puts him in role of common-law spouse. Legal document clarifying parental rights and duties is advised!	Little potential for custody conflict if casual lover never learns that you are pregnant. If lover does find out, anger at being deceived may motivate custody conflict.

- *Privacy.* Couples often have a hard time keeping their infertility treatment a secret. But if friends and coworkers do find out, they tend to react by supporting the married couple's desire to have a child. Not so for the single woman. Unwanted personal comments and intrusive questions are par for the course, single mothers report; so is gossip behind the woman's back. But if you are a strong person and either don't give a hoot what people say, or you are able to come back with a sharp, comment-stopping retort, then you will be well equipped to withstand the assaults on your privacy that you undoubtedly will experience.
- *Hardship.* Infertility treatment is often painful and emotionally draining. It's hard enough for a couple to go through it together. A single person will find it helpful to have a good friend to rely on, someone who has a shoulder you can cry on and a steady hand to hold. Think carefully who would be the best person to ask to stand by you when you're feeling down. If no one comes to mind, ask yourself now how much stress and strain you think you can take on your own.
- *Loneliness.* Going to an infertility clinic is a trip to couple-land. They're all around—in the waiting room, in group meetings, in seminars, and in the lobby. You've got to be prepared to be the only solo player in a hall full of duets.

If you have the inner strength and determination to tackle all these problems head on, then you undoubtedly have what's needed to get through a pregnancy as a single woman and be a great single mom.

The Single Man

CAN I BE HELPED?

Maybe yes . . . and maybe no. The answer hinges on your ability to find a woman to bear your child. If you are healthy and have normal sperm production, that should be your only problem. However, if it turns out that you have any of the types of male infertility identified in Chapter Four, then you must first have your problem treated by any of the methods currently in use before attempting to impregnate a woman. Your chances of success in treatment are the same as for any married man.

WILL IT BE HARD TO FIND DOCTORS WILLING TO WORK WITH ME?

In some circumstances, yes. You should have no difficulty finding a urologist to correct a varicocele or clear a blockage in your sperm ducts or reverse a vasectomy; these are straightforward surgical procedures, and if questioned as to your motives for wanting the procedure now, when still single, you can simply say that you are concerned about preserving your reproductive potential for the future.

But oftentimes the most effective approach is not to try to increase the man's sperm production but to try to make his partner produce many eggs, to increase the chance of union between egg and sperm. Here's the stumbling block. It may be possible for a single man of normal fertility to persuade a close female friend to have a child with him—but a less than fully fertile man will be very hard pressed to find any woman willing to undergo the rigors of a fertility drug regimen if she doesn't have to.

What about surrogacy? A single man could advertise or use a surrogacy attorney to find a woman willing to participate in a fertility program with him for a set fee—but even if he could find the perfect candidate, he might still have a hard time finding a fertility clinic to work with him and his "hired help." Why would a doctor turn a single man away when that same doctor is willing to help a single woman to get pregnant using sperm from a donor or a male friend that she brings along? Society is not gender blind, and doctors are often understanding of a single woman's desire to have a child (it's her "maternal instinct" at work) when they are perplexed or disapproving of the same parental urge in a man. The law will also be an obstacle. All states currently recognize the child born to a single woman as hers, without question. In many states she can even arrange for the adoption of her child by others without obtaining a release from the child's father. Unwed fathers have far fewer rights. A single man might well arrange for a woman to have his child; and he might find a doctor who is willing to assist in the endeavor; and then a child might be conceived as a result of fertility treatment—only to end up in a terrible custody dispute when the woman suddenly decided she wants to keep the baby. A single man will be at a great disadvantage in any legal tangle with his newborn baby's mother, and even if he prevails, the court time and expense will be more than most men could bear.* Doctors generally shy away from cases that could well result in litigation, and so despite the high fees

---

*In the one court case I found that fits these circumstances, a divorced man battled his hired surrogate for custody in California. The judge ultimately ruled that the two strangers should have joint custody of the daughter they had created together. Part of the baby's week would be spent in her mother's cramped apartment in a crime-ridden part of Los Angeles, the other part would be spent in her father's expensive, suburban house. Both parents voiced bitter disappointment with the judgment.

for fertility treatment, they will usually refuse to get involved.

It is, of course, possible to go to a fertility doctor with a hired surrogate mother and represent her as your girlfriend—though such a dishonest course of action cannot be recommended.

How do i go about finding help?

There are several ways you might go about finding a woman to enter into a childbearing agreement with you. You might ask a very close female friend. You might try contacting an attorney who specializes in surrogate motherhood and ask for help in recruiting and screening candidates. You might try placing ads in the "personals" columns of magazines (though the request is so offbeat, you would undoubtedly have a greater chance of getting a response if you tried a magazine with an out-of-the-mainstream sort of readership). Or try contacting Single Mothers by Choice—you might be able to learn of a single woman who is contemplating pregnancy and is looking for a partner in the venture. If it worked out, you could form an agreement to create and raise a child together, providing the benefits of a two-parent home for your child (though you may continue to live apart).

However you find the woman you will work with, you should arrange to have her thoroughly screened, and you should have her sign a contract drawn up by a good lawyer spelling out how she will be compensated, how child custody is to be arranged, and how many other important matters are to be settled (for further information on this subject, see the section on Surrogate Motherhood).

As for going about finding a willing medical team, you might first try calling different clinics and describing the type of childbearing arrangement you'll be making, but in a hypothetical way—and without identifying yourself. If the doctor does not automatically rule out treating a couple fitting the description you supply, then go ahead and schedule a consultation.

Options

To be frank, the best option for a single man who is not living with a woman is to put aside the idea of having a biological child and pursue adoption. It is not so unusual these days for an adoption to occur in a

Single Fathers by Choice

*T*he August 31, 1992, issue of *People* magazine featured the stories of five single men who had each chosen to become a father and bring up a child on his own. Christensen von Wormer of Michigan hired a surrogate mother to bear his daughter for him. He lives with her and a full-time nanny in a ten-room house that he bought shortly before her birth. Sherman Hamilton of Colorado and Joe Young of Connecticut each had a child with a former girlfriend and then took custody of the child that the mother chose not to raise herself. Rocky Story of Texas had a baby with a girlfriend; when he later found out that she was addicted to cocaine, he sued for custody and won. Brad Akin of California, a gay man, adopted an infant girl of mixed nationality. All five men interviewed for the magazine article appeared to be happy and fulfilled by the choices they had made.

household made up of other than the traditional heterosexual married couple. There are even adoption agencies that specialize in bringing about such nontraditional placements. Of course, the child adopted by the single man is rarely a newborn. Most commonly placed are older boys and children with "special needs" (this is a term used to describe children with disabilities, illnesses, emotional problems, or children who may have been abused or abandoned by their parents). Governments of some foreign countries will also permit a homeless child or baby to be adopted by a single man. An adoption counselor can brief you on your choices.

If, however, you are determined to become the father of a biologically related child, and you have found a woman to assist you in this endeavor, then you have basically two choices: (1) you can produce a sperm specimen to artifically inseminate the woman; or (2) you can have the woman calculate her time of ovulation (see Chapter One for description of method) and have intercourse with her two or three times within that two-day window of opportunity.

SPECIAL CONSIDERATIONS

All of the methods discussed, with the exception of adoption, are so fraught with pitfalls that it's hard to know where to begin. There is a general societal bias against the single father raising a baby. There are social, moral, legal, and financial constraints upon the use of any surrogacy arrangement to produce a child. There is the difficulty (perhaps impossibility) of finding a fertile woman to help you who is neither mentally unbalanced nor totally venal, and who can be trusted to keep her side of the bargain. There is the issue of childcare: who will look after the baby when you are at work? And that of secrecy: what do you tell the child about how it came to be born? I'm sure there are twenty or thirty other major problems to be considered, but the five I've mentioned here should be enough to think about for starters.

The Unmarried Heterosexual Couple

Can we be helped?

Yes, there is no reason why you should not be treated the same as any couple who are married.

Will it be hard to find doctors willing to work with us?

No. There may be a few old-fashioned doctors who will reject you because of your unmarried status, but there are many more good doctors who will not pass judgment on the nature of your relationship. Even so, you should expect the doctor to ask you some personal questions that might not be asked if you were married. How long have you been living together? Do you have a joint bank account and shared expenses? Do you have any kind of a contractual relationship (a living-together agreement drawn up by an attorney)? Have you designated each other as beneficiary in case of death and have you given each other a power of attorney in case you fall into a coma? By asking these or similar questions, your doctor will only be trying to protect himself from the legal mess that could result if at some point during treatment one of you should die, fall ill, or (worst of all, from the doctor's point of view) default on your bills.

How do we go about finding help?

When checking out fertility clinics as suggested in Chapter Two, be sure to ask if there is a general rule regarding unmarried couples. If you sense an air of disapproval—even as you're being told of the doctors' willingness to take you on—then keep looking, until you find an office whose staff members come across as welcoming and supportive.

Options

Treatments available are no different from those available to married couples.

Special considerations

The section above on finding a doctor includes some important questions about your legal situation if you should die or become incompetent during the course of treatment. The unmarried couple, devoted to each other though they might be, are still well advised to have an expert in family law draw up an agreement stating what will happen to any children, or embryos, created as a result of successful treatment, if their relationship should end. If you haven't already done so, you should also write a will, so that the inheritance rights of a child born outside of marriage will be fully protected. These measures are designed less to protect you against the claims of your partner as to prevent any other members of your family (such as parents from whom you have become estranged) from stepping in and attempting to take custody of your child or deprive your partner of any money you would leave for your child's support. With a little forethought now (despite your natural reluctance to contemplate such depressing scenarios), you can prevent years of painful litigation over your child's fate. A few notorious child custody cases pitting the decreased partner's parents against the surviving partner demonstrate the wisdom of following this advice.

The Gay Male Couple

Can we be helped?

There is no reason why you cannot have treatment to correct problems in your reproductive tract, the same as any heterosexual would. The main obstacle you face is in finding a woman to bear a child for you.

Will it be hard to find doctors willing to work with us?

That depends on what your fertility problem turns out to be and how you present yourself to the doctor. If you have a physical defect, such as an obstruction in one of your ducts, you should have no difficulty finding a surgeon to repair the problem. You need not go into any detailed discussion of your life-style and how you intend to add children to it.

But what if you have the sort of problem that is best treated by giving fertility drugs to the woman to make her ovulate a large number of eggs? Then you will first have to recruit a woman who is willing to undergo the necessary series of shots and daily monitoring appointments—but even if you did find someone willing to do all that for you, you would still have the problem of finding a doctor willing to help to create a child under your particular set of circumstances. There may be some doctors who will work to create a surrogate pregnancy resulting in a baby to be brought up by its biological father and his wife; there may even be a few doctors who will work to create a surrogate pregnancy resulting in a baby to be brought up by its biological father and his live-in female lover; but you will have a *very* hard time finding one to help create a surrogate pregnancy resulting in a baby to be brought up by its biological father and his live-in *male* lover. Perhaps you would need to find a gay fertility doctor to view your desire to have a biological child with the same understanding that would be shown as a matter of course to a heterosexual couple. If that is not possible, then you and the woman you recruit will probably have to present yourselves to the doctor as a heterosexual couple, hiding the fact of your male lover's existence. However, there are important ethical and emotional arguments against embarking on such a course.

How do we go about finding help?

Your first place to start looking for a woman willing to bear a child for you should be among your own friends and family. There have been children born to gay male couples by means of the following arrangement: The partner who will not be the biological father asks his sister to agree to be artificially inseminated with the sperm of his lover. During her pregnancy she is given emotional and financial support, both from her brother and from his lover, the father of her child. After the birth she gives the baby to the male couple to be brought up as their child— or she might even move in with the pair to create a household composed of a child and *three* parents.

If neither of you has a sister who would consider such a plan, you might start raising the idea with any close female friends that you have (best to start broaching the subject very gently, and retreat at the first indication of a rebuff).

It is *not* recommended that you start a deceptively heterosexual relationship with a woman with the idea that she will get pregnant and you can win custody of the child. That is a recipe for heartbreak for all concerned.

However, if you can't find a female friend willing to go into the venture with you, you might try advertising in a gay/Lesbian newspaper or magazine. You just might be able to find a single Lesbian who would like to become a mother, who would consider a shared-custody arrangement with you and your lover, or you might even find one partner in a Lesbian couple who would like to get pregnant by you, resulting in a baby who would be born with *four* adults occupying parental roles. (A family created in just such a fashion was the subject of the *Geraldo* show broadcast on September 3, 1992. The four parents and their young daughter all appeared happy with their rather unusual living arrangement.)

As for finding a doctor who would help to bring about a pregnancy in any of the above circumstances, you might try contacting a gay men's health clinic or gay family support group to find a referral to a fertility doctor who is either gay himself or who is known to be sympathetic to gay family issues.

OPTIONS

Once you have found a woman to bear your child, unless you are bisexual, you will undoubtedly wish to rely on artificial insemination to bring about a pregnancy. If you are having difficulty finding a doctor willing to carry out the procedure, you may wish to consider doing the insemination in the privacy of your own home. If you have normal sperm production, and if the woman keeps track of her ovulation so that she is able to identify the fertile peak of her cycle, your chances of bringing about a pregnancy in this manner are only slightly lower than if attempted with a doctor's assistance. Instructions on how to perform home insemination may be found in a book called *Having Your Baby by Donor Insemination: A Complete Resource Guide* (for further information on this book, see the Suggested Reading List).

For most gay male couples there is a much easier way to create a family than the ones outlined above, and that is by adoption. Especially in major cities where there is a politically strong gay minority, many of the legal hurdles that formerly barred such adoptions have been cleared, allowing gay couples to take in children in need. Often teenage or even younger boys will become homeless when they first exhibit signs of gay orientation and their intolerant parents evict them from their homes. When a troubled boy is placed in a nontraditional household, some counseling to help ease the transition for all concerned is usually in order. But a family formed in this way can end up being most rewarding for all involved, since it was formed entirely by the choice of all its members.

SPECIAL CONSIDERATIONS

As with any couple lacking the state-sanctioned protection of marriage, it's wise to have a legal agreement between the parties stipulating what would happen to the child or children in the event of various misfortunes (see section on unmarried heterosexuals for contingencies to be covered).

In any situation involving the transfer of bodily fluids from one person to another—but especially one involving gay men—the possibility of transmission of AIDS needs to be ruled out. At least six months prior to insemination, and then a few weeks prior to the time of insemination, the partner who wishes to father a child should have himself tested for the human immunodeficiency virus (HIV).

One serious issue the couple ought to examine is that of the social pressure that their child will certainly experience. Other children will tease and make cruel jokes about anyone whose home life is different from the norm. Before you assume full parental responsibility for a child you should consider your ability to foster your child's confidence and self-esteem in the face of name-calling and other inevitable acts of intolerance.

The Lesbian Couple

CAN WE BE HELPED?

Yes. There is no reason why your chance of conceiving should not be the same as those of a heterosexual woman undergoing fertility treatment.

WILL IT BE HARD TO FIND DOCTORS WILLING TO WORK WITH US?

Possibly. As described in the section above dealing with gay male couples, you may encounter widespread resistance to the idea that a same-sex couple deserves medical help in having a child, just the same as an opposite-sex couple. The partner who desires the pregnancy may possibly find it easier to find a doctor to help if she presents herself simply as an unmarried woman rather than as someone in an ongoing, stable

Lesbian Parents Go Public

*O*n December 3, 1991, the *Sally Jessy Raphaël* show featured a Lesbian couple, Tiffany and Carol, who talked about the choice they had made to have a child. First they found a male friend, Jim, who was willing to contribute the sperm. He agreed to be tested for HIV, and after his tests came back negative, he provided a sample that was used to artificially inseminate Tiffany. She became pregnant and had a daughter, Sophie. Jim intends to be a father to his daughter throughout her life, although he does not live in the same house with her. Sophie will grow up in a household with two "mommies."

Lesbian relationship. On the other hand, if it turns out that the medical care you need is a relatively simple, straightforward matter (for example, all you need is a prescription for Clomid to enhance your ovulation, or a hysteroscopic procedure to repair a uterine septum) then it shouldn't be necessary for the doctor to concern herself with the nature of your relationship; she should simply do what is necessary to increase the odds that you will conceive, and leave up to you how that conception will be arranged.

HOW DO WE GO ABOUT FINDING HELP?

The woman who wants a child without a male partner has the advantage over the man who wants one without a female partner. She and her female lover have control over their own bodies, and may choose which one of them will get pregnant and bear the child. Finding a male to supply the sperm is not a major stumbling block; if a brother or other male relative of the nonchildbearing partner cannot be persuaded to donate a sample, nor can a male friend be recruited, then anonymous donor sperm may be used. You can select your donor from a catalog and have the sample shipped directly to you, along with complete instructions for home insemination, or you can make arrangements for the procedure through your doctor's office.

To find a doctor who is sympathetic and supportive of your desire to bring a child into your life, try asking for a referral from any organizations you may belong to that support Lesbian/gay rights, or see if there is a feminist women's health collective or a clinic that specializes in Lesbian patients in your local area.

OPTIONS

Artificial insemination will be the preference of most Lesbians.

A bisexual woman who has an ongoing relationship with a man may wish to attempt to conceive through intercourse, but she should be up-front with him about her intentions, and before dispensing with the use of birth control, discuss what if any parental role he would be expected to play. To fail to inform him of her plan to conceive by him would almost certainly create an atmosphere of mistrust and hostility that will be harmful to the child born of such a relationship.

Adoption, mentioned above in the section about gay male options, is also a valid, and very popular choice.

SPECIAL CONSIDERATIONS

All of the legal and social issues raised in the section under The Un-married Heterosexual Couple and The Gay Male Couple should be con-sidered by the Lesbian couple as well.

The Postmenopausal Woman

CAN I BE HELPED?

Yes, technology today can make it possible for you to have a child— but it will not be genetically related to you. See the section on Donor Egg (page 281) for description of how pregnancy can be possible for postmenopausal women.

WILL IT BE HARD TO FIND DOCTORS WILLING TO WORK WITH ME?

Yes, for two reasons: first, there are few clinics with the technological capability for success with egg donation in a woman whose hormonal output is so low; second, of the relatively few doctors able to perform the procedure, a high percentage are unwilling, on ethical grounds, to help bring about a pregnancy in a woman whose childbearing potential has been ended by the normal process of aging. Some say that treatment for such a woman is "unnatural," while others focus their fears more on the child who will grow up having a mother in her fifties and sixties, who may lack the energy and stamina (and possibly the lifespan) needed to care for a child from infancy through young adulthood.

Yet there *are* doctors who have successfully worked with postmenopausal women and who continue to do so with generally good results. In New York City, especially, but also in some other major cities, it may not be too difficult to find the help you need.

HOW DO I GO ABOUT FINDING HELP?

First, find out how many fertility clinics in your area run donor egg programs. You might want to order the latest survey put out by the Society for Assisted Reproductive Technologies (SART), which lists success rates for participating clinics across the nation. Contact as many as are within your reasonable traveling distance and ask if they have any restrictions as to the age or condition of the women who will receive donor eggs. If no egg donor program in your local area will take you on, you may have to be willing to relocate for a period of time to work with a clinic that will admit you as a patient.

OPTIONS

Pregnancy through use of a donor's egg is not the sole means available to the postmenopausal woman who wants a baby. She might also attempt to become pregnant through the embryo transplant procedure, or she might seek to become the adoptive mother of her husband's biological baby by a surrogate mother.

Adoption of a healthy American infant will be very difficult for the postmenopausal woman to arrange, as most agencies and birth mothers consider a woman beyond the age of forty to be "too old" (no matter how active and energetic you really are) to be a mother. But some foreign governments have liberal rules regarding adoption of orphaned babies. You might also be interested in having an older child or one with a disability who is in need of your special love and care. Such adoption can be arranged with far fewer restrictions as to the adoptive parents' age or other factors.

SPECIAL CONSIDERATIONS

It takes a considerable physical and emotional toll on any woman (regardless of her age) to go through pregnancy, labor, and delivery and then be primary caretaker for a baby for the first two or three very demanding years of its life. You must ask yourself squarely, "Am I really prepared to get up four or five times a night for three months to feed my crying newborn?" and "When I am on my thousandth diaper change, will I still be thrilled that I made the choice to have a child?" To help you get a sense of how you would feel if you succeed in your quest, spend as much time as you can with friends or relatives who have infants, including some overnight baby-sitting, if possible.

Sometimes the postmenopausal woman does not need to examine her motives so minutely. She has a driving reason to want a child. Perhaps she once had a child who died. Or she might have spent all of her fertile years in a marriage with a man who did not want children but now she is remarried to a man who shares her intense desire to become a parent. Perhaps she had to forgo parenthood while she was younger to take care of an elderly or incapacitated parent but has now been freed of her obligation through that parent's death. She herself may have been suffering from a disease or disability, the treatment for which closed off the possibility of pregnancy during her fertile years. These are all circumstances beyond the postmenopausal woman's control, and her urge to pursue parenthood should be seen in a different light than that of the woman who postponed childbearing until too late, out of her own uncertainty or sense of unreadiness for motherhood.

Regardless of the reason for the delayed pursuit of pregnancy, societal disapproval remains an issue. Can you deal with people coming up to you, saying, "Oh, what a cute grandchild you have!" Can you deal with the stares and comments of strangers while you are pregnant? Do you have any reservations about having a child who is not genetically related to you? Do you have confidence that your health and stamina will remain strong enough for you to fulfill your parenting obligations for the next eighteen or twenty years? Do you have the financial wherewithal to take on the costs of an "experimental" (that is to say, uninsurable) medical procedure, and then pay all the bills involved in feeding, clothing, housing, and educating your child? If you have answered yes without reservation to each of these questions, then you very likely have what it takes to be a good parent, even though you may be over forty-five or even over fifty.

Disabled or Seriously Ill

CAN I BE HELPED?

In many cases, yes. Fertility doctors have performed procedures that have made parenthood possible for

- a man who is undergoing cancer chemotherapy which has destroyed his ability to produce sperm
- a man who is paralyzed from the waist down and is unable to have intercourse with his wife
- a woman who is undergoing radiation therapy for breast cancer
- a woman who has lost both ovaries to cancer
- a woman who has had a hysterectomy
- the widow of a man who knew that his illness would be terminal
- a couple who both carry the genes for a serious genetic disease that they do not wish to risk passing down to their child.

WILL IT BE HARD TO FIND DOCTORS WILLING TO WORK WITH ME?

When one is struggling against an illness or disability and at the same time struggling to have a child, one must have great determination, grit, and faith in the future. These are also the qualities needed in your search for the right doctor to assist you in your quest. The specific type of condition you have and its relationship to your reproductive system will determine the type of fertility skills you will require. In some simple cases the ordinary fertility specialist will be able to help you, but for those already receiving medical treatment for cancer or some other life-threatening or disabling condition, you will need to find a fertility doctor who can work as part of a team with the other doctors on your case.

The usual difficulty is not in finding cooperative fertility specialists. They tend to be encouraging of the hopes of most couples, no matter what their condition, to have a baby. The main opposition, as reported in numerous letters from patients to RESOLVE on the subject, tends to come from the doctors treating the illness or condition. They tend to doubt both the patient's physical and emotional ability to have a child under the circumstances. Fertility treatment during other medical treatment is also an extra thing to keep track of, and many doctors like their patients to keep their lives simple and concentrate on getting well first. They may say things like: "Just be glad you are still alive," and "Don't think about having a child until after this is all over." Of course, oftentimes by then it is too late.

But despite near-universal discouragement from their regular doctors, patients have managed to become parents under the most trying of circumstances. To see some wonderful examples, you need only tune in to television talk shows for a period of time. *Geraldo* had the story of a multiply handicapped woman whose doctor told her it would certainly kill her to try to have a child. She was there with her beautiful and perfectly healthy two-year-old girl. *Sally Jessy Raphaël* featured a panel of "Celebrity Miracle Babies," including the actress Ann Gillian, who had had a baby at age forty-one, her pregnancy occurring after she had lost both breasts to cancer.

How do I go about finding help?

Start with your own doctor, but expect him to react negatively at first. Be prepared to have to educate him as to the feasibility (both physical and psychological) of childbearing for a person in your situation. You may want to do some research in a medical library to find other cases like yours in which conception was accomplished and a pregnancy successfully carried to term. Ask the librarian to assist you in locating case studies of the sort you need. Once your doctor is persuaded that what you seek to do is possible, then let him suggest the name of a fertility doctor to work with.

Another approach would be first to find a fertility doctor willing to take you on, and then to ask that doctor to brief your regular doctor on the forms of treatment available to you. To go about finding a fertility doctor on your own, follow the recommendations of Chapter Two, but be sure to ask the doctor if he has had any experience in working with someone in your condition. If he hasn't, then ask him if he is familiar with any similar cases in the medical literature and whether he thinks he would be able to diagnose and treat you effectively.

Options

What you can do to solve your fertility problem will, of course, depend a great deal on the nature of your illness or disability and its effect on your reproductive system. However, the following are just some examples of the kinds of treatment others have used to become parents despite some formidable physical obstacles:

For the man with spinal paralysis, a procedure called *electroejaculation* is highly effective (success rate of up to 80 percent). The penile nerves can be electrically stimulated and a sperm sample collected which is then used to artificially inseminate the man's wife. This method has helped thousands of men to become fathers—many of whom had been told by their doctors that they must give up hope of ever having a child.

The man diagnosed with cancer who must undergo sperm-destroying chemotherapy or radiation treatment must take steps to preserve his fertility before treatment begins. Unfortunately, cancer specialists seldom warn men of the sterility-inducing side effects of many anticancer drugs, nor do they advise men of the very simple way they can get around this problem. All the man needs to do is to produce a number of sperm samples to be "washed" and frozen for later use. If he leaves enough samples in storage and his wife is normally fertile, the couple could well have a large family, if they so desired.

Similarly, the woman who must undergo egg-destroying radiation or chemotherapy could first go through a fertility-drug stimulating cycle to produce as many eggs as possible that will be retrieved, and hopefully will be fertilized with her husband's sperm in vitro. The resulting embryos can then be frozen, to be thawed and implanted in her uterus when her cancer treatment is over and her disease is in remission. This option will not be available to all female cancer patients, as the use of fertility drugs could possibly speed up the growth process of certain types of tumors. But it is certainly worth asking your doctor or a fertility specialist whether egg retrieval and embryo freezing could be attempted in your case.

The woman who has lost both ovaries due to cancer is an excellent candidate to be helped by a donor egg program.

The woman who has had a hysterectomy, but whose ovaries were left intact, is an excellent candidate for egg retrieval, leading to the creation of an embryo to be placed inside a host uterus. If you have been told you need a hysterectomy but have not yet had the surgery, and you are intent on preserving your option to become a mother, you must impress upon your surgeon your desire to keep your ovaries so that you can produce eggs to be fertilized in vitro. If your surgeon routinely removes the ovaries of all uterine cancer patients, then find another who does not! The ovaries should be removed only when there is some indication that they are diseased as well.

For the couple who have a genetic disease that they fear passing down to their child, there is now a new medical technology called **BABI**, or **blastomere analysis before implantation**. Let's say that a husband and wife both carry the gene for Tay-Sachs disease (or sickle cell anemia, or hemophilia, or another chronic or terminal illness). Prior to the arrival of the BABI technique the only way the couple could be sure that their child would not be born with the fatal disease would be to wait until the fetus was between nine and sixteen weeks of gestational age and have a genetic test performed (by chorionic villae sampling or by amniocentesis) to determine if the fetus carried the gene. If it did, the couple could choose abortion, to avoid bringing a child into the world only to watch it suffer and die. The loss of a much-wanted fetus after the first trimester is of course emotionally devastating for the couple.

With BABI, the woman produces eggs to be fertilized in vitro in an IVF or ZIFT cycle. A single cell is removed from the *blastomere* (the four- or eight-celled pre-embryo) and tested, and if the results are positive the pre-embryo is simply not inserted into the woman's uterus. She is thus never pregnant and never experiences the loss of a well-formed fetus. If several embryos are produced and some are genetically normal and others are not, only the normal embryos will be returned to her uterus, hopefully to implant. In England the BABI technique has resulted in at least seven healthy girls born to parents who were carriers of the hemophilia gene. In the United States, the Genetics and IVF Institute of Fairfax, Virginia, has announced that it has begun recruiting patients for its experimental BABI program.

Even when one partner knows that his condition is terminal, the couple may wish to plan for a pregnancy that will occur after his or her death, leaving a child behind as a genetic legacy. While still healthy enough to produce sperm, the man will have several samples frozen, to be used by his wife to attempt pregnancy when she feels ready.

The key to all the fertility solutions cited above is forethought. If you will discuss with your doctor your strong desire to do everything possible to keep your reproductive options open, then your doctor in many cases will be able to devise a treatment for your condition that is both effective and compatible with your long-term goals. But if you fail to bring the subject up, you will find that few doctors will even mention it, and you could easily end up losing your fertility potential before you are fully aware of your choices.

One caution from former patients: never accept the first no as the final answer. If one doctor tells you it is impossible for you to become a parent, seek another opinion—and if need be, another and another. If you hear a whole chorus of nos then you will know it is time to accept the limitations of your own body and seek some other resolution of your infertility. Remember, too, that medical technology is advancing rapidly in this field. In the not-so-distant past all diabetic women were routinely told they must not attempt pregnancy. Now, with the proper medical guidance all the way through, such pregnancies are not only possible—they're commonplace. The future for you could be as bright.

SPECIAL CONSIDERATIONS

You need to think beyond what is involved in bringing about conception in your case, and seriously examine your own capability to care for a baby, should fertility treatment succeed. Your medical prognosis should be good enough for you to feel great confidence about your physical strength and energy level, both short-term (during the critical first few months of your baby's life) and long-term (until your child is through the often troublesome teenage years). The temptation of most determined patients is to grit their teeth and say, "I can handle anything"—and most of these patients can. But first sit back and review thoroughly what will be involved in daily childcare for someone in your condition. If you find yourself feeling strong doubts, listen to them now before taking any irrevocable steps.

Cost is also an important factor to be given due weight in your deliberations. Living with an illness or disability can be financially draining. You probably won't be able to go insurance policy shopping because of the pre-existing condition exclusion written into most policies, so if your present policy does not cover fertility treatment, you will be stuck. In persons suffering from certain forms of illness or disability, fertility treatment will automatically be considered experimental and so will be excluded from coverage, even if your policy normally does cover most forms of fertility treatment for others. Disabled parents in some cases may need to employ others to assist them in caring for the baby, and that is yet an additional heavy expense. This is not to say that a couple will be unable to find some way over these hurdles—just to emphasize that you need to take a clear-eyed, unsentimental view of the course that lies ahead before you enter the race.

The Couple Who Already Have One Child (Secondary Infertility)

CAN WE BE HELPED?

Yes, and you are the fertility doctor's favorite kind of patients because you have already demonstrated by having produced a child that you are not a hopeless case. Many doctors believe on the basis of anecdotal evidence that "if you've done it once, you can do it again"—though they'll still want to put you through the complete battery of tests to find out what's holding up conception this time around.

WILL IT BE HARD TO FIND DOCTORS WILLING TO WORK WITH US?

Not at all. The only factor that may limit your acceptance into certain infertility programs is age (many clinics have a cutoff of forty for women attempting IVF or GIFT).

How do we go about finding help?

The same as you would if seeking help in trying to have a first child (called *primary infertility*). When searching for the right specialist for you, be sure to ask the doctor about his experience in treating patients with secondary infertility. Ask what percentage of patients, approximately, fit this category. A doctor who does little besides ultrahigh-tech treatment for women who have never conceived may be inclined to view a secondary infertility case as a low priority. You will generally receive greater attention and feel more comfortable going to a practice that frequently works with patients like yourself.

Often it is only the woman in secondary infertility cases who seeks help. Men have a tendency to feel that, having fathered one child, their fertility has been proven for all time. Not so. Any number of conditions that can affect sperm production might have developed in the intervening years, and the only way to be sure is to have a sperm analysis done.

Options

All the treatments available to the couple with primary infertility will be available to those with secondary infertility. The chief difference usually lies in the response of the secondary infertility couple when hearing of those options. Whereas the couple without any children will often prefer the most aggressive program to attempt pregnancy, the couple who already have a child will generally be far more reluctant to embark on a program requiring daily shots and monitoring, or undergo surgery that must be followed by a long period of recovery. When you've got to spend a part of each morning getting your child up and dressed for school, it's hard to find time to get to those early-morning clinic appointments. When you have a small child, it can be even harder to make love at the time specified by your doctor. Before selecting a treatment approach, be sure to ask your doctor how each option would affect your life-style, including the time you normally spend each day taking care of your child.

Special considerations

The most common problem that secondary infertility patients report is the lack of understanding from friends, family, and colleagues. "You've already got a wonderful child," they tell you. "Why don't you just count

> $\mathcal{M}$y family had very little sympathy or interest in my miseries. They said, "You have one baby—why are you bothering with all this? Just enjoy your baby." I tried to educate them, but my medical problems are complex, and they didn't grasp enough about the subject even to ask the right questions.
>
> $\mathcal{J}$oan from Massachusetts

your blessings?" If it will bother you to hear these kinds of comments, then give special attention to keeping your treatment a secret. Or come up with some snappy retort to let people know you won't put up with any interference in your personal life. If you can't do either one, then be prepared to endlessly defend your right to use high-tech methods to try for more than one child.

The second most commonly reported problem is coping with feelings of separateness from other infertility patients you meet. The other women in the sonogram waiting room, the couples you meet at RE-SOLVE functions, and even many professional counselors will seem less than sympathetic. They think (and may even tell you to your face), "I'd be thrilled to pieces to have a child. I'd never go through all this if I already had one." After you've heard lines like these, it's easy to start feeling a little unwelcome in the waiting room (and sometimes even a little guilty for taking up your space). What may help is to spend some time among others in your situation. If there is a RESOLVE chapter near you, call to find out if there is a subgroup composed of couples with secondary infertility; attend the meetings and get the support you need from the only ones able to understand exactly how you feel.

If there is no secondary infertility support group in your area, start one!

Member of a Religion That Restricts or Forbids Fertility Treatment

Devout Roman Catholics who are infertile long to have children just as much as anyone else. So do Christian Scientists, Orthodox Jews, and Muslims, along with people of every other religious faith. But many believers are held back from treatment by the fear that any medical meddling with procreation runs counter to the tenets of their faith. The truth, however, is quite often different from what the couple thinks.

SECONDARY INFERTILITY CAN CAUSE SOME PRETTY TRICKY SITUATIONS!

*W*hen you are being treated for secondary infertility, your doctor probably doesn't stop to think how difficult it can be for you to make love at the time and date of his choosing. When you already have a young child in the house, it's not so easy anymore.

My wife had had her hCG shot at eleven P.M. and the doctor said we should have intercourse thirty-six hours later, which put it at eleven A.M. Our preschooler was home with the baby-sitter at the time, and neither of us liked the idea of going to the bedroom, locking the door, and trying to make love with our little girl playing in the next room—nor did we feel like explaining the situation to the sitter. So we decided to go to a nearby motel instead.

That might have been fine, except that the motel room we got was on a floor that the maids were cleaning at that hour. All while we were trying to enjoy ourselves we heard the deafening roar of an industrial-sized vacuum cleaner just outside the door. To make matters worse, we couldn't find a Do Not Disturb sign to hang on the doorknob. I wrote out the words in pencil on a piece of motel stationery, but then had no tape to stick the sign up with. I had to shove it in the doorjamb and hope it wouldn't fall down. Later on, at a crucial moment in our lovemaking, I heard the maids asking each other (in very loud voices) why that piece of paper was stuck in our door, and should they open the door to get the paper out. Fortunately for us, they decided not to!

We have learned some useful lessons from our little hotel adventure which I'd be glad to pass along.

1. If possible, find a *nice* hotel, with staff who can read signs.
2. Just in case you can't find a Do Not Disturb sign, bring along some paper, a marking pen, and a roll of Scotch tape.
3. When you check in, tell the desk clerk you've been driving all night and intend to go to sleep. Say you need a quiet room where you will be left alone.
4. Just to be on the safe side (so that no one jumps to the conclusion that you are bringing a hooker into the room!), bring along a small overnight bag or suitcase.
5. Turn the ringer off the phone, uncork the bottle of champagne you've brought along, and have fun!

*J*ay from New York

To find out how fertility treatment is regarded, theologically speaking, I conducted interviews with religious leaders from four very different faiths. I spoke to a Roman Catholic priest, an official of the Christian Science church, an Orthodox rabbi, and an expert on Islamic law. I asked questions about all forms of treatment, from simple use of fertility drugs to the ultrahigh-tech procedures such as embryo freezing and micromanipulation of sperm. I made a special point of finding out the official view of forms of treatment involving a third party, such as a donor of sperm or eggs, a host uterus, or surrogate mother.

I chose only the four religions mentioned above because there is not space enough to allow for discussion of how fertility treatment is viewed by leaders of the many hundreds of other faiths in the world. The four selected, however, do appear to reflect a broad range of attitudes toward the use of the medical arts in aid of reproduction. Though your own religion may not be represented here, you will very likely be able to find points of similarity between the views of the religious figures quoted here and those of leaders of your own faith. The sections below should at the very least serve to provide you with some points to cover when discussing the matter with the leader of the congregation you belong to.

Working within the moral boundaries imposed by your religion is quite different from working within the physical limitations imposed by your own body. Therefore the questions asked in this category must be different from those asked in the previous sections dealing with other types of patients. Instead of finding out *Can I be helped?* you need to know *Can help be arranged in a way that does not violate the teachings of my particular faith?* After answering this question separately for each of the four religions I researched, I will briefly consider three other questions of general interest to members of all faiths that place restrictions on fertility treatment. These three questions are *Will it be hard to find doctors willing to work with me? How do I go about finding help? Are there any considerations special to my situation that I should bear in mind?*

CAN HELP BE ARRANGED IN A WAY THAT DOES NOT VIOLATE THE TEACHINGS OF THE ROMAN CATHOLIC FAITH?

For an answer to this question I turned to Father James A. Coen, director of the Catholic Information Center located at the Catholic University of America in Washington, D.C. He told me that in Roman Catholic theological thinking there is no problem at all with the use of surgery or drugs to correct a physical defect in either the male or female reproductive tract. Nor is there any restriction on the use of fertility drugs to induce ovulation or bring about the production of multiple eggs per cycle.

The line as it is currently drawn forbids the use of any medical technology that brings about conception outside of the natural environment of the woman's body. Thus, IVF, GIFT, ZIFT, and other variants are not to be attempted by any Roman Catholics who wish to stay true to the teachings of their faith.

"What about artificial insemination of a wife by her husband's sperm?" I asked Father Coen. Technically, he informed me, such a procedure would be considered immoral, but as its intended purpose is to further procreation within a lawful marriage, few priests would consider it "a sin of any consequence."

Father Coen went on to add that there *are* some priests who would like to see the Church accept as morally permissible such procedures as IVF and GIFT—though those who now speak out in favor of such a doctrinal change are, in Father Coen's words, "singing outside the chorus." What I understood from Father Coen's remarks is that the devout Roman Catholic couple who have nevertheless decided to do IVF might well be able to find a priest who would not be disapproving of their quest—if they will only be persistent in their search for pastoral guidance.

Concerning the method a good Roman Catholic man should use to collect semen for laboratory analysis, Father Coen saw "no real moral dilemma" involved in the use of masturbation for such purpose. However, for those Roman Catholics who would prefer to avoid any occasion of sin, no matter how mitigating the circumstances, it is also possible to collect semen through the act of marital intercourse. The husband may withdraw just at the point of ejaculation and allow the semen to flow into a collection cup. Since a few drops of semen are always released just prior to ejaculation, and these drops theoretically could cause a pregnancy, the procreative nature of the sexual act is preserved, and sin avoided.

Concerning the use of a third party's sperm or eggs, Father Coen's words were strong and unambiguous. Involvement of a donor, whether male or female, he said, "interferes with the natural relationship of husband and wife." The use of a host uterus or a surrogate mother he characterized as "anathema" to the Church.

Though the ultrahigh-tech methods are unequivocally outside the realm of acceptability, it is clear that the devout Roman Catholic couple still has a large number of options for treatment available to them. It is also not unreasonable to think that at some time in the future, as some of those priests who are currently "singing outside the chorus" rise within the Church hierarchy, there could well be a reevaluation of some of the prohibitions, and that certain techniques (such as GIFT, which does not involve creation of human embryos in a lab dish) might well become available to members of the faith.

CAN HELP BE ARRANGED IN A WAY THAT DOES NOT VIOLATE THE TEACHINGS OF THE ORTHODOX JEWISH FAITH?

Rabbi Barry Freundel of Kesher Israel Congregation of Washington, D.C., was a source of much insight into the Orthodox Jewish view of infertility treatment. Bringing children into the world is recognized as one of the highest values in life for the Jewish married couple, so many forms of infertility treatment are not only accepted but, when needed, welcomed. There are no restrictions imposed on any drug treatments or surgeries intended to enhance the ability of the husband to father a child or the wife to conceive and carry one. If the normal act of intercourse cannot produce a child, there is no barrier to the practice of artificial insemination using the husband's sperm.

Collection of the sperm sample through masturbation, however, does present a problem. The observant couple should instead engage in intercourse and the semen collected from the woman's body afterward.*

If conventional treatments are unavailing, the couple may then turn to one of the assisted reproductive technologies for further attempts at conception. IVF, GIFT, ZIFT, and other variants using the wife's egg and husband's sperm are all accepted treatments.

All these forms of treatment require the woman to go to her doctor's office every morning for tests, for up to seven to ten days in a row, including the sabbath and religious holidays. I asked Rabbi Freundel if that would present the observant woman with a moral dilemma. Judaism permits violations of the sabbath for medical reasons that cannot be avoided, he answered, but "to the extent possible the woman should try to minimize" the violation. If her series of office visits happens to coincide with the time of the High Holy Days, then she should postpone treatment until the following cycle to fulfill her religious obligations.

"What about the use of third-party sperm or eggs?" I asked next. I was informed that these techniques raise many serious questions, although some Orthodox rabbis prefer a "lenient response" in such cases. If the couple are determined to go ahead, then they are advised to

---

*In fact, there is a brand of condom designed especially for use as a means to collect semen during intercourse. Called SCD and produced by the HDC Corporation of San Jose, California, it is available only by your doctor's prescription.

choose a Gentile donor whose identity is known. In order to have a wedding according to Jewish law the bride and groom must both be able to certify that there is no incest in the union. That would be an impossible requirement for the child of an anonymous donor to fulfill, because there would be no way to guarantee that that child was not a half-sibling of his or her intended spouse. The use of a known donor who is not Jewish seems the clearest way for the parents to protect the future marriageability of the child who will be born from a donor's egg or sperm. To ensure that the child of a Gentile donor will be recognized as Jewish, the child should undergo a conversion ceremony at a relatively young age.

Though steps may be taken to keep use of donor sperm or eggs within the boundaries of acceptability, there are no comparable measures to make either the use of a host uterus or a surrogate mother permissable under Jewish law. Rabbi Freundel explained that parenthood is "a relationship of responsibilities" and that to conceive a child with the intention of giving it away at birth violates the faith's most fundamental teachings about parental duty. Despite these two prohibitions, the Orthodox Jewish couple will still have an encouragingly wide range of treatment options available to them.

Can help be arranged in a way that does not violate the teachings of the Islamic faith?

For an informative response to this question I called the Islamic Center of Washington, D.C., and was referred to Mohamed Hagmagid, the center's librarian and an expert in Islamic law. I began by asking about the use of fertility drugs and/or surgery to help overcome the cause of infertility. Mr. Hagmagid replied that there was no restriction on the use of the medical arts to cure a physical problem.

I then explained the process of monitoring required when certain powerful infertility drugs are used. The woman must travel to her doctor's office each morning for up to ten days in a row, including religious holidays. "Would this schedule conflict with the woman's religious obligations?" I asked. His answer was no—she would simply need to make up her religious obligations on other days.

I next asked about the feasibility of continuing fertility treatment during Ramadan, the Muslim month of atonement. Since Muslims are required to abstain from all eating, drinking, and sexual activity during the daylight hours of the holy month, should the couple drop out of treatment until Ramadan is over? Not necessarily, according to Mr. Hagmagid. Although the couple must refrain from intercourse during the day, they are under no such restriction after sundown. "What if the man had to produce a sperm sample in the morning that would be used to artificially inseminate his wife later that same day?" I asked, and then was told that "The man cannot give sperm during the day—only at night."

As the subject of artificial insemination had already been raised, I next wanted to know whether there was any restriction on the method by which the sperm sample was obtained. The answer was no. Then I raised the question of artificial insemination by donor—was that permitted? No, that is not, Mr. Hagmagid replied, explaining that the involvement of any outsiders (other than medical doctors) in the creation of a child would be viewed as a violation of the essence of marriage under Koranic law. Following the same reasoning, egg donation, host uterus, and surrogate motherhood are all forbidden to the observant Muslim couple.

Next I asked about artificial methods of conception that use only sperm from the husband and eggs from the wife (such as IVF, GIFT, and ZIFT). "There is no problem with this kind of medical assistance," Mr. Hagmagid informed me.

Knowing of the traditional sexual segregation practiced by most Islamic societies, I asked whether it would violate the code of propriety for an infertile woman to be treated by a male doctor. An observant woman is allowed to accept medical treatment from a male doctor, Mr. Hagmagid observed, but "it would be better for her" to find a woman with the medical skills required.

Despite the few restrictions outlined above, Muslim couples have been among the most willing to try out new technologies to solve their infertility. At some of our most advanced treatment centers it is not at all unusual to see Muslim couples who have traveled to this country from Egypt, Saudi Arabia, Pakistan, Indonesia, and many other Muslim countries to avail themselves of the techniques that science has devised to help bring about conception for couples who would otherwise have no hope.

CAN HELP BE ARRANGED IN A WAY THAT DOES NOT VIOLATE THE TEACHINGS OF THE CHRISTIAN SCIENCE FAITH?

Mr. David Williams, a public information officer with the title of Federal Representative of the Christian Science Committee on Publications advised me as to the general views held by members of his faith. Christian

Science teaches that the healing of "all kinds of inharmonious bodily functions" is accomplished "through prayer alone." However, Mr. Williams quickly added that "the Church doesn't tell the practicing Christian Scientist what he may or may not do. The Church has no sanction."

I asked what would be the next step recommended for the couple who have been praying to have a baby but remain unable to conceive. Is there any form of treatment that might be considered "natural" and thus permissible?

Mr. Williams answered that the couple should keep praying and "stick with it—but if they come to believe that a medical procedure is justified, then they can do that." Although characterizing such medical intervention as "not consistent with Christian Science beliefs," Mr. Williams emphasized again that each Church member is free to follow the dictates of his individual conscience.

I remarked that I had in the past met believing Christian Scientists who wore glasses or used hearing aids. This suggested to me that infertile couples might be able to avail themselves of treatments that are accomplished through the wearing of a mechanical appliance. I had in mind the use of a testicular cooling device by a man whose infertility was caused by excessive testicular heat, or the use of a GnRH pump by a woman who needed additional hormonal support.

Mr. Williams explained that since glasses are not a cure for poor vision, nor are hearing aids a cure for partial deafness, these "temporary aids" are seen as acceptable. That struck me as an interesting and useful distinction for the Christian Science couple to consider. Many of the available forms of fertility treatment give a very temporary measure of relief at best. Taking drugs for five to ten days certainly does not "cure" anyone of infertility. The couple simply ends up with a reasonable chance to have conception occur within a very limited number of days each month, rather than no chance at all.

Though it seemed to me that the practicing Christian Scienctist couple could be able to fit certain forms of fertility treatment into their system of religious beliefs, it also seemed clear that they should not count on Church approval for the decision they have reached.

FOR MEMBERS OF ANY RELIGION THAT RESTRICTS FERTILITY TREATMENT:

WILL IT BE HARD TO FIND DOCTORS WILLING TO WORK WITH ME?

No, if you will simply explain to your doctor the nature of the religious restrictions you wish him to respect, he should be able to devise a treatment in accordance with your values and beliefs. It may not be the most effective treatment of all the technologies available, and the doctor may tell you so bluntly, but beyond giving you the medical facts, a good doctor will not pressure you to choose a treatment that you find unacceptable for religious reasons.

How do I go about finding help?

You will be at a distinct advantage if you have any friends of the same religion who have been through treatment before you. Find out where they went for help, and you will be sure to be getting a doctor who has had some experience in working with a couple of similar beliefs. If you don't know anyone who has been in treatment, you might try asking around, discreetly of course, as you meet other couples at social functions and other nonreligious activities sponsored by your church or religious institution. You will probably discover you don't have to search too hard to find someone else with your same problem.

Another approach (for those too shy to mention their infertility to casual acquaintances) would be to ask your regular doctor to make a recommendation. Perhaps he will even be able to refer you to a specialist of the same religion as you. If not, he will at least be familiar with your views and values and so have some insight as to the kind of personality most suited to your case.

Yet another way of finding the right doctor is through RESOLVE. Become active in your local chapter; you probably will meet some other couples through the organization who not only share your physical problem but your religious values as well. You could also place a "request for contact" in the RESOLVE newsletter describing the religious restrictions you are under and asking to hear from other couples who have successfully been treated in the same situation.

You may not want to spend much time soliciting the experiences of others. You might prefer to go at the problem immediately, and start setting up look-see consultations with doctors you have selected according to the general recommendations of Chapter Two. In addition to the normal list of questions you will bring, be sure to tell the doctor about any religious restrictions you would need to observe vis-à-vis your treatment, and see how he reacts. If he starts to argue with you over your religious views or seems annoyed to be told at the outset what treatment he can't use, then keep looking. But if he is respectful of your right to restrict what is done to your own body and if he is reassuring and optimistic about the treatment options that remain available to you, then go ahead and get started with your tests.

Special considerations

It could well turn out that the only medical treatment that would give you a reasonable chance to have a child would be one forbidden by your religion. Then you must search your own conscience and talk things through completely with your spouse. Ask yourself the following:

Could I live easily with my conscience if I went outside the dictates of my faith to try to have a child?

If I remained true to my faith and did not try this technique, would I always look back on my lost chance to conceive with regret?

If I went against the teachings of my faith and used this technique but still failed to conceive, would I end up feeling my childlessness was a punishment for my sin?

If I went against the teachings of my faith and used this technique to have a child, would I look upon my child with feelings of guilt over the manner of her or his conception, or perhaps even view my child as tainted because she or he was the product of a sinful act?

If you answered yes to the first two questions and no to the second two, then you will probably feel comfortable doing whatever is necessary to have a child, and worry about reconciling your religious beliefs with your actions afterward. But if you hesitated in your answers or were troubled by the questions, you should keep in mind that there are more ways to become a parent than through medical intervention. You can remain true to your beliefs and even help to extend them by adopting a child to whom you can pass on your religious values.

CHAPTER ELEVEN

PREGNANCY AFTER INFERTILITY

After one and a half years of IVF and GIFT, and five IUIs, I had been preparing for one more GIFT cycle, scheduled for January 8. I found out I was five weeks pregnant on January 6. No drugs, no IUI, nothing. We feel very blessed. I guess miracles *do* happen.

Marcia from New Jersey

Are You or Aren't You?

It's been two weeks since the date of ovulation. Your doctor said your egg follicles looked good on the ultrasound. Sperm quality was also fine. Everything seems to be going according to plan. Every day before you get up you take your temperature. It's still high, above 98.3°. You're beginning to feel a little strange. . . . Is it the aftereffects of the drugs you've been taking, or could it possibly be that you're pregnant? You're starting to get hopeful, but at the same time trying not to think about it, and worrying about how let down you will feel if this time, just like last time, nothing happens.

When you've hung on for as long as you can, then you're ready to take your first home pregnancy test. You go to the drugstore and start reading all the information on the back of the test boxes. Some say you can test the same day of an expected period, others say test the first day after you would expect your period; some say test anytime during the day, others say use only your first morning urine. One brand costs $15, another is $13.50, and then there's the brand that offers two days' tests for $26. Which one should you buy and what day should you start?

As far as accuracy goes, they all are fairly good—every brand on the shelf claims over 99 percent accuracy in laboratory tests. As for timing, I recommend waiting at least fifteen days after your LH surge. If you were given a single shot of hCG to trigger ovulation, then test on the fifteenth day after the shot. If given a series of hCG shots as a form of treatment, *do not use a home pregnancy test kit;* the home tests all work by detecting the level of hCG in your urine, and so if you have recently had a shot, you will *always* test positive, whether you are pregnant or not. Regardless of what it says on the test package, test your first morning urine—the concentration of hCG will be strongest then (unless you had something to drink or got up to urinate in the early-morning hours). If not using first morning urine, then try to go at least four hours without urinating or drinking anything before you test.

The various brands of tests take different times to perform and have different advantages and disadvantages. To help you decide which type to buy I purchased eight of the most popular and widely available brands and tried each out. My findings are recorded on the table on pages 404–405.

Now let's suppose you've just done your first pregnancy test. Let's say you're using the one that shows you a plus sign if you're pregnant and a minus sign if you're not. Well, the horizontal line of the plus sign is there, all right, but the vertical line . . . it's hard to say. You can just barely make out where that line *would* be if it was going to be anywhere. What does that mean? You call the toll-free number included in the instructions and you ask that question of the registered nurse who answers the phone. She tells you that you *could* be pregnant, but to be sure, wait forty-eight hours and test yourself again.

Sure. You're supposed to just hang around biting your nails for another two days. Well, you know just what you're going to do. You will run out to the nearest drugstore and buy two or three more test kits. You will hold in your pee for four or five hours if you have to, and try again just before your bladder bursts. Maybe this time the brand you're using will be a little more sensitive. Maybe in the last six hours your hCG level will have risen enough to make the results more readable. Maybe this time you will count off the three-minute waiting time precisely to the second, and that will make a difference.

But after you do all that you find you still get another ambiguous result. Better to wait until evening before you retest. Or better yet, test again the next morning, with your first urine of the day. If you *are* pregnant, your hCG level will double every forty-eight hours, and so by twenty-four hours later, your level should be 50 percent higher— and perhaps just high enough to give you a definite yes or no.

If your second test looks positive—even if the positive indicator is still extremely faint—call your doctor at once and schedule an hCG test of blood taken from your vein. Blood tests are extremely sensitive, and can sometimes pick up a detectable level of hCG only twelve or thirteen days after ovulation. Go in early in the morning so that the blood sample will be ready in time for the early pick up for the lab (assuming that your doctor sends his lab work out, rather than using an in-office lab). You should be able to find out your results that same afternoon.

If your doctor uses a blood lab that does not give same-day results, complain to him about the slowness. There is no good reason why your doctor can't work with a lab that is able to perform this very quick and simple test and have results back the same day. If it turns out that you must wait more than a day for your results, then you might start think-ing about going someplace else that is more efficiently run. The few hours you wait each month to find out if your treatment worked can seem like the longest time in your life. Compassionate doctors under-stand this and will put the term *stat* (meaning "rush") on their infertility patients' pregnancy tests to make sure that the lab technicians speed the news to you as soon as possible.

Finding the Right OB

The phone rings. It's your fertility specialist. He sounds jolly from the very first syllable of his hello. He says he has your test results back from the lab. Your heart is in your throat, until you hear him pronounce the words: "Congratulations! You are pregnant!"

Okay . . . now what?

You need an obstetrician—and not just any obstetrician. You need one who is used to treating pregnant former infertility patients. You need one who won't be impatient with your anxieties, your gnawing fear of miscarriage, your endless list of questions, and your acting as if you are the only woman in the world who has ever had this experience before.

If your fertility specialist is also an OB-GYN and you have been happy with that doctor's care, then you will probably want to stay with him. But if his practice is limited to infertility, or if you thought him highly skilled at infertility treatment but think you would be happier with a different sort of personality (perhaps someone with a friendlier manner) for the next nine months' worth of appointments, then by all means ask for a recommendation to see someone else. Be very specific if you can about what you are looking for. Younger or older? Male or female? Are you interested only in a graduate of a top medical school? Do you

COMPARISONS OF PREGNANCY TESTS

BRAND OF TEST	Number of Steps	Total Test Time	Positive Indicator	When to Test	Remarks
First Response*	4	2 min.	Pink circle appears in test well	Day of missed period; anytime during that day	A very faint pink result may be ambiguous, since test does not provide a "color comparison area"
Fact Plus	1	5 min.	Plus sign appears in test well	Day of missed period; anytime during that day	Thirty min. after test is completed, a negative result might turn faintly positive, causing false hope
QTest	6	17 min.	Bottom pad of test stick turns blue	Day of missed period; anytime during that day	Though this test requires more steps and takes longer, I found it the most sensitive of the ones I tested. It detected my pregnancy with a clearly positive result the day *before* my missed period
1-Step Advance	2	5 min.	Double pink line appears in test window	Day of missed period; anytime during that day	Simple to perform and relatively quick result that is easy to interpret

(continued)

BRAND OF TEST	Number of Steps	Total Test Time	Positive Indicator	When to Test	Remarks
Answer Quick & Simple	4	3 min.	Lower dot on test stick turns pink	Day after missed period; anytime during that day	Easiest test to interpret. Has comparison window to show what negative color looks like, and control window that turns red to let you know you have performed test correctly. One drawback: It's hard to fill urine dropper to exact amount shown on line
Clearblue Easy	1	3 min.	Blue line appears in test window	Day of missed period; use first A.M. urine	No urine collection cup. You urinate on end of test stick. Test is invalid if you get any urine on test window
E-P-T	1	4 min.	Pink circle appears in test window	Day of missed period; anytime during that day	No urine collection cup. You urinate into tiny test cap. Easy to miss or invalidate test by getting urine on test window
1-Step First Response	1	3 min.	Pink line in test window	Day of missed period; wait at least one hour after last urination	No urine collection cup. You urinate on end of test stick—but there is no chance of splashing urine on the test window because it is covered with a clear protective tape

*An identical test by the same manufacturer is sold under the brand name Answer Plus.

only want someone in a group practice? Before you ask your fertility doctor for a recommendation, draw up a list of the qualities in an OB that are most important to you.

Whoever you see should have experience in dealing with "high risk" cases. Now, don't panic at the use of the term "high risk." The great majority of pregnant former infertility patients will enjoy a perfectly normal pregnancy. But you *are* in a different category from someone whose reproductive system is more easily able to conceive. This pregnancy is extra-precious to you because it could well be the only one you will have. You need a doctor who knows all the very latest techniques that can be used to try to preserve a pregnancy at the first sign of trouble.

It will also be important to choose someone whose office is located in a convenient place and who has coverage for all hours of the day, seven days a week, so that you can get a fast response in case of emergency. If your fertility specialist cannot name someone who fits your main criteria, then you could try asking infertile friends who have been pregnant about their OBs, or you might call RESOLVE to get the name of a suitable doctor who has often treated former infertility patients.

You should doctor-shop for your OB with the same care you brought to your search for your infertility doctor. Ask plenty of questions over the phone before making an appointment. You might even want to make appointments to meet more than one doctor, and then select the one you feel would be most compatible with your personality.

What should you ask at your first visit to help you decide if this OB is for you? You will want the doctor to answer your questions on the following subjects:

- scheduling of appointments, frequency of appointments
- coverage for off-hours and during the doctor's vacation
- what hospital(s) are used for labor and delivery
- what to do in an emergency
- handling of routine questions—whom to call and when
- doctor's past experience with infertility patients
- doctor's past experience with older first-time mothers (if applicable)
- rate of cesarean section in doctor's practice
- doctor's views on the use of anesthesia, fetal monitors, and episiotomy during childbirth
- genetic fetal testing: who should be tested? when and where are tests performed?
- views on prenatal vitamins, nutrition, exercise

- doctor's experience with patients with complications (e.g., pre-eclampsia, placenta previa, gestational diabetes)

After you have found someone you feel is right for you, make sure she gets a complete case history of your infertility treatment, including all drugs taken (during all past cycles as well as this last cycle), any reproductive-tract operations you have undergone, and information about any past miscarriages or ectopic pregnancies.

You will probably see your OB no more than once every four weeks at the start—unless you feel something out of the ordinary is happening. Then you should call right away to see if a same-day appointment is needed to check out your symptoms. Your doctor will undoubtedly brief you on what to look out for, but certainly any vaginal bleeding (even if it's only slight spotting) should be reported right away, as should any lower abdominal pain or cramping or any colored or profuse vaginal discharge.

The Critical First Three Months

The first twelve weeks of pregnancy are called the *first trimester,* and it is the time of most rapid change in your developing baby. It goes from a pinpoint-sized bundle of cells to a tiny version of a human being, attached to its own life-support unit, called the *placenta,* within your womb. All its major organs are well on their way to being formed. It is also during this time that 85 percent of all miscarriages occur. Of course you will find that statistic worrisome, but just keep in mind that once you have safely passed the first-trimester mark, your chance of miscarriage has decreased by 85 percent. To show how you would figure your new, reduced odds of miscarriage, let's say that you have learned that 30 percent of all pregnancies conceived with the help of the fertility drug you took will end in miscarriage. After the first trimester you can figure 85 percent of 30 (25.5) and then subtract that number from 30 to arrive at the miscarriage rate of a mere 4.5 percent for women like you in their thirteenth week of pregnancy or later.

Most often when a first-trimester miscarriage occurs, nothing can be done to prevent it. A mistake in the genetic code conveyed by either the egg or the sperm is the cause, and the embryonic tissue simply ceases to develop as it should. But assuming that the forces of random selection have created a genetically normal embryo, then the new life will be spending this time establishing itself inside your womb, taking nourishment from your body, and rapidly doubling and redoubling in size until it becomes (somewhere between twenty-four and twenty-eight weeks gestational age) *viable*—that is to say, capable of surviving outside your womb. You want to do everything possible to make your uterus into the sort of environment that will foster the baby's growth and good health.

Women who can conceive easily probably will think you are being overconcerned, or even paranoid about your pregnancy, but they didn't go through what you went through to get to this point. It may be okay for other pregnant women to keep jogging five miles a day, or work overtime at nights and on weekends, or have a couple of cups of caffeinated coffee a day, but you will want to be more cautious. To give yourself maximum peace of mind, you will probably want to take it easy as much as possible during the first trimester. That means no strenuous exercise, only low-impact aerobics and other activities as approved by your OB; no sports with risk of falling (no rock climbing, bicycling, gymnastics, or horseback riding); and no raising your heartbeat above 140 beats per minute while exercising.*

And, like all other pregnant women, you will be advised to

- abstain from alcohol
- quit smoking and try to avoid others' smoke
- restrict or eliminate your intake of caffeine (which is in coffee, tea, and cola drinks)
- avoid all prescription and over-the-counter medicines unless specifically approved by your OB
- eat a well-rounded diet, avoiding excessive sugar and fat
- drink eight glasses of liquid a day
- get plenty of folic acid (found in green, leafy vegetables and essential for normal brain and spinal development)
- take prenatal vitamins as directed by your OB (don't take vitamins on your own, and especially avoid megadoses of any vitamin)
- avoid airplane travel, if practical (the greater radiation levels at high altitudes increase risk to fetal development); if you must fly, keep the number and length of trips to a minimum
- avoid dental X rays
- get plenty of sleep

When you know you have been taking care of yourself, even if something does go wrong, you can be assured that nothing you did was the cause. Miscarriage is, unfortunately, a common event. You need to un-

---

*During a break in your exercise routine, take your pulse for ten seconds and multiply the result by six. If your pulse count is above twenty-three, then reduce the tempo of your exercise pace.

derstand that *it's not your fault.* Despite all our wonderful scientific advances, we still know very little about the early weeks of pregnancy—why one embryo develops perfectly when another will not.

However, science has given us a few techniques to help us unravel the mysteries of nature. Genetic testing is now in widespread use, allowing us to find out if the fetus has been affected by such diseases as Down's Syndrome, Tay-Sachs disease, sickle-cell anemia, thalassemia, cystic fibrosis, Huntington's disease, and a host of other hereditary illnesses. Either an amniocentesis or a CVS (stands for *chorionic villae sampling*) will be recommended for the pregnant women over age thirty-five or when there is any family history to indicate a need for testing. In many obstetrical practices the CVS test, usually performed between nine and eleven weeks, has all but come to replace the older test, amniocentesis, which cannot be performed until several weeks later (usually between fourteen and nineteen weeks gestational age). Fetal tissue for CVS testing is obtained by taking a tiny scraping from the inside of the uterus; the results take about a week to come in. The sample for amniocentesis is obtained by inserting a needle through the woman's abdomen, and inside the amniotic sac and drawing about an ounce of fluid out; results can take two to three weeks to come back.

Which test should you have? There is no question in my mind that a former fertility patient should *not* have a CVS, but should choose amniocentesis instead. Why? The rate of miscarriage after CVS is between 1 and 5 percent, depending on the skills of the person performing the procedure. Amniocentesis in skilled hands has a miscarriage rate of 0.5 to 1 percent. That means that CVS is *two to ten times more likely to result in miscarriage.* If you felt assured that you could easily get pregnant again, then you might prefer to take the higher risk of miscarriage in order to have the genetic testing completed and results in hand early in your pregnancy. That way if the news is bad, and you chose to end your pregnancy rather than bring a seriously impaired or terminally ill child into the world, you would be spared the additional trauma of a second-trimester abortion. But the woman who knows it will not be easy to get pregnant again will think less about the potential tragedy of a late abortion than the here-and-now increased threat of miscarriage. After all, the risk of Down's Syndrome, even if you are in your late thirties, is still only about one in a hundred—still lower than the risk of miscarriage from the average CVS.

Before making a decision on this very sensitive ethical and emotional issue, you should, of course, talk over the pros and cons carefully and completely with your husband and your OB, and then do what *you* feel is the right thing for you.

Coping with the Fear of Miscarriage

Though you are taking excellent care of yourself and you keep reminding yourself that the great majority of pregnant former infertility patients go on to have healthy deliveries, you may still find yourself worrying a lot. It's only natural—you suffered so much to get to where you are now, and if anything goes wrong, you're not sure you'll ever be able to conceive again. Every little twinge makes you think about premature labor. Every time you hear other women talk about their pregnancies, they're always bringing up some new danger, some new thing to worry about. Newspapers, magazines, and TV new reports seem to be full of announcements from scientists that this or that environmental hazard or drug will cause miscarriage or birth defects. How are you ever going to make it through the next nine months and still be sane? Here are ten strategies for coping:

1. *Feel good about feeling bad.* If you're waking up with terrible nausea each morning and generally feeling rotten for the rest of the day, take heart: you have a fairly reliable indicator that all is going well with your pregnancy. Studies have shown that women who experience nausea and other discomforts during pregnancy are extrasensitive to the hormones secreted in pregnancy. Therefore you know that your hormone levels are steadily rising as they should, and that your fetus is developing well.

2. *Feel good about feeling good.* But what if you never have a moment of morning sickness? What if you feel absolutely normal, and you don't have any sense that big changes are going on inside you? Does that mean that nothing is happening? Not at all. You just aren't as sensitive as some to your changing hormone levels. If your blood tests show that your hormone levels are rising as they should in early pregnancy, that's all you need to know. Enjoy the early months before your increased girth begins to slow you down. If anything was wrong, you'd feel cramping or see spotting or show some other sign, but as long as you feel all right, then you can trust that you *are* all right.

3. *Keep your mind focused on the present.* If you *must* worry, then limit your worries to the stage you are in at the moment. Don't start thinking about things that can go wrong in the second trimester when you're still in your first. Don't even start reading about labor and delivery until you're past the first sixteen weeks. And abso-

lutely avoid doing anything early on to prepare your home for the arrival of a baby. Don't order any nursery furniture till you're at least twenty-four weeks along; don't start arguing over names until you're at least at the point at which you can feel the baby move and can begin to think of it as a distinct personality (and possibly know what sex it is, too).

4. *Tell those you think will be supportive, and don't tell anyone else.* You know what your friends and family are like. If you think anyone is likely to say thoughtless things or in any way add to your worries, then postpone giving that person the news for as long as possible. But those you can count on to say just the right thing, who will share your joy and help alleviate your fears, can be informed as soon as you'd like. Just be sure that they know whom they're allowed to tell, and whom they're not.

5. *Keep control of the flow of events.* You don't want to feel pushed around too much during this very emotionally charged time of your life. Already, much of what will happen in the next nine months is beyond your control; you need to keep a strong grip on those things that are still left up to you. That means that you won't agree to requests from your boss to fill in for an absent coworker on a date that is not good for you, nor will you let yourself be drafted to organize your civic association's annual block party if you don't have the time or the energy for it, nor will you run errands or do other favors for friends and acquaintances if they conflict with your own inclinations. Now is a good time to be a little selfish—nine months from now you'll be spending more than enough of your time putting someone else's needs ahead of your own.

6. *Have confidence in your doctor.* If miscarriage does threaten, remember that a highly skilled doctor will be able to take many steps to save your pregnancy. There are safe, highly effective drugs that your doctor can give you to supplement your hormone production or suppress premature labor. Your doctor can put a stitch in your cervix to keep it from opening up before it's time. Or he can check you into the hospital so that your condition can be monitored closely and immediate steps taken if a miscarriage seems to be in progress. Just be sure you know how to get in touch with the doctor at all hours in case anything does seem to be going wrong (memorize your doctor's emergency off-hours number!) and don't be shy to call at the first sign of distress. Your OB would *want* you to!

7. *Reassure yourself with facts.* Did you know that once a fetal heart-beat has been detected by ultrasound, 94 percent of all pregnancies proceed to a safe delivery? Did you know that an older mother who has undergone genetic fetal screening has no greater chance to have a baby with a birth defect than a younger mother does? Did you know that over 80 percent of the women who have had one miscarriage will go on to deliver healthy babies (as will 75 percent of those who have had two miscarriages)? When you read pregnancy books and magazine articles, look for facts that boost your confidence. There is no shortage of studies proving that pregnancy after infertility tends to be a normal, uneventful experience.

8. *Pamper yourself.* If you never found time to relax and take a nice vacation while you were in infertility treatment, do it now, before the baby comes and there's very little time to yourself at all. Since you're no longer paying big bills for infertility treatment, use some of the money that might have gone for one more Pergonal cycle to book a room at a quiet, cozy inn somewhere. Enjoy sex whenever you like, without having to consult a calendar or call your nurse for permission. Sleep late or take afternoon naps. Indulge yourself in whatever little ways you like. You'll feel more relaxed, and when you're relaxed, you tend to be optimistic and free of worry.

9. *Use relaxation techniques.* If a nice back rub or a weekend in the country is just not enough to keep your mind off your fear of miscarriage, then you need stronger measures to help you cope. I talked to one patient who saw a hypnotist to help her work through her fear of miscarriage. Others have benefited from relaxation techniques learned in meditation classes, or have read books describing how you can get your brain to produce more calming alpha waves, or tried floating in water in an isolation tank. If there is any physical effort involved, just make sure your OB okays the activity.

10. *Join a support group.* RESOLVE, as always, can be a great resource. Your local chapter may already have a subgroup made up of former infertility patients who are now pregnant, who meet to socialize and give each other support and advice. Many couples have found belonging to such a group the perfect way to work through their fears. You always feel better when you know you are not alone in your situation but among people who understand and don't need everything spelled out for them in capital letters.

How Many Are There?

Pregnant former infertility patients differ from other pregnant women in at least one important way. They are much more at risk for multiple gestation—that is, for having twins, triplets, or more. The rate is 20 percent for users of Pergonal, with 80 percent of those multiple births being twins. The rate for users of Clomid is just 6 percent. Though it is more of a strain on the body to carry twins, oftentimes pregnant patients are thrilled at the news because they always wanted to have more than one child, and now know they won't have to go through treatment again to have another.

If the woman has been properly monitored while taking potent fertility drugs, the risk of having a number larger than triplets should be very small. Responsible doctors in charge of IVF or ZIFT cycles should not put back more than four viable embryos in your uterus or fallopian tubes (only rarely will all four "take"). If you are simply taking fertility drugs and your ovaries respond by producing too many eggs, or your blood test indicates too high an estradiol level, your doctor can simply cancel the cycle by withholding the ovulation-triggering shot of hCG. The couple should abstain from intercourse for several days to avoid the chance of a large number of eggs fertilizing and starting a pregnancy of quadruplets or more.

Despite these precautions, occasionally four or more embryos will implant and grow. Such a pregnancy is not only difficult for the mother to carry without endangering her health, it is dangerous for the fetuses as well. Virtually all multiple gestations of more than triplets will result in extremely premature birth, with consequent, usually serious, problems of insufficient development of the babies' lungs, brains, digestive tracts, and other organs. Stillbirth is also a distressingly frequent outcome.

To prevent such a tragedy, the woman pregnant with four or more embryos may be advised to undergo a procedure known by the rather horrible euphemism of *selective reduction*. It's difficult for both doctors and patients to state straight out what the procedure really is: an abortion done on several of the fetuses so that the remaining ones (usually twins or triplets) will have a chance to continue to develop normally, without endangering the mother's health.

Very few doctors in this country are trained to perform this type of abortion, and if you do not happen to live near one of the major hospital centers where such doctors practice, then you will have to travel, possibly some distance, to find a doctor who is both skilled and willing to help you.

Because of the medical necessity of abortion in this situation, IVF and other ART patients should be warned in advance of the possibility (though remote) that they may have to undergo the procedure. Patients who are unable to contemplate the destruction of any of their fetuses in order to secure the birth of two or three probably should not participate in a drug-stimulated ART cycle. Even for a woman who ends up with healthy twins, the trauma and heartbreak of having to lose any of her deeply wanted offspring will be emotionally devastating.

Fortunately, the situation described above is rare. Most women pregnant after fertility treatment will have a sonogram at about six weeks' gestation, during which the sonographer should be able to discern the embryonic sac and tell you if there is more than one. The sonogram is the most reassuring evidence you can get early on that you will have a normal pregnancy. You can even observe the embryo's heartbeat, which appears as a tiny flickering light on the dark screen. Seeing this miraculous sight is enough to make you think that all you went through to get to this point was well worth it, and give you confidence that the remainder of your pregnancy will be a happy, healthy, rewarding experience.

Parenthood After Infertility

For infertility patients, parenting is different than for ordinary couples. Quite possibly your baby will be an only child. You may well be older than most of the other parents of infants that you meet. Your baby may be treasured, worshiped, and worried over to excess. If you and your spouse are in your late thirties or forties, your own parents are more likely to be deceased, and so your child may have little extended family to advise and help out the new parents. In these circumstances it is easy to get the sense that you are alone when coping with the everyday challenges and difficulties of parenthood.

These are all things for the pregnant infertile couple to consider. You may not necessarily experience any of them; I mention them now because if you've come this far, you are probably ready to start turning to some other books for advice. There is a book, *The Long-Awaited Stork,* by Ellen Sarasohn Glazer, written especially for former infertility patients who are now parents, and I highly recommend it.

In one way (at least for me) the infertility treatment experience made my job as a new mother much easier. It was no hardship for me to adjust to the routines involved in caring for a newborn baby (diapering, night feedings, dealing with spit-up, etc.) because those chores were nothing compared to the chores involved in bringing about her conception (the nights spent mixing and receiving injections, and the pre-dawn hours spent driving to the clinic for monitoring, and the times I spent on the examining table having my uterus scraped and prodded during tests). Other women might groan to hear the baby cry at two in the morning; to me it was the most beautiful sound in the world.

Becoming a parent through infertility treatment seems to be a guarantee that you will never take your child for granted. I am constantly awed by the miracle of my daughter's existence, and one day I intend for her to learn (in exhaustive detail, if she's interested) just how science worked to bring her into being.

CONCLUSION

After spending the past year talking and listening to former and current infertility patients from all over the United States, I have come to believe the following about fertility treatment: that it is, on the whole, painful (both physically and emotionally), much too expensive, far too often unproductive, and unfortunately in many cases practiced by doctors who are uncaring, greedy, insufficiently skilled, and/or outright incompetent.

Having said all that, it seems to follow that I would not recommend it for anyone. But that is not my conclusion. For the couple who are willing and able to undertake the risks and difficulties to have a baby, treatment will certainly be worth trying. But *only* if you are willing to do some work. You've got to be well prepared. If you do your research, if you know what to expect in the way of tests and treatments, if you know how to search for a good doctor (and are willing to switch doctors if your first choice turns out to be a mistake), if you exercise prudent judgment and common sense about your care (and do not simply defer to the doctor on the assumption that he knows best), and if above all you *listen to your own instincts,* question anything that causes you concern, and keep a close guard on your own rights and dignity, then you should be able to emerge from the treatment process knowing that you did everything possible to give yourself the best odds of having a baby through medical intervention.

If treatment works to bring a baby into your life, you will never doubt that what you went through was worth it. If it doesn't, then you will be able to move on to your chosen nonmedical alternative secure in the knowledge that you are following the right course for you at the right time.

One thing I asked of all the women and men that I interviewed or surveyed: if you were to meet someone who has just discovered a fertility problem, what one piece of advice would you give that person? Former patients were remarkably united in their responses: virtually everyone (with a handful of exceptions) gave one of the three pieces of advice listed below. They are

Number One: See a fertility specialist. Don't waste time with your regular OB-GYN or internist. Find a clinic that does infertility and only infertility; have all the tests and procedures you need done by someone whose livelihood and reputation depend on good success rates. My respondents were full of regret for months (in many cases, years) wasted seeing someone who misdiagnosed the problem or prescribed inadequate or incorrect treatment.

Number Two: Use the resources of RESOLVE. My respondents got much more than emotional support from this volunteer self-help network. They got doctor referrals, information, ideas for new approaches, as well as companionship of others in the same situation, bringing an end to their feelings of isolation and despair.

Number Three: Educate yourself. Read medical journals, follow any news about infertility in the general media, learn to understand doctors' jargon, be assertive and unafraid to criticize aspects of your treatment. My interviewees told story after story of confronting doctors who had done something wrong, and receiving more attentive care as a result.

To these three points I add my own piece of advice: *Decide in advance how much of your life you will spend in pursuit of a medical solution.* Set a reasonable time limit, given your age, personality, physical condition, and number of years of marriage or relationship. Remind yourself frequently that the ordeal is finite, and you will find it easier to live through.

One way or another your time spent wandering in the netherworld of infertility will come to an end. You will become pregnant and have a child, or you will successfully adopt a child, or you will make a decision to consider your life complete without taking on the full-time responsibility of parenthood.

When you have finally put your infertility behind you, by whatever method, you can be said to have become "resolved." That's the idea behind the name of the RESOLVE organization, and it's what all couples who are working on their infertility problem should be trying to achieve. Yes, for most of us it will be a long and difficult road, but it is also one that takes us along a path of self-realization, making us aware of what is truly important in our lives.

Whatever the outcome, if you emerge from your journey a more thoughtful, compassionate person, one who is capable of appreciating the awesome mystery surrounding the creation of a new life, then you can tell yourself that what you did was worthwhile, and in that sense, your quest was truly a success.

GLOSSARY

All **boldfaced** terms used within definitions are also listed as separate glossary items.

Adhesion Scar tissue that forms a joint between structures in the abdominal cavity, such as scar tissue connecting the fallopian tube to the ovary.

Agglutination Clumping together of sperm, which makes the sperm unable to swim well.

AI/D Artificial insemination by donor.

AI/H Artificial insemination by sperm from the recipient's husband.

Amenorrhea Medical term meaning "not having menstrual periods."

Androgens Male sex hormones.

Anovulation Medical diagnosis of female infertility, meaning, "not ovulating" (not producing an egg).

Antisperm antibodies A diagnosis of infertility based on the finding that chemical substances are being produced that either attack the sperm and leave it incapable of fertilizing an egg, or create hostile conditions in the cervical mucus, making it impossible for sperm to swim through it.

ART *See* **Assisted reproductive technology**

Aspiration Medical term for "sucking out," as when fluid is sucked out of a follicle during the egg-retrieval stage of an IVF procedure.

Assisted reproductive technology (ART) Any of several procedures to bring about conception without sexual intercourse. ARTs include IVF, GIFT, ZIFT, POST, and PROST, as well as any other alphabet-soup combinations that may be developed in the future.

Azoospermia Medical diagnosis of male infertility, meaning, "not producing any sperm."

BABI *See* **Blastomere analysis before implantation**

Basal body temperature (BBT) The temperature of the body at its lowest point of the day, just upon waking. Normal BBT is "biphasic," that is, having a low phase (during menstruation until the time of ovulation) and a high phase (after ovulation and just prior to the onset of menstruation).

BBT *See* **Basal body temperature**

Bicornuate Divided into two parts; a medical term used to refer to a uterine abnormality.

Blastomere analysis before implantation (BABI) A test for genetic diseases that is performed on a four- or eight-celled pre-embryo that has been created in a laboratory dish after an IVF or ZIFT cycle. BABI was first performed in England in 1991 as a means for parents who carried the hemophilia gene to avoid the risk of having to abort a fetus that was found to have the defect. After the results of a BABI test, only the genetically normal embryos are implanted, so that the parents are assured, even before pregnancy begins, that the child will not have a genetic disease.

Cervical cerclage An in-office surgical procedure used to help prevent miscarriage, in which the doctor puts a stitch or two in the cervix to prevent it from opening up and starting premature labor.

Cervix The part of the uterus that extends down into the vagina, and which has an opening (called the os) through which sperm may enter or through which menstrual fluid may exit.

Chlamydia A sexually transmitted disease caused by the bacterium *Chlamydia trachomatis*. The disease can lead to infertility in women.

Clomid The brand name of clomiphene citrate, a commonly prescribed fertility drug. Also marketed under another brand name, **Serophene.**

Corpus luteum The name given to the egg follicle after ovulation, when it turns a yellowish color (*corpus luteum* is Latin for "yellow body") and produces the hormone **progesterone.**

Cryopreservation A technique of preservation of embryos, sperm, or other tissue, by dehydration and freezing.

Cul-de-sac The name for the space located between the uterus and the rectum.

Danazol A drug (brand name: Danocrine) commonly prescribed as a treatment for **endometriosis.**

D and C Universally used abbreviation for the procedure *dilation and curettage,* in which the cervix is dilated and the contents of the uterus are removed (for example, following a miscarriage).

DES *See* **Diethylstilbestrol**

Diethylstilbestrol (DES) A drug often prescribed in the 1950s as a miscarriage preventative, which frequently caused damage to the reproductive organs of the daughters (and sometimes the sons) born to the women who took it.

Dyspareunia Medical term for "painful intercourse." Often used by doctors when questioning patients about a possible diagnosis of endometriosis. Example: Instead of asking the patient, "Does it hurt when you have sex?" the doctor will say, "Have you ever experienced dyspareunia?"

Ectopic pregnancy Medical term for a pregnancy that is "out of place"—that is, somewhere other than the uterus, usually in the fallopian tube, but occasionally elsewhere in the abdominal cavity.

Electroejaculation A process that can be used in many cases to allow a man who is paralyzed below the waist to produce a semen sample that can be used in artificial insemination.

EMB *See* **Endometrial biopsy**

Embryo transfer The movement of embryos that have been created in a test tube (or laboratory dish), whether fresh or thawed after **cryopreservation,** to the uterus (or fallopian tubes) of a woman who desires to become pregnant.

Embryo transplant An **ART** in which one woman becomes pregnant through artificial insemination with the sperm of another woman's husband, and then the resulting embryo is flushed out of her uterus and transferred to the uterus of the wife who wishes to become pregnant and give birth to her husband's genetic offspring.

Endometrial biopsy (EMB) A test performed to check for **luteal-phase defect** by taking a small tissue sample from the lining of the uterus and analyzing it to see if it is "in phase"—that is, at the proper thickness for the day of the menstrual cycle on which it was obtained.

Endometriosis A disease of uncertain cause occurring when overgrowths of menstrual tissue are found outside the uterus, usually around the ovaries and fallopian tubes. Symptoms include painful menstrual periods, pain during intercourse, and painful bowel movements, though in some cases the patient is completely unaware of the presence of the disease.

Endometrium The medical term for the lining of the uterus. The endometrium is normally built up with nutrients, hormones, and blood during the latter half of the menstrual cycle. If pregnancy does not occur, much of the lining is shed in the form of menstruation.

Epididymis The long, coiled tube behind the testicles where sperm are stored.

Epididymitis Inflammation of the epididymis caused by an infection, a possible source of male infertility.

Estradiol A form of **estrogen.** The blood test most commonly used to measure estradiol is called "E_2—Rapid Assay." (If you are being **monitored** while on Pergonal or any other fertility drug, you will probably undergo many tests for estradiol blood levels.)

Estrogen The principal female sex hormone.

Fallopian tubes The tubes that extend from the uterus toward the ovaries. At least one open fallopian tube is necessary for fertilization to occur naturally in a woman's body.

Fibroid tumor A benign (noncancerous) growth found in the uterus, commonly associated with miscarriage or infertility.

Fimbria The finger-like projections at the ends of the fallopian tubes that reach out and grab the egg after it has been released from the ovary, sweeping it into the fallopian tube.

Follicle A fluid-filled sac inside the ovary that contains an egg.

Follicle-stimulating hormone (FSH) A hormone produced by the pituitary gland which in women causes the egg follicle to develop and in men stimulates the production of sperm.

Follicular phase The phase of the menstrual cycle prior to ovulation, during which a new egg is developing within its follicle and is being prepared to be released. Normally the follicular phase takes between twelve and fourteen days.

FSH *See* **Follicle-stimulating hormone**

Gamete Scientific term for a reproductive cell (an egg or a sperm).

Gamete intrafallopian transfer (GIFT) An **ART** in which eggs are removed from the ovaries, mixed with sperm, and reinserted in the woman's fallopian tubes during a minor surgical procedure.

GIFT *See* **Gamete intrafallopian transfer**

GnRH *See* **Gonadotropin releasing hormone**

Gonadotropin releasing hormone (GnRH) A hormone that encourages the production of **FSH** and **LH,** which in turn cause the ovaries to produce eggs or the testicles to produce sperm.

Habitual abortion The medical term for **recurrent miscarriage.**

hCG *See* **Human chorionic gonadotropin**

hMG *See* **Human menopausal gonadotropin**

Host uterus Also called *surrogate gestational mother.* A means of childbearing in which the woman who desires to have a child has her eggs fertilized in a lab dish with her husband's sperm, and the resultant embryo is transferred to another woman who will carry the pregnancy to term and then give the baby back to its genetic parents immediately after its birth.

HSG *See* **Hysterosalpingogram**

Human chorionic gonadotropin (hCG) A hormone released naturally after conception has occurred. HCG may also be given by injection to women to trigger ovulation after a course of fertility drugs has been used, or it may be given to men to stimulate the production of testosterone.

Human menopausal gonadotropin (hMG) A combination of the hormones **FSH** and **LH,** which is extracted from the urine of postmenopausal women and marketed under the brand name Pergonal.

Hyperprolactinemia A cause of infertility in which excessive levels of the hormone prolactin are produced.

Hyperstimulation A dangerous reaction to powerful fertility drugs (Pergonal or Metrodin) in which the woman's ovaries become enlarged and produce a superabundance of eggs, and her blood hormone levels skyrocket. Fluid may also collect in the lungs or abdominal cavity, and cysts that have formed within the ovaries may rupture, causing internal bleeding. Rarely (and most seriously) blood clots can develop. Symptoms of hyperstimulation include sudden weight gain and abdominal pain. Warning signs of hyperstimulation should be evident if the woman is being properly **monitored** during her drug-stimulated cycle.

Hysterosalpingogram (HSG) An X ray of the pelvic organs using a radio-opaque dye, usually performed to check for open fallopian tubes.

Hysteroscopy A procedure in which the doctor inserts a fiber-optic viewing device inside the woman's uterus to check for abnormalities. Minor surgical repairs may also be accomplished during the procedure.

Implantation Occurring about ten days after conception, the moment at which the pre-embryo attaches itself to the uterine wall, establishing a pregnancy.

Incompetent cervix Medical term for one of the causes of recurrent miscarriage—though many women find it unnerving to have one of their body parts given such a pejorative label. *Incompetent cervix* refers to the fact that the cervix opens up prematurely during pregnancy and causes the loss of the fetus.

Intra-uterine insemination (IUI) The most commonly performed method of artificial insemination, in which the doctor inserts a "washed" (specially processed) sperm sample directly into the woman's uterus. The other forms of artificial insemination are *intratubal (ITI),* in which the sperm are inserted into the fallopian tube, and *intracervical (ICI),* in which the sperm are placed in a caplike device that the doctor fits over the cervix.

In vitro fertilization (IVF) A procedure in which eggs are removed from the ovaries and mixed with sperm. Any embryos that form are transferred to the uterus in the hope that implantation will occur and a pregnancy will result.

IUI *See* **Intra-uterine insemination**

IVF *See* **In vitro fertilization**

Laparoscopy A surgical procedure in which the doctor inserts a fiber-optic viewing device through a small incision, made usually in the woman's navel, to look for endometriosis and other abnormalities in the pelvic organs. Oftentimes, any endometrial adhesions that are found will be lasered away during the laparoscopy. Egg retrieval for **IVF** or **GIFT** is also occasionally performed during a diagnostic laparoscopy.

Laparotomy Any major surgery performed through an incision in the abdomen.

LH *See* **Luteinizing hormone**

Luteal phase The part of the menstrual cycle following ovulation but prior to menstruation. A normal luteal phase should last between ten and sixteen days.

Luteal-phase defect A cause of infertility in which the time between ovulation and menstruation is too short for the endometrium to be sufficiently built up to allow a fertilized egg to implant. LPD (as it is often abbreviated by doctors) is generally detected by an **EMB.**

Luteinizing hormone (LH) The hormone released just prior to ovulation. Home ovulation test kits are designed to detect the "LH surge" by turning the end of a test stick blue on the day when LH becomes most concentrated in a woman's urine.

Menarche Medical term for the first menstrual period. A doctor's questionnaire may contain the question, "Age of menarche?" instead of asking "How old were you when you got your first period?"

Monitoring Daily medical tests (usually an ovarian ultrasound and a blood test) performed when a woman is taking Pergonal or other powerful fertility drugs, allowing her doctor to gauge the progress of the drug, set the day's dosage, and prevent ovarian **hyperstimulation.**

Morphology Doctor's term for "shape." A man may be told that his sperm have "poor morphology," meaning that a high percentage of them are mis-shapen and thus are incapable of fertilization.

Motility Doctor's term for the swimming ability of sperm. A man may be told that his sperm have "poor motility," meaning that a high percentage of them are unable to swim in a forward direction and so are less likely to be able to reach a woman's egg.

Myomectomy A surgical procedure to remove fibroid tumors from a woman's uterus, leaving the uterus intact. If a doctor recommends hysterectomy and the woman has any interest in retaining her ability to become pregnant, she should always ask about the possibility of having a myomectomy instead.

Occlusion Medical term for blockage. If your doctor says your fallopian tubes are occluded, he is telling you they are blocked.

Oligomenorrhea Medical term meaning "having infrequent menstrual periods."

Oligospermia Medical term meaning "having few sperm"—a common diagnosis of male infertility.

Oocyte An egg cell (a term used most often for the egg before it has matured).

Oviducts Another term for the fallopian tubes.

Ovulation The release of the mature egg (or eggs) from the ovary.

Ovum (*plural,* **ova**) an egg cell.

Patent Doctor's term for "open." If your doctor tells you that you have patent tubes, he is telling you that they are open, without any **occlusion.**

PCO *See* **Polycystic ovarian disease**

PCT *See* **Postcoital test**

Pelvic inflammatory disease (PID) An infection of any of the pelvic organs (the ovaries, fallopian tubes, or uterus) that if left untreated, or if not treated correctly, may result in infertility.

PID *See* **Pelvic inflammatory disease**

PMS *See* **Premenstrual Syndrome**

Polycystic ovarian disease (PCO; *also called* Stein-Leventhal Syndrome) A cause of infertility characterized by excessive production of androgens by the ovaries, the presence of cysts in the ovaries, and lack of ovulation. Outward symptoms can include weight gain, acne, excessive hair growth, and absence of menstrual periods—though PCO may also be completely symptomless.

Postcoital test (PCT; *also called* Sims-Huhner test) An examination of the woman's cervical mucus performed between two and twelve hours after intercourse, to determine if sperm are able to swim within the mucus.

Pre-embryo The term for the fertilized egg until about fourteen days after conception.

Premenstrual Syndrome (PMS) A set of symptoms including irritability, depression, breast discomfort, bloating, and personality changes, generally occurring in the two weeks prior to the onset of the menstrual period. PMS has been associated with low levels of the hormone progesterone, and thus also linked to infertility.

Progesterone The hormone produced during the **luteal phase** that thickens the lining of the uterus to prepare it to accept the **implantation** of a fertilized egg.

Prolactin The hormone that stimulates the production of milk in breastfeeding mothers. Excessive production of prolactin in a woman who is not breastfeeding may result in infertility.

Recurrent miscarriage The term most people use for what doctors call **habitual abortion.**

Retrograde ejaculation A cause of male infertility, most often found in some diabetics and in men who have undergone prostate surgery, in which the semen flows backward into the bladder instead of forward into the urethra.

Secondary infertility The inability of a couple who already have a biological child to have another.

Septate uterus An abnormality in which the uterus has a dividing piece of tissue. The division itself is called a *septum.*

Serophene A brand name of clomiphene citrate. (The more commonly prescribed brand of this fertility drug is **Clomid**.)

Sexually transmitted disease (STD) A term for a wide variety of diseases, including gonorrhea, syphilis, chlamydia, herpes, and AIDS.

Sonogram *See* **Ultrasound**

Speculum The device a doctor inserts into the vagina during a pelvic exam to hold apart the vaginal walls, allowing him to view the cervix or insert instruments needed to perform tests or treatments.

Spinnbarkeit Medical term used to identify the quality of clear, thin stretchiness that cervical mucus exhibits when it has become most hospitable to swimming sperm, around the time of ovulation.

Spontaneous abortion The medical term for miscarriage.

STD *See* **Sexually transmitted disease**

Surrogate mother The term for a woman who has agreed to become pregnant with the sperm of the husband of a couple who desire to have a child. The surrogate mother agrees that shortly after her baby is born she will give it to be brought up by its genetic father and his wife.

Teratogen Any substance that causes birth defects.

Testosterone The principal male sex hormone.

Ultrasound (U/S; *also called* sonogram) A medical test performed by bouncing inaudible sound waves off an organ (such as an ovary or uterus) to project an image of that organ on a viewing monitor.

Unexplained infertility The diagnosis that is left over when all testing on the couple is complete and no specific cause of infertility has been identified.

Unicornuate uterus An abnormality in which the uterus is "one-sided," and smaller than normal, usually making pregnancy impossible.

U/S *See* **Ultrasound**

Uterine lavage A procedure in which the uterus of a pregnant woman is flushed out, to allow the embryo to be recovered and reimplanted in the uterus of another woman who wishes to bear and raise a child. The woman undergoing uterine lavage is thus a very short-term surrogate mother.

Varicocele A varicose vein in the testicle, a condition often associated with male infertility.

Vas deferens The tubes through which sperm and semen travel before ejaculation.

Vasogram An X ray taken after a radio-opaque dye has been injected into the male reproductive system to determine if a blockage exists.

ZIFT *See* **Zygote intrafallopian transfer**

Zona pellucida The outer layer of the egg.

Zygote The fertilized egg.

Zygote intrafallopian transfer (ZIFT) An **ART** in which eggs are removed from a woman's ovaries, fertilized with the man's sperm in a laboratory dish, and any resulting embryos are transferred to her fallopian tube(s) during a minor surgical procedure.

SUGGESTED READING LIST

Note: Some books by small or specialized presses may be difficult to find in general-interest bookstores. In such cases the publisher's address is included so that the reader can contact the publisher directly.

ON FERTILITY AND THE REPRODUCTIVE SYSTEM

Bellina, Joseph H., M.D., Ph.D., and Wilson, Josleen, *You Can Have a Baby*, Bantam, 1985, 442 pp. Though somewhat dated in its descriptions of the technologies available today, the book is still valuable for its clear, readable accounts of how the male and female reproductive systems work and what can go wrong.

Berger, Gary S., M.D., Goldstein, Marc, M.D., and Fuerst, Mark, *The Couple's Guide to Fertility*. Doubleday, 1989, 442 pp. A good, all-purpose doctors' guide to infertility treatment. Though sometimes overtechnical and often oversanguine about the discomforts and difficulties involved in treatment, many of my interviewees cited this book as informative and worthwhile. An appendix lists fertility specialists state by state.

Birke, Lynda, Himmelweit, Susan, and Vines, Gail, *Tomorrow's Child: Reproductive Technologies in the 90's*. Virago Press, Ltd., 20–23 Mandela Street, Camden Town, London, NW1 0HQ, England, 1990, 340 pp. Includes brief descriptions of how various ARTs are performed; however, the greater part of the book is devoted to a spirited defense of the ethics of high-tech medical intervention for infertility. The three British feminists strongly rebut the argument advanced by some prominent American feminists that reproductive technologies will be used to exploit poor women and keep all women defined primarily as childbearers.

Franklin, Robert R., M.D., and Brockman, Kay, *In Pursuit of Fertility: A Consultation with a Specialist*. Henry Holt and Co., 1990, 348 pp. Comprehensive guide covering all aspects of infertility treatment. Most information is conveyed through stories the doctor tells of past patients he's treated and cured. Can be a little grating to read about couple after couple who gratefully thank the doctor for help in making their babies, but at least the guide is not too technical or difficult for the lay reader to follow.

Hammond, Mary G., M.D., and Talbert, Luther M., M.D., editors. *Infertility: A Practical Guide for the Physician.* Medical Economics Books, Oradell, New Jersey, 07649, 1985, 197 pp. For the reader who wants to know what doctors read when learning to evaluate and treat fertility patients. Contains papers on diagnosis, the doctor-patient relationship (from the doctor's point of view), the role of the nurse in infertility treatment, and discussion of a few specific infertility problems and treatments.

Hotz, Robert Lee, *Designs on Life: Exploring the New Frontier of Human Fertility.* Pocket Books, 1991, 290 pp. Profiles and stories about the scientists, doctors, and patients involved in the high-tech world of ARTs. Includes descriptions of what fertility researchers and doctors do in IVF and other specialized procedures. Reads like fiction, though full of technical information for readers interested in the scientific aspect of fertility treatment.

Llewellyn-Jones, Derek, M.D., *Getting Pregnant: A Guide for the Infertile Couple.* Delta Books, 1990, 220 pp. Although aimed at a general audience, this book by a noted Australian fertility expert is full of technical terms, and rather tough going for the lay reader. However, it does contain some very useful tables on the success rates of different types of treatment for each of several infertility problems—of interest to the couple trying to decide what would be the most effective treatment option for them.

Menning, Barbara Eck, *Infertility: A Guide for the Childless Couple.* Prentice Hall, revised ed., 1988, 201 pp. The founder of RESOLVE provides a readable (though rather brief) overview of the diagnoses and treatments of many fertility problems. Strong chapters on the emotional fallout of infertility and on choosing a nonmedical alternative.

Sher, Geoffrey, M.D., Marriage, Virginia A., R.N., and Stoess, Jean, M.A., *From Infertility to In Vitro Fertilization.* Pinnacle Books, 1988, 256 pp. A mass market paperback that describes in easy-to-follow language the steps involved in IVF. Limited information about other infertility treatments.

Silber, Sherman, M.D., *How to Get Pregnant with the New Technology.* Warner Books, 1991, 390 pp. A well-known fertility expert gives both a technical account of how ARTs are performed and a defense of his very strongly held and controversial views on such fertility problems as endometriosis, varicocele, oligospermia, and unexplained infertility. A must-read book for anyone being treated for one of these conditions.

Steinbock, Bonnie, *Life Before Birth: The Moral and Legal Status of Embryos and Fetuses.* Oxford University Press, 1992, 256 pp. Those confused by the ethical issues arising in IVF or other high-tech fertility treatments will find this book helpful in defining problems and analyzing the moral choices faced by the infertile couple. The author is a philosophy professor specializing in medical ethics.

Toth, Attila, M.D., *The Fertility Solution: A Revolutionary Approach to Reversing Infertility*. Atlantic Monthly Press Books, 1991, 174 pp. In this hotly debated book, a specialist in the treatment of pelvic and urinary tract infections argues that up to 50 percent of all infertility can be cured by antibiotic therapy.

Wisot, Arthur L., M.D., and Meldrum, David R., M.D., *A Guide to In Vitro Fertilization and Other Assisted Reproductive Methods*. Pharos Books, 1990, 260 pp. Best for its description of what happens in an IVF cycle, though frequent use of medical jargon makes it less helpful than it might have been. Still, very worthwhile reading for the couple about to begin IVF.

GENERAL MEDICAL BOOKS, INCLUDING USEFUL SECTIONS FOR THE
FERTILITY PATIENT

American Medical Association, *The Essential Guide to Prescription and Over-the-Counter Drugs*. Random House, 1988, 576 pages. Includes descriptions of many of the drugs used in fertility treatment, with valuable information on drug interactions, side effects, and dosages.

Boston Women's Health Collective, *The New Our Bodies, Ourselves*. Simon and Schuster, 1984, 647 pp. A wonderful resource for the woman who wants to understand how her own body works, with many helpful essays about how most mainstream doctors are trained in medical school to regard "female complaints."

Gross, Amy, and Ito, Dee, *Women Talk About Gynecological Surgery*. Clarkson Potter Publishing, Inc., 201 East 50th Street, New York, NY 10022, 1991, 353 pp. In easy-to-follow question-and-answer format, the authors provide an excellent, comprehensive guide to all forms of surgical procedures in use for female patients today. Describes D and C, laparoscopy, ovarian surgery, tuboplasty, pelvic repairs, myomectomy (fibroid tumor removal) as well as many operations not related to infertility. Highly recommended for any woman contemplating a surgical procedure.

Shtasel, Philip, D.O., F.A.O.C.R., *Medical Tests and Diagnostic Procedures*. Harper Perennial, 1991, 316 pp. A guide for the general reader to medical tests, including most of those used in male and female infertility workups.

Springhouse Editorial Staff, *The Physician's 1992 Drug Handbook*. Springhouse Publishing, Springhouse, PA, 1992, 1174 pages. Produced by a medical publishing company for doctors and available only at medical textbook and scientific bookstores. More comprehensive than the AMA drug-guide, though more difficult for the lay reader to understand.

BOOKS ABOUT SPECIFIC PROBLEMS/BOOKS AIMED AT
SPECIFIC TYPES OF PEOPLE

Ballweg, Mary Lou, *Overcoming Endometriosis: New Help from the Endometriosis Association*. Endometriosis Association, 8585 N. 76th Place, Milwaukee, WI 53223, 1987 (reissued, 1992), 329 pp. A cofounder of the self-help group, the Endometriosis Association, tells about treatment options, impact on fertility, and tips for coping with the emotional side effects of the disease.

Curry, Hayden, and Clifford, Dennis, *A Legal Guide for Lesbian and Gay Couples*. Nolo Press, 950 Parker Street, Berkeley, CA 94710, new edition, 1991, unpaged. Includes section titled, "So you want to become a parent?" Essential information about legal contracts, custody, adoption procedures, and other options for having a child.

Dalton, Katarina, M.D., *Once a Month: A PMS Handbook*. Hunter House, P.O. Box 847, Claremont, CA 91711, 1990, 250 pp. Informative discussion of the relationship of cyclical hormones to appearance of PMS symptoms.

Hepburn, Cuca, Ph.D. and Gutierrez, Bonnie, R.N., *Alive and Well: A Lesbian Health Care Guide*. The Crossing Press, Freedom, CA 95019, 1988, 243 pp. Includes helpful information on Lesbian options for motherhood, including instructions for AI/D through self-insemination.

Noble, Elizabeth, *Having Your Baby by Donor Insemination: A Complete Resource Guide*. Houghton Mifflin, 1987, 461 pp. *The* book for the anyone, whether married, or single, considering this method of conception. Discussions on every related topic, including self-insemination, choosing a sperm bank, finding a doctor, and ethical, legal, and practical considerations. Highly recommended.

Norris, Ronald L., M.D. and Sullivan, Colleen, *A Doctor's Proven Program on How to Recognize and Treat PMS*. Berkeley Books, 1983, 338 pp. Takes a refreshingly straightforward medical approach; does not theorize about social or psychological factors but offers practical prescriptions for relief.

Schwartz, Lita Linzer, Ph.D., *Alternatives to Infertility: Is Surrogacy the Answer?* Brunner/Mazel Publishers, 19 Union Square West, New York, NY 10003, 1991, 207 pp. *The* book for couples considering surrogacy. Thoughtful discussion of pros and cons of surrogacy, as well as other solutions to infertility. Includes suggestions for surrogacy contracts and other legal matters.

Winstein, Merryl, *Your Fertility Signals: Using Them to Avoid or Achieve Pregnancy, Naturally*. Smooth Stone Press, P.O. Box 23911, St. Louis, MO 63119, 1989, 159 pp. For the couple who wish (for personal or religious reasons) to continue trying to have a baby without medical intervention, this book explains in clear, nontechnical language how to recognize the most fertile time of a woman's cycle and contains self-help suggestions for natural means (such as diet, exercise, elimination of harmful habits) of maximizing the chance for conception.

SELF-HELP FOR EMOTIONAL OR SEXUAL PROBLEMS CAUSED BY INFERTILITY

Achtenberg, Jeanne, *Imaging in Healing*. Shambala Books, 1985, 251 pp. Explains methods developed to help patients suffering from cancer, immune system disorders, and other serious illnesses stay hopeful and feel positive about themselves. Techniques can be adapted for infertility. Also includes discussion of the relationship of mental activity to the body's biochemistry. May be easier to find this book in "New Age" bookstores than in general interest stores.

Becker, Gary, Ph.D., *Healing the Infertile Family*. Bantam, 1990, 310 pp. Recommended by several of my interviewees. How to strengthen your relationship and cope with pressures from friends and family as you seek a resolution to your infertility.

Benson, Herbert, M.D., and Stuart, Eileen M., R.N., M.S., *The Wellness Book: The Comprehensive Guide to Maintaining Health and Treating Stress-Related Illness*. Birch Lane Press, 1992, 493 pp. Includes a section on infertility and stress. The stress reduction techniques described in this book will not, of course, repair blocked tubes or eradicate a varicocele, but they *will* help you live a healthier, happier life while waiting for medical treatment to take effect.

Comfort, Alex, M.D., D.S.C., *The New Joy of Sex*. Crown, 1991, 253 pp. When infertility treatment creates stress that detracts from the couple's sexual pleasure, this book may be of help. Contains descriptions of a multitude of erotic practices and positions, each given a tantalizing title. Photos and drawings are helpfully explicit but not offensive.

Johnston, Patricia Irwin, *Understanding: A Guide to Impaired Fertility for Family and Friends*. Perspectives Press, P.O. Box 90318, Indianapolis, IN 46290-0318, revised ed. 1987, 28 pp. $4.50 per booklet (includes postage and handling fee). If you'd like your family and friends to stop making unwelcome comments about your infertility, or you're thinking of telling them what your treatment has been like, but you're not sure what to say, just hand them this booklet. It says it all.

Rush, Anne Kent, *Romantic Massage: 10 Unforgettable Massages for Special Occasions*. Avon Books, 1991, 145 pp. Recipes for ten relaxing, stress-erasing evenings, including menus for meals, and suggestions for setting the ambiance. Perfect for the couple suffering from too much doctor-directed sex. Also good for those times when the couple desire intimacy but doctor says to avoid intercourse.

Stoppard, Miriam, M.D. *The Magic of Sex.* Dorling Kindersley, Inc., 1991, 256 pp. This sex manual also includes essays about men's and women's differing expectations from sex, advice on dealing with sexual problems, information on sex during pregnancy, sexually transmitted diseases, and a host of other topics. Also includes questionnaires so that each partner can evaluate his or her own sexual needs and better understand the other's needs, too. Color pictures. Highly recommended for the couple experiencing loss of libido or other sexual difficulties.

Tannen, Deborah, Ph.D. *You Just Don't Understand: Women and Men in Conversation.* Ballantine, 1990, 330 pp. If you and your spouse are having trouble talking about your infertility, or you can't agree on how much to tell others about the problem, it could be that you have gender-based differences in the way each of you uses language to describe the problem. This book sheds much light on the hows and whys of miscommunication between the sexes. Highly recommended.

PREGNANCY AFTER INFERTILITY

Glazer, Ellen Sarasohn, L.I.C.S.W., *The Long-Awaited Stork: A Guide to Parenting After Infertility.* Lexington Books, 1990, 224 pp. Helpful advice, information, and stories about the experience of parenthood following fertility treatment. Received a glowing review in the February 1991 RESOLVE newsletter.

Noble, Elizabeth. *Having Twins.* Houghton Mifflin, 2nd ed. 1991, 429 pp. When fertility treatment results in double the joy, this is the book to buy! Includes information on fertility treatment and twinning, and a section on triplets. Great resource guide.

Scher, Jonathan, M.D., and Dix, Carol, *Preventing Miscarriage.* Harper Perennial, 1991, 240 pp. Written in down-to-earth language that encourages precautions about pregnancy without inducing panic.

Semchynshyn, Stefan, M.D., and Colman, Carol, *How to Prevent Miscarriage and Other Crises of Pregnancy.* Macmillan, 1989, 242 pp. Though the title promises more than any book can deliver, the authors still have much helpful information to impart on maximizing the chance for a healthy pregnancy and delivery.

ADOPTION AND OTHER NONMEDICAL ALTERNATIVES

Ademec, Christine A., *There Are Babies to Adopt: A Resource Guide for Prospective Parents*. Pinnacle Books, revised ed. 1990, 352 pp. Covers all forms of adoption with section on advantages of each. Several useful appendices, including lists of state agencies, independent agencies, adoptive family support groups, and private adoption attorneys. Of special value is a table summarizing adoption laws state by state.

Burger, Linda Cannon, *The Art of Adoption*. W. W. Norton, revised ed. 1981, 156 pp. Written by an adoption agency director and most useful for the couple intent on pursuing a traditional agency adoption only.

Carter, Jean W., and Carter, Michael, *Sweet Grapes: How to Stop Being Infertile and Start Living Again*. Perspectives Press, P.O. Box 90318, Indianapolis, IN 46290-0318, 1989, 144 pp. The authors explain their own choice to become a "child-free" couple, rather than continue invasive medical procedures or seek a child to adopt.

Cohen, Joyce S., and Westhues, Ann, *Well-Functioning Families for Adoptive and Foster Children*. University of Toronto Press, 1990, 162 pp. Although written for child-welfare workers, this book gives the prospective adoptive or foster parent a detailed account of what social service agencies are looking for when evaluating a home for placement of a child.

Faux, Marilyn, *Childless by Choice,* Anchor Press, 1984, 216 pp. Worthwhile reading for the couple interested in the "child-free" life-style option.

Gilman, Lois, *The Adoption Resource Book*. Harper Perennial, revised ed. 1992, 421 pp. A comprehensive guide covering all forms of adoption, and including a state-by-state directory of adoption agencies and support organizations.

Jewett, Claudia L., *Adopting the Older Child*. Harvard Common Press, 535 Albany Street, Boston, MA 02118, 1978, 308 pp. Includes both how-to advice and case studies of couples who have adopted older children. Clear-headed descriptions of both the challenges and the advantages of adoptions of older children.

Melina, Lois Ruskin, *Making Sense of Adoption,* Harper & Row, 1989, 276 pp. A one-of-a-kind book that discusses what to tell the child who has been brought into the family in an unusual way, and how to introduce the subject and at what age. Perfect for parents of children by donor egg, surrogate mother, and other high-tech procedures, as well as adopted children of parents of different ethnic or racial groups, and children whose birthmothers are known to the adoptive parents.

Michelman, Stanley B., and Schneider Meg, with van der Meer, Antonia, *The Private Adoption Handbook: The Complete Step-by-Step Guide to Independently Adopting a Baby*. Dell, 1989, 228 pp. Explains in clear nonlegalistic language how to arrange a private adoption in accordance with laws of each state. Gives reasons for choosing private over agency or other forms of adoption.

Morton, Cynthia D., Ph.D., *Beating the Adoption Game*. Harcourt Brace Jovanovich, revised ed. 1988, 362 pp. If I had to recommend a single book on adoption, this would be it! The author covers all aspects of the subject thoroughly, and without the usual saccharine, over-encouraging view. In fact, she is angry about much of the bureaucratic hassling most adoptive couples must go through to get a child. Especially useful for those who do not fit the usual agency picture of the "perfect" adoptive couple: e.g., older couples, low-income couples, singles, homosexual couples, couples of mixed religions or races, and others. Also covers transracial adoption, adoption of children with disabilities, foster parenting, surrogate motherhood, substitute parenting (which I call "partial parenting") and deciding to live child-free.

Rappaport, Bruce M., Ph.D., *The Open Adoption Book*. Macmillan, 1992, 195 pp. Discusses reasons for choosing this form of adoption over other types, gives how-to advice, covers legal, emotional, and practical problems involved.

Visher, Emily B., Ph.D., and Visher, John S., M.D., *How to Win as a Step-family*. Brunner/Mazel, 19 Union Square West, New York, NY 10003, 1991, 207 pp. Written by the founders of the Stepfamily Association of America, this book is a wonderful resource for the former fertility patient who has decided to make the stepparent/stepchild relationship the central parenting experience of his or her life.

MAGAZINE ARTICLES OF EXCEPTIONAL INTEREST

Carey, Benedict, "Sperm, Inc.," *In Health* magazine (now known simply as *Health* magazine), Vol. 5, No. 4, July-August 1991. Well-researched article about operations and procedures at major sperm banks, includes a list of questions that any prospective customer should ask before deciding on a sperm bank. Valuable information for anyone contemplating AI/D.

Ethics Committee of the American Fertility Society, "Ethical Considerations of the New Reproductive Technologies," *Fertility and Sterility,* June 1990, Vol. 53, No. 6. The entire issue of the monthly magazine is devoted to articles discussing the ethics of each of the types of reproductive technologies in use today. If you have any doubts about the morality about any type of ART that your doctor has recommended, then send off for a back-issue of this magazine. Send $10 check to the American Fertility Society (see Resource Guide for address).

Gordon, Meryl, "Inconceivable? Medical Breakthroughs Have Made Pregnancy Possible After Menopause, Even Chemotherapy." *Mirabella,* July 1991. Excellent article about new treatments available for postmenopausal women, cancer patients, and others who have previously been told that pregnancy was impossible. Includes information about fertility clinics willing to treat patients in these hard-to-help categories. Get hold of this issue if you are having trouble finding a fertility clinic that will take you on.

Hopkins, Ellen, "Tales from the Baby Factory," *The New York Times Magazine,* March 15, 1992. An investigative reporter looks closely at IVF and other ARTs and delivers grim findings about success rates. This very discouraging piece should be read by everyone who has already tried six or more IVF cycles without success; it will finally convince you that the time has come to say "enough is enough."

Raymond, Janice G., Snitow, Ann, Rowland, Robyn, Williams, Patricia J., Chesler, Phyllis, Russ, Joanna, and Wolf, Naomi, contributors to "Special Report: Women as Wombs," a set of seven articles, all critical of reproductive technologies, in *Ms.* magazine, Vol. I, No. 6, May-June 1991. Those who consider themselves feminists but who also wish to avail themselves of medical help to have a baby may be angered or disturbed by the vehement attacks on fertility treatment in this issue—but the views expressed are intellectually challenging and worthy of serious debate.

Rothman, Barbara Katz, Ph.D., "The Frightening Future of Baby-Making," *Glamour,* June, 1992. A somewhat alarmist account of the dangers (known and as-yet-unrevealed) of IVF, GIFT, and other high-tech methods of reproduction. The author contends that the unregulated fertility industry has been allowed to experiment on thousands of women, who in years to come may well suffer cancer or other ominous aftereffects. If you have qualms about undergoing a high-tech form of treatment, you may find it helpful to copy this article for your doctor and have him respond to the assertions it contains.

RESOURCE GUIDE

American Association of Tissue Banks
1350 Beverly Road, Suite 220A
McLean, VA 22101
(703) 827-9582

Publishes a list of sperm banks that follow the safety guidelines established by the AATB. Send stamped self-addressed return envelope to receive free list.

American College of Obstetricians and Gynecologists Resource Center
409 Twelfth Street, SW
Washington, DC 20024
(202) 638-5577; to order publications, call (800) 762-2264

Professional organization of OB/GYNs; puts out publications for doctors and patients on variety of subjects, including infertility.

American Fertility Society
2140 Eleventh Avenue South
Suite 200
Birmingham, AL 35205-2800
(205) 933-8494

Source of *Fertility and Sterility* magazine; The "Annual Clinic-Specific Report" on success rates for IVF, GIFT, and other ARTs; many pamphlets and book-

lets on specific problems of infertility.

American Society of Andrology
301 West Clark Street
Champaigne, IL 61820
(217) 356-3182

A professional society of doctors who treat male reproductive-tract disorders. Will give patient referrals.

Center for Surrogate Parenting, Inc.
8383 Wilshire Blvd., Suite 750
Beverly Hills, CA 90211
(213) 655-1974
(213) 852-1310 fax

A for-profit clinic that specializes in "third-party reproduction," including surrogate mother, egg donor, and host uterus programs. Publishes a newsletter with many articles of interest for the couple considering any of these methods of creating a child.

DES Action—USA (East Coast Office)
Long Island Jewish Medical Center
New Hyde Park, NY 11040
(516) 775-3450

DES Action—USA (West Coast Office)
1615 Broadway, Suite 510
Oakland, CA 94612
(510) 465-4011

A nonprofit organization providing information to the public and to medical professionals about DES exposure.

Endometriosis Association
8585 N. Seventy-sixth Place
Milwaukee, WI 53223
(800) 992-ENDO
In Canada (800) 426-2END

A support network made up of women who have the disease and others interested in its diagnosis and treatment. Many local chapters around the country. Provides information, publishes a newsletter, collects research, engages in patient education, offers crisis call help, and many other services.

GEnie System Computer Bulletin Board
Medical Roundtable, Subgroup—Infertility

If you have a PC with a modem and subscribe to the GEnie System, you can join in on an ongoing discussion group on infertility. Support, advice, and often valuable new information comes to you via your computer screen—great for those who have no time for meetings.

National Committee for Adoption
1930 Seventeenth Street, NW
Washington, DC 20009-6207

(202) 328-1200—general information
(202) 328-8072—helpline

Provides information and referrals for couples interested in adoption. Call the helpline to receive the "Starter Kit" packet of materials about becoming an adoptive family.

Obstetrics and Gynecology Update
Lifetime Cable Television half-hour show
Consult your local cable guide for airtimes

This weekly television program aimed at doctors frequently deals with various causes and treatments of infertility; oftentimes a useful source of information about breakthroughs in research and newly available treatments.

Perspectives Press
P.O. Box 90318
Indianapolis, IN 46290-0318

Founded by a former RESOLVE activist, this small publishing house specializes in books and pamphlets about infertility, adoption, and child-free living. Catalog available on request.

RESOLVE, Inc.
1310 Broadway
Somerville, MA 02144-1731
HelpLine (617) 623-0744
Business Office (617) 623-1156

An amazingly comprehensive resource for information about all aspects of infertility treatment, as well as alternatives to treatment such as child-free living and adoption. Publishes a quarterly newsletter; puts out fact sheets and briefs on over fifty different subjects from A (for "Anovulation") to Z (for "Zona Free Hamster Egg Test"). Local chapters all across the country put on lectures, seminars, get-togethers, and group counseling sessions, and refer patients to infertility doctors and therapists.

Serono Symposia
100 Longwater Circle
Norwell, MA 02061
(800) 283-8088

The manufacturer of Pergonal, Metrodin, and other fertility drugs publishes pamphlets on a wide variety of infertility topics, including insurance coverage and emotional aspects of treatment. Serono also sponsors conferences and educational programs on all aspects of infertility treatment. Call the toll-free number to order publications or to ask questions of a Serono representative.

Single Mothers by Choice
P.O. Box 1642
Gracie Square Station
New York, NY 10028

A support group for mothers (and those considering single motherhood) that puts members in touch with others in the same area; also puts out a newsletter.

Society for Assisted Reproductive Technologies

Professional organization, a subgroup of the American Fertility Society (see above)

Society of Reproductive Endocrinologists

Professional organization, a subgroup of the American Fertility Society (see above)

Society of Reproductive Surgeons

Professional organization, a subgroup of the American Fertility Society (see above)

INDEX